Birth and Power

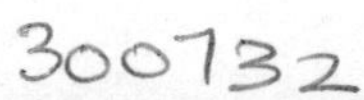

Birth and **Power**

A Savage Enquiry revisited

Wendy Savage

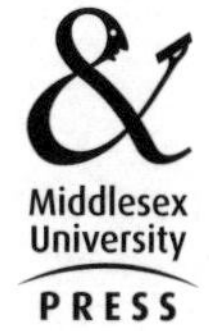

First published in 2007 by Middlesex University Press

A Savage Enquiry was first published in 1986 by Virago Press Ltd

ISBN-10: 1 904750 58 3

ISBN-13: 978 1 904750 58 1

A CIP catalogue record for this book is available from
The British Library

Design by Helen Taylor

Printed in the UK by Cambridge Printing

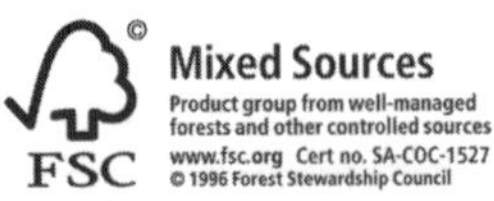

Middlesex University Press
North London Business Park
Oakleigh Road South
London N11 1QS

Tel: +44 (0)20 8411 5734: +44 (0)20 8411 4162
Fax: +44 (0)20 8411 5736

www.mupress.co.uk

Contents

	Author Biographies		vii
	Preface	*Luke Zander*	xiii
	Introduction	*Wendy Savage*	1
	My Return to Work	*Wendy Savage*	5
Section 1	**Birth and Power**		
	Birth and Power	*Wendy Savage*	27
	Birth and Power	*Marsden Wagner*	35
	Behind Every Midwife is a Doctor Trying to Stop Her	*Joan Donley*	45
Section 2	**Accountability**		
	Accountability of Doctors and the District Health Authority	*Wendy Savage*	59
	The Health Authority: Accountable for What, to Whom and How?	*John Eversley*	65
	The Accountability of Doctors	*James Drife*	83
Section 3	**Incompetence**		
	Incompetence	*Wendy Savage*	93
	Ensuring the Competence of Doctors	*Ron Taylor*	99
Section 4	**Disciplining Doctors**		
	Disciplinary Procedure for Doctors and Dentists in the NHS	*Wendy Savage*	109
	Employers' Discipline of Doctors in the NHS	*John Hendy QC*	119
	Disciplinary Procedures in Health Care: Use and Abuse	*Michael Goodyear*	133
	A Personal Account of Suspension in the Twenty-first Century	*Anonymous Surgeon*	149
Section 5	**Academic Freedom**		
	Academic Freedom	*Wendy Savage*	157
	Academic Freedom and Blowing the Whistle	*Anne Maclean*	161

Section 6 What Women Want

What Women Want — *Wendy Savage* — 171

What Services do Women Want and Who Decides on the Kind of Care that is Offered to Them? — *Beverley Beech* — 179

Who Decides What Women Get in Childbirth? — *Jane Sandall* — 187

Summary and Policy Implications — *Wendy Savage* — 199

Appendix — 203

A Savage Enquiry — **Wendy Savage** — 207

Index to *Birth and Power* — 357

Author Biographies

Beverley Beech

Beverley Lawrence Beech is a freelance writer, researcher, campaigner, and mother of two and has campaigned to improve maternity care since the birth of her second child in 1976. For six years she was a lay adviser to the National Perinatal Epidemiology Unit at Oxford and is currently a lay member of the Professional Conduct Committee of the Nursing and Midwifery Council (NMC) and a member of the Midwifery Committee of the NMC. She was also a lay member of the Royal College of Obstetricians and Gynaecologists Maternity Forum, and is currently a committee member of the Maternity Forum of the Royal Society of Medicine and a founder member of CERES (Consumers for Ethics in Research).

She lectures, both nationally and internationally, on consumer issues in maternity care and the medicalisation of birth. She is the honorary chairman of the Association for Improvements in the Maternity Services (AIMS), which is a leading campaigning pressure group on maternity care in the UK. Beverley has authored and co-authored a number of publications including: *Who's Having Your Baby?* (Camden Press, 1987), *Choosing a Water Birth* (AIMS, 1994), *Birthing Your Baby – the Second Stage of Labour* (AIMS, 2001) and Am I Allowed? (AIMS, 2003).

Joan Donley

Joan Donley was born in Canada in 1916 and moved to New Zealand in 1964. She trained as a midwife and became one of only three domiciliary midwives practising in the country. Joan became one of the pioneers in the revival of the home birth movement and a founding member of the New Zealand Homebirth Association, and later the New Zealand College of Midwives. Her services to midwifery were further acknowledged when she was awarded an OBE in 1989. This was the first time such an award had been given for services to midwifery.

Joan was a mentor and role model to many and her wisdom and expertise were highly valued both nationally and internationally. She was often invited to speak at international meetings and events and was an international midwifery advisor to the Canadian government where she travelled to the far north to help set up a service for the Inuit people. Joan was active in the restoration of midwifery education and her regular presentations to the students were memorable occasions. In 1997 she was awarded an honorary degree by the Auckland Institute of Technology for her contribution to midwifery education. This was the first time AIT had ever awarded an honorary degree.

She was also an author of three books, the last of which, *Joan Donley's Compendium for a Healthy Pregnancy and a Normal Birth*, was published in 2003. She died 4 December 2005 having written this chapter in 1999. Sadly she suffered a stroke and spent her last two years incapacitated by this.

James Drife

Professor James Drife graduated in Edinburgh in 1971 and after junior posts became an MRC research fellow, writing his MD thesis on the effects of the menstrual cycle and the Pill on the breast. He held posts in Bristol and Leicester before becoming Professor of Obstetrics and Gynaecology at the University of Leeds in 1990. He was first elected a member of Council of the RCOG in 1993 and was junior vice-president in the late 1990s. From 1985 to 1994 he was a member of the Cases Committee of the Medical Protection Society and from 1994 to 2005 an elected member of the General Medical Council. Since 2002 he has been chairman of the Association of Professors of Obstetrics and Gynaecology. He is a central assessor for the

Confidential Enquiries into Maternal Deaths and assisted in setting up a similar enquiry in South Africa. Recently he has visited countries of the former Soviet Union as consultant to the WHO's *Making Pregnancy Safer* initiative. He has lectured in Europe and the USA and has published widely. He writes a regular column in the *BMJ*. Since 2003 he has been Co-Editor-in-Chief of the *European Journal of Obstetrics Gynecology and Reproductive Biology*. His hobby is songwriting and he has appeared several times on the Edinburgh Festival Fringe as part of 'Abracadabarets'.

John Eversley

John Eversley has worked in the voluntary sector, for the trade union movement and policy think tanks, in local government, the health service and further and higher education. At the time of Wendy's reinstatement, John was the trade union nominee on Tower Hamlets District Health Authority. Later on he became an Executive Director of East London and the City Health Authority.

John now researches and teaches in the field of public policy and management. He is currently a part-time Senior Lecturer in the School of Health Sciences at City University, visiting Senior Lecturer at London Metropolitan University and managing director of a not-for-profit social research company, ppre Limited.

Michael Goodyear

Michael Goodyear is an Assistant Professor in the Department of Medicine at Dalhousie University, Halifax, Nova Scotia. A native of New Zealand he was educated in England and Australia, where he received his medical degree at Monash University in Melbourne before moving to Canada in 1980. In Canada he has also held positions at the University of Toronto and McMaster University. He holds fellowships in the Australasian, Canadian and American Colleges of Physicians. His clinical interests are in medical oncology, clinical trials, clinical epidemiology, biostatistics, public health, and the ethics of research. Other interests include women's health and studies, health law, social justice and human resources. He serves on the editorial board of the *Journal of Clinical Oncology*, is a reviewer for several ethics journals, and an auditor for the National Cancer Institute of Canada, and the Radiation Therapy Oncology Group in the US, where he is also co-chair of Medical Oncology. A former chair of the district research ethics board, he is active in organisations involved in research ethics governance including being a member of the Board of Directors of the Alliance for Human Research Protection. His major ethics activities currently involve restoring normative values in science and shifting from a culture of competitiveness and secrecy in research to one of collaboration and transparency. A member of the editorial board of the Ottawa Group which develops the Ottawa Statement on trial registration and open cultures in research, he has also worked with the Canadian Institutes of Health Research, Health Canada, the International Committee of Medical Journal Editors, the Cochrane Collaboration and the World Health Organization on policies and standards for clinical trial registries.

John Hendy

John Hendy QC was called to the Bar in 1972 and took silk in 1987. He is a Bencher of Gray's Inn, practising predominantly in the fields of industrial relations and employment law together with personal injury and medical negligence cases. He has a particular area of practice in representing many consultants and other clinical staff in relation to allegations of misconduct or lack of capability.

Since representing Wendy Savage in 1986, he has regularly appeared in trust disciplinary hearings and at the GMC. He has successfully obtained many injunctions to restrain dismissals in breach of contractual procedure. He has also appeared at a number of significant public enquiries including the Ladbroke Grove train crash enquiry (on behalf of the bereaved and injured). He led ground-breaking test case litigation establishing liability for 'vibration white finger' on behalf of British Coal mineworkers which resulted in 1999 in a Scheme now valued in excess of £2.5 billion and which remains under the supervision of the court.

John Hendy is a visiting Professor in the School of Law, King's College London and Chair of the Institute of Employment Rights. He is a Senior Commissioner of the International Labour Rights Commission. He is Standing Counsel to nine trade unions. He is a Fellow of the Royal Society of Medicine.

David McAvoy

David McAvoy read Philospphy, Politics and Economics at Pembroke College, Oxford. He taught Politics at the University of Salford and English at the University of Freiberg, Germany, and was Senior Lecturer in Social Studies at the Royal Military Academy, Sandhurst. He spends much of his retirement walking the Cumbrian fells with Wendy Savage, when he isn't helping her to edit papers or to finish the Guardian crossword puzzle.

Anne Maclean

Anne Maclean read Philosophy at Swansea and Oxford (Somerville) and taught the subject at the Queen's University of Belfast, Newcastle University and the University of Wales Swansea, where she was for three years a Fellow of the Centre for the Study of Philosophy and Health Care. She took early retirement in September 2004. She has written a number of articles and one book, *The Elimination of Morality: Reflections on Utilitarianism and Bioethics* (Routledge 1993).

Jane Sandall

Jane Sandall is Professor of Midwifery and Women's Health and leads the Women's Health Research Group in the Division of Health and Social Care at King's College London. Her first degree is in Social Science, her MSc is in Medical Sociology, and her PhD in Sociology. She has also practiced as a midwife in the UK and in Africa. She was a member of the UK National Service Framework for Children, Young People and Maternity Services Evidence Group and of the Maternity Working Group, and is a member of the UK National Stem Cell Bank Steering Committee. Her research has been funded by the ESRC/MRC Innovative Health Technologies programme, Department of Health, NCCSDO, Wellcome Trust, and a range of Medical and Health Charities, and has come to be concerned with two questions:

> How does the social and cultural shaping of maternal health policy influence the organisation and delivery of healthcare work, and the services that women and their families receive?
>
> How are professional knowledge and practice shaped by, and mediated through, new reproductive technologies and what are the social, ethical and organisational implications of these?

Her current interests are focused on developing greater sociological understanding of the relationship between context and health care practice using complex intervention frameworks for evaluation and the use of institutional ethnography. She is currently leading a Cochrane Review of midwifery-led care, the evaluation of a programme of community-based midwifery-led continuity of care for women in disadvantaged areas, and an ethnographic study of transfer and handover in midwife-led units. She is working with others on a national evaluation of outcomes for low-risk women in midwifery-led and obstetric-led units; the development of access, quality, optimal outcome indicators in maternal health care, and the social and ethical implications for staff working with Pre-implantation Diagnostic Technologies.

Wendy Savage

Professor Wendy Savage qualified as a doctor in 1960 and in 1977 became Senior Lecturer in Obstetrics and Gynaecology and Honorary Consultant at the London Hospital Medical College. She was suspended from her post in 1985 accused of incompetence in the management of five obstetric cases. The subsequent debate and public enquiry became a cause célèbre. The allegations were not upheld and she was reinstated in 1986 and retired in 2000. She wrote about this experience in *A Savage Enquiry: Who Controls Childbirth?* Wendy Savage is the author and co-author of over forty-five papers on a number of topics including induced abortion, sexually transmitted disease, childbirth and caesarean section. She was an elected member of General Medical Council 1989–2005.

Ron Taylor

Ron Taylor was born in Bootle in 1932. In that community the three most important professional individuals were the Doctor, the District Nurse/Midwife and the Schoolmaster, in that order. He was the first in the family in recent times to seek entry to a profession and decided to go for the top. Thus he qualified MBChB from Liverpool in 1957. He had considered a career in teaching and never lost his interest in it. Thus, when the opportunity arose to teach medicine, he accepted it with delight.

Being mechanically minded he was initially attracted to orthopaedic surgery but the practice of obstetrics proved even more enticing. Problems in labour in the 1950s were commonly mechanical ones so the move from setting bones and joints to assisting the birth of a baby was not as great as it might have seemed. More rewarding was the fact that a doctor could start with one sick patient and, with a little skill and good fortune, finish with two healthy ones. He recalls getting the same feeling of relief and satisfaction when he delivered his last mother in 1989 as he did when he carried out his first forceps delivery forty years earlier.

He completed a research project on the mechanism of action of oestrogen and demonstrated the way in which progesterone blocked many of its effects on target cells in the female genital tract. This provided a rational basis for modern hormone replacement therapy.

He retired from active obstetric practice because of ill health in 1989 and has devoted a great deal of time to medico-legal work since then. He is in no doubt that the scrutiny by independent medical experts of cases where the outcome is sub-optimal has been and will remain very important in raising standards of practice.

Marsden Wagner

Marsden Wagner completed his medical education at University of California at Los Angeles (UCLA) including clinical specialty training in perinatology and an advanced scientific degree in perinatal epidemiology. Following several years of full-time clinical practice and some years as a full-time faculty member at UCLA Schools of Medicine and Public Health, he was a Director of Maternal and Child Health for the California State Health Department. Then after six years as Director of the University of Copenhagen–UCLA Health Research Center, he was for 15 years a Director of Women's and Children's Health for the World Health Organization. He is now an independent consultant.

With extensive experience in maternity care in industrialized countries, including midwifery and the appropriate use of technology during pregnancy and birth, he has consulted and lectured in over 50 countries and given testimony before the US Congress, British Parliament, French National Assembly, Italian Parliament, Russian Parliament, Danish Parliament and Israeli Knesset. His publications, in English, German, French, Spanish, Russian, Italian, Japanese, Chinese, Swedish, Hebrew, Danish, include 143 scientific papers, 23 book chapters, 15 books. Honors include UCLA School of Medicine Alumnus of the Year.

Luke Zander

Dr Luke Zander was for over 30 years a general practitioner in a London inner city practice and Senior Lecturer in the Department of General Practice at St Thomas's and Guy's Hospital Medical School. He had a particular interest in the role of the general practitioner in the provision of maternity care and in furthering the integration of hospital and community-based services, and held a firm belief in patient-centred medicine. As a direct result of this approach to his clinical care, he became a strong advocate and supporter of women expressing the wish to have their baby in the setting of their own home, and provided care for over 500 domicilary confinements.

He has written widely on many aspects of pregnancy care, being co-author with Michael Klein of 'The Role of the Family Practitioner' in *Effective Care in Pregnancy and Childbirth* (ed. Chalmers, Enkin and Keirse), and co-editor with Geoffrey Chamberlain of *Pregnancy Care in the 1980s* (1984) and *Pregnancy Care in the 1990s* (1992).

Luke Zander was the founder of the multidisciplinary Forum on Maternity and the Newborn at the Royal Society of Medicine; a founder member of the Association of Community Based Maternity Care; an advisor to the Parliamentary Select Committee on Health under the chairmanship of Nicholas Winterton, for their report on the Maternity Services; an advisor to the National Perinatal and Epidemiology Unit in Oxford; and an advisor to the National Childbirth Trust. He is a past President of the General Practice Section at the Royal Society of Medicine, and is currently a Trustee of the Iolanthe Midwifery Trust.

Preface

In April 1985 Wendy Savage was summarily suspended from her post as Senior Lecturer and Consultant Obstetrician at the London Hospital Medical College where she had, over many years, developed a maternity care service sensitively orientated to the special needs of the population it served. In 1986, four months after the enquiry of the Tower Hamlets Health Authority, she was exonerated of all charges made against her and reinstated.

Thus ended, in part, a saga that had for over fifteen troubled months been the subject of publicity and interest which were remarkable for their breadth and intensity. Wendy had became a national figure, and twenty years later remains a household name, as a result of the stand she took, the principles that guided her course of action and her determination to defend them.

The essence of the case centred round the justification or otherwise of providing a form of maternity care that she felt most appropriately met the needs and wishes of a particular group of women. Significantly, the case against her was brought not by her patients but by her own colleagues, with whom there was clear evidence of a dysfunctional personal and professional relationship.

The details of the enquiry have received widespread publicity and been fully described from a subjective perspective by Wendy herself in her book very appropriately entitled *A Savage Enquiry – Who Controls Childbirth?*

Her case aroused an extraordinary degree of interest, and the support that she received was truly remarkable, both because of its extent and its origins. First and foremost it was drawn from women and their representatives, who clearly felt that the care that she was defending was of a nature that met their perceived needs.

She also received great support from midwives who saw that what she was endeavouring to do was to provide a woman-centred approach to care, one that underpins the essence of midwifery, yet is frequently in conflict with the medical model or disease-centred approach to care – so often the orientation provided in much of our present day health care system.

A third, and very significant element of her support came from the general practitioners within the local community. The relationship between primary and secondary care, between the general practitioner and the specialist, is complex and, as in any interpersonal activity, a sensitive understanding of the competencies and role of the other is necessary if the potential contribution of each is to be fully realised.

Wendy clearly recognised the contribution that general practitioners could make to maternity care because of their role as doctors providing personal, generalist and continuing care to individuals and their families in the setting of their own homes. She was very unusual in the degree to which she found many ways, both clinical and educational, to encourage and enable them to realise this potential.

It was for this reason that her suspension was so greatly opposed.

As a general practitioner myself, with a very particular interest in the provision of domiciliary maternity care, I came to know her well, first as a professional colleague and increasingly as a very good friend.

I became deeply concerned about what was taking place, not just because it was happening to a personal friend, but more significantly, because it challenged a form of pregnancy care based on a belief in the importance of patient autonomy and the appropriateness of a woman's involvement in the clinical decisions about how she gives birth.

What had transpired raised fundamental questions of medical ethics and professional behaviour which had wide implications for the profession as a whole. Many of these concerns were considered in depth at a meeting of the Maternity Forum of the Royal Society of Medicine in 1986 entitled 'The Savage suspension – its significance and implications', which interestingly took place against the expressed wishes of the Society's President. Its proceedings were submitted to the President of the RCOG and to the GMC in the hope that they might facilitate some positive action.

Over the twenty years since that time much has changed on the medical scene, and although some initiatives have given initial hope for optimism, all too frequently subsequent events have been less than helpful in pushing them forward. Thus, in spite of the widespread and enthusiastic response given to the suggestions made by the Winterton report (1992) and the Cumberlege report which followed, both of which were seen by so many to be an imaginative and eminently appropriate way forward, little has been achieved.

The reasons for this are clearly manifold, but important amongst them lies the fact that many of the fundamental issues that lay at the heart of the suspension of Wendy Savage remain as relevant and unresolved today as they were then.

With her depth of personal experience and her many years as one of the elected members on the General Medical Council, it is to be warmly welcomed that Wendy has seen fit to undertake a detailed exposition of these issues, together with the help of a number of colleagues highly qualified to undertake this task. If the book is able to make a contribution towards the resolution of some of these areas of conflict, something very important and positive will have been derived from a most unfortunate and unnecessary event that occurred so many years ago.

Luke Zander
Former Senior Lecturer
Department of General Practice
Guy's, King's and St Thomas' Medical School

Introduction

Wendy Savage

In April 1985 I was suddenly suspended from my post as Senior Lecturer in Obstetrics and Gynaecology at the London Hospital Medical College and honorary consultant at the London Hospital because it was alleged that I was incompetent. An NHS enquiry, which was held in public and generated sustained press interest, rejected the allegations, and I was reinstated by the Tower Hamlets Health Authority in July 1986, though I did not return to work until four months later.

The book I wrote about the affair told the story up to the time of my reinstatement. *A Savage Enquiry: Who Controls Childbirth?* was published by Virago in October 1986 and sold almost 30,000 copies but has been out of print for some years. Many of the issues raised by my case are still relevant today and doctors often ask me for a copy of the book when they find themselves in the limbo of suspension.

Although 20 years have passed since Andrew Veitch of the *Guardian*, Nick Timmins of *The Times* and Clare Dyer of the *BMJ* were reporting on the saga, at some points daily, people have not forgotten the case. I am often asked, for example, what happened when I returned to work. I feel I owe it to the many thousands who supported me by letters, postcards and donations to describe what did happen when I returned to the London Hospital as I think it shows how difficult institutions find it to deal with such problems even today.

This book has chapters relating to the six issues I identified at the end of the 1986 book:

- Birth and power
- What kind of services do women want and who is to decide on the kind of care that is offered to them?
- Accountability – of District Health Authorities and of doctors
- Incompetence – What does it mean? How does one measure it?
- Can disciplinary procedures for doctors in the NHS be improved?
- Academic freedom and the roles of professors and senior lecturers.

Much has happened in the intervening decades. The Winterton Committee[1] and the Cumberlege report[2] aimed to give women more say in how maternity care was provided and to put the woman at the centre of that care. Sadly, the high hopes that women and midwives had in 1993 have not been realised.[3]

Clinical governance has been introduced into the NHS and in this century a plethora of new bodies has been set up to try to ensure high standards, such as the National

1 House of Commons Health Select Committee (1992)

2 Department of Health (1993)

3 Sharples Weston (2005)

Clinical Assessment Authority (NCAA) and the National Care Standards Commission (NCSC). These have now been amalgamated as the National Clinical Assessment Service (NCAS) under the umbrella of the National Patient Safety Agency (NPSA) and the Commission for Health Improvement (CHI) (later the Commission for Audit and Health Improvement (CHAI) and now the Health Commission). Successive re-organisations have meant changing staff and, in many cases, hospitals and health authorities are no more accountable to their patients than they were in 1986.[4]

The finding of serious professional misconduct by the GMC's Professional Conduct Committee against the chief executive in the Bristol paediatric cardiac surgery case[5] can be seen as affirming the principle that doctors should be accountable for their actions.[6] However, it is my opinion that the GMC finds it difficult to act in cases where doctors disagree amongst themselves.

The definition of incompetence is still problematic. The introduction of performance procedures by the GMC in 1997[7] has helped in the assessment of poor performance, but the procedures are cumbersome and there is evidence that they can be manipulated by unscrupulous doctors who wish to be rid of a colleague.[8]

Norman Fowler set up a working party in October 1986 to look at disciplinary arrangements and a new procedure, HC(90)9, was introduced in 1990 to replace HM(61)112.[9] This directed that enquiries into disciplinary cases should be held in private. Since then the reforms of the NHS have meant that some hospitals have opted out of the national procedure and doctors' rights have been further eroded. In December 2003 new guidelines were issued by the Chief Medical Officer and in 2004 unjustified suspensions dropped for the first time to 20 a quarter from an average of 29 in 2000.[10]

Ian Stone audited gardening leave in 2002 and believes that this practice has now ceased.[11] The Audit Commission has been a positive force for change. Its report on suspended clinicians[12] certainly highlighted the need for more appropriate and cost-effective ways of disciplining doctors and for improved systems for holding health authorities to account.

Academic freedom has received less attention than it warrants in the media and medical journals, but the chapter by Anne Maclean is a salutary warning of the dangers of the changing ethos of our universities. Professors should not be able to stifle the expression of unorthodox opinions by their junior academic colleagues.

I hope this exploration of the issues will be of particular interest to practitioners, teachers and students of sociology, law, medicine and other health care subjects, and to NHS administrators and managers. I hope that it will also be accessible to the general public, whose taxes keep the NHS going.

I thought it was important to reprint the original book here. After my suspension, lots of people, including my GP colleagues, childbirth organisations, AIMs (Association

---

4 National Audit Office (2003) p.28 case 3

5 Kennedy (2001)

6 Privy Council (1999)

7 The Medical (Professional Performance) Act 1995

8 Privy Council Appeals (2003) and personal communications 1999–2002

9 Department of Health (1990) Annex B paragraph 11

10 National Clinical Assessment Service (2006)

11 Personal communication (2006)

12 National Audit Office (2003)

for Improvements in the Maternity Services), the NCT (National Childbirth Trust) and individual women, many of whom had been my patients, came together and organised an effective campaign for my defence. By so doing they helped to ensure that I was reinstated. From the chapter about disciplinary procedures for doctors you will see that I was very fortunate in being able to resume my career. Many other doctors have not been so lucky.

Despite the rhetoric about 'choice' for women in childbirth, and 'openness and transparency' in governance, there is still a lot to do to if women are to be able to give birth in the way they wish to and if all those involved in health care are to be truly accountable to the wider society they serve.

I would like to take this opportunity to reiterate my thanks to all those who supported me through my ordeal in 1985–6 and my core group of supporters who continued to do so when I returned to work. I want to thank all the contributors to this book who worked hard on the issues allocated to them and delivered their chapters on time. I am particularly grateful to David McAvoy who, as co-editor, has read through, corrected and commented on all the draft chapters. He has done so through several drafts of my own chapters where he has improved my English and clarified obscure passages. His perspective as a non-medical, non-legal person has been invaluable in making this book comprehensible to the general reader. I am also grateful to Michael Cotton and Adrian McAndrew of the General Medical Council (GMC) who provided me with old GMC papers and up-to-date figures, Alastair Scotland and Ian Stone of the National Clinical Assessment Service for their time and some unpublished data, and the CMO for sending me a copy of *Supporting Doctors, Safer Patients.* Lastly I would like to thank Colin Francome for his support as a member of the Middlesex University Press editorial board who has read much of the book, John Lisners who gave legal advice and all the staff of Middlesex University Press who have worked so hard to produce the book.

References

Department of Health (1990) 'Disciplinary procedures for hospital community medical and dental staff'. London: Department of Health. (HC(90)9).

Department of Health (1993) *Changing Childbirth: Report of the Expert Maternity Group* (The Cumberlege report). London: Her Majesty's Stationery Office.

House of Commons Health Select Committee (1992) *Second Report on the Maternity Services* (The Winterton report). London: Her Majesty's Stationery Office.

Kennedy I (2001) *Learning from Bristol. The report of the Public Inquiry into children's heart surgery at the Bristol Royal Infirmary 1984–1995.* Bristol Enquiry Publications CM 5207 (1) http://www.bristol-enquiry.org.uk

National Audit Office (2003) *The management of suspensions of Clinical Staff in NHS Hospital and Ambulance Trusts in England.* Norwich: The Stationery Office.

National Clinical Assessment Service (2006) *Analysis of the first four years referral data.* London: NCAS. http://www.ncas.npsa.nhs.uk

Privy Council (1999) *Dr John Roylance vs the General Medical Council. Oral judgement upon petition.* Privy Council Appeal No.49 of 1998. http://www.privycouncil.org.uk

Privy Council (2003) *Anthony Peter Sadler vs General Medical Council 15.7.03* Privy Council Appeal No.59 of 2002. http://www.privycouncil.org.uk

Sharples Weston R (2005) 'Liberating Childbirth', *AIMS Journal*, Vol.17, No.3, pp.6–9.

The Medical (Professional Performance) Act 1995. London: The Stationery Office.

Stone I (2006) personal communication (Ian Stone is an advisor to CMO (England) and HR advisor to NCAS), Market Towers, 1 Nine Elms Lane SW6 5NQ.

My Return to Work

Wendy Savage

A Savage Enquiry was published in October 1986 after a magnificent effort by the Virago team and my friend Jane Leighton to get it finished on time.

The District Health Authority (DHA) decided unanimously to re-instate me at its July meeting,[1] but I did not return to work until 3 November 1986. I saw my first patient a day later in the Florida Street practice community antenatal clinic. The only fellow consultant to welcome me back was David Oram, who came especially to Mile End to do so. The first time I met together with the other consultants was later that month at an interview for a new registrar. The person who was in my opinion the undoubted best candidate, a woman who has gone on to have a distinguished research career, was not supported. I felt that nothing had changed.

The Munro panel

The DHA set up a panel to make recommendations on the future working of the Department of Obstetrics and Gynaecology (O&G). It was chaired by Dame Alison Munro, a distinguished retired civil servant with experience in maternity services (and the sister of Ian Donald, a quote from whose book *Practical Obstetric Problems*[2] I had used for the frontispiece of *A Savage Enquiry*). She interviewed all the obstetricians in September. The Dean, Mike Floyer and a previous Dean, Sir John Ellis, both of whom I had known since I was a student, submitted written evidence. It was hard being questioned without the support of my lawyers but I could deduce what my colleagues had been saying from the content of the interview. The other panel members were Bob Atlay, an obstetrician from Liverpool and Honorary Secretary of the Royal College of Obstetricians, and Gynaecologists (RCOG) and Mr John Alway the district general manager (DGM). Their report had 13 points.

These included statements about the situation, the organisation of the service, agreement to adhere to joint policy decision, an increase in consultant sessions and clear understanding between the Medical College and NHS about how sessions should be deployed to meet the clinical requirements of patients and the teaching needs of the College, continuing perinatal mortality meetings and a suggestion that the O&G division be merged with the surgical or medical divisions.

Their recommendations included the following:

3. All consultants should adhere to the Labour ward protocol of April 1986.
4. As required by their Conditions of Service, all consultants should cover for each other. There should be a published rota. This is widely accepted practice.
6. The consultant on call will assume full responsibility for the Obstetric and Gynaecology patients in the hospital and would normally follow the agreed management plan for a

---

1 Savage (1986) p.172

2 Donald (1955)

woman's care. But in an emergency or if circumstances change in a way that was not anticipated, the consultant on call will take whatever decision he or she deems necessary in the interests of the mother and baby.

7. If a consultant wishes to manage a case in an unusual or unfamiliar way, he or she will take personal and direct responsibility for the patient throughout and so inform the consultant on call and junior staff concerned. This should be made explicit in the Labour Ward Protocol.

11. If difficulties of interpretation of these working arrangements should arise, they should in the first instance be discussed by the division of Obstetrics and Gynaecology. If they are unable to be resolved, they should be referred to the Chairman of the Medical Council, who in consultation with the Dean, will convene a small group of eminent colleagues who will act in the best interests of patients, the Hospital and Medical College.

12. Any questions of unresolved differences in clinical philosophy may be referred to the RCOG.

13. As required by the General Medical Council in its guidance to the profession, medical practitioners involved in these arrangements must refrain from depreciating the professional skills and services of each other.

The preamble pointed out that generally professionals agreed working arrangements themselves, but the situation in the O&G division had reached a point where it could not resolve its own problems. After the 13 points, a concluding paragraph included the words:

> It provides a framework within which the interpersonal difficulties which have become magnified in the last year could be resolved. It may well take a little time to establish professional working relationships… Success will require the sincere determination of all parties to work in harmony with tolerance and respect for each other's viewpoints. We trust that in the interests of the women of Tower Hamlets they will do so.[3]

In the mid-nineties I was sent, anonymously, some papers relating to my case. I read the submissions from the two Deans to the Munro panel with amazement and sadness and with renewed admiration for the panellists who had genuinely sought to assist. The late Sir John Ellis started his background to the problems in the department with the words 'During its first 100 years the governors of the London Hospital strictly forbade the admission of pregnant women'. This strongly resonated with my own sense at the time that there was a deep-rooted culture of misogyny within the hospital and medical college.

When I returned to work I hoped we could put the past behind us and work together, if not amicably, at least reasonably; but when I discussed my timetable in October 1986 with the unit general manager (UGM) Vicki Hardman (who did her best to make things work) the omens were not good.

My inpatient list had been changed from midweek to Monday morning. Monday is not popular as one needs to do a pre-operative ward round on a Sunday. My outpatient list, which had been on Friday morning, was now on Friday afternoon – unpopular with doctors in training as it leaves no chance of getting away early for the weekend. There was no space in the outpatient department at Whitechapel for my senior house officer

3 Munro (1986)

(SHO) and I to do a pre-admission clinic, so we had to use a side-room in the gynaecology ward, which was cramped and lacked privacy. Later, Norman Williams, the Professor of Surgery, allowed me to use two rooms in the academic wing, which improved things for the women and gave space for students to take histories and examine patients.

During my suspension, Gynaecology had been moved from Mile End to Whitechapel, although Obstetrics was still split between the two sites. There were six senior house officers in post (SHOs), and each consultant was allocated one. My SHO had to travel between the two sites to look after my patients, whereas the others had all their duties on the Whitechapel site. Also, they worked a one-in-four on-call rota whereas my SHO worked a one-in-two (that is, working for 24 hours and the next working day, followed by one night off). His opposite number worked solely at Mile End doing antenatal clinics for those consultants who had clinics there in the mornings, and had the afternoons off. These were considerably less onerous duties. Sam Everington, doubly qualified as a doctor and barrister and active in the BMA juniors' committee, was my first SHO. He was very supportive, later became a GP in Tower Hamlets and is now Deputy Chair of the BMA Council. Nevertheless, the arrangements for junior staff were such that, in my opinion, those working on my firm were significantly disadvantaged.

A key recommendation of the Munro panel was that the O&G division should be merged with either Medicine or Surgery. However, the other divisions did not want to do this, although the Medical Council had voted 44 to 11 to accept the Munro panel's recommendations (although, only a little more than a quarter of the consultants had voted). The compromise, which I accepted, was that we would have a facilitating Chair. The first was Professor Colin Berry, a morbid anatomist who had always been very pleasant towards me. However, I learned that he was a Mason and, since I knew that at least two of my colleagues were Masons,[4] I was concerned that impartiality should be maintained. When I pointed out that I considered this rota was clearly unfair and seemingly designed to make my SHO post unattractive, he agreed to discuss it with Sam Everington. It did not change, and the next SHO went off sick after a few weeks. After two years, Professor Berry was replaced by Peter McKelvie, an ENT surgeon. His first task was to sit on an appointments committee for a new Head of Midwifery and he was told that all the consultants supported the internal candidate, who got the job. Only two people had applied and I had said to some of my colleagues that we should re-advertise as I considered that neither candidate had sufficient experience.

By July 1989, I was so demoralised that I called a meeting of my supporters, who included all those who had appeared at the enquiry in my defence, two of whom had commented on the cases, Michael Moore and John MacVicar, Peter Diggory, John Hare, Luke Zander and John Hendy. One of these wrote the *Lancet* editorial reproduced with permission below.[5]

Bitter reinstatement

At a major London teaching hospital the division of Obstetrics and Gynaecology is chaired by an otorhinolaryngologist. Four years ago at that same hospital a consultant obstetrician of eight years' standing was suspended without warning. In the interim the

4 Ferriman and Leigh (1985)

5 Editorial, *Lancet* (1989a)

consultant, whose professional competence had been challenged, was reinstated after a long and expensive enquiry, an advisory panel made recommendations about the establishment of professional working arrangements in light of the enquiry's findings and a senior figure at the Royal College of Obstetricians and Gynaecologists was called upon to pronounce because the recommendations of the panel were not being implemented. Many of our readers will instantly perceive that we are talking about the London Hospital and Mrs Wendy Savage. Why should we wish to revive the subject? Unfortunately, this miserable saga shows no signs of ending satisfactorily. When the disciplinary enquiry headed by Mr Christopher Beaumont QC made the final part of its report public almost exactly three years ago we commented that 'it would be naive to assume that all will now be harmony and light'.[6] *Anything but!*

The advisory panel established after the Beaumont enquiry (the first such enquiry to be held in public) was chaired by Dame Alison Munro (Chairman, Chichester Health Authority) and reported in October, 1986. The panel suggested several modifications to the working arrangements and organisation of the division of Obstetrics and Gynaecology at the London Hospital. In all there were thirteen recommendations. Members of the panel seem to have been aware of the depths to which inter-professional relationships had sunk because one of the recommendations, number eleven, stated 'If difficulties of interpretation of these working arrangements should arise they should in the first instance be discussed by the division incorporating Obstetrics and Gynaecology. If they are unable to be resolved, the matter should be referred to the Chairman of the Hospital Medical Council who in consultation with the Dean, will convene a small group of eminent colleagues who will act in the best interests of patients, the Hospital and the Medical College'. Among other suggestions was that the division of Obstetrics and Gynaecology should be merged with either the medical or the surgical division 'to give a wider perspective to its deliberations'; although such a merger has not come about, a 'neutral' Chair of the division of Obstetrics was appointed, hence the otherwise rather unlikely position occupied by an ear, nose, and throat surgeon.

The Munro panel's fears were realised. When Mrs Savage returned to her post in July 1986, after her reinstatement she found that she was virtually ostracised and unable to work properly. She eventually started seeing patients in November but, although she was a senior lecturer, she was effectively barred from teaching. She threatened to sue the London Hospital Medical Council (LHMC) and was once more given teaching responsibilities in March 1987.

Nevertheless, the working atmosphere within the division of Obstetrics was such that it was agreed that she should be assigned to the Academic Department of General Practice under Professor Mal Salkind. She joined the department in November 1987.

In May 1988, finding that it was impossible to achieve any consensus with her colleagues in the obstetric division, Mrs Savage asked the Chairman of the Council to proceed according to 'Munro eleven' and convene a group to discuss the outstanding problems. The Chairman thought it was a matter for the District Health Authority, who in the event deemed it to be a medical problem and referred the case back to the Council. In August last year, the Council decided to involve the Royal College of Obstetricians and Gynaecologists to suggest a suitable adjudicator.

Sir Malcolm MacNaughton was duly chosen and saw all the relevant consultants in

6 Editorial, *Lancet* (1986)

December. In January of this year, Sir Malcolm continued his deliberations and saw selected members of the junior staff; Mrs Savage was not asked to nominate any of the junior doctors. In April, Sir Malcolm reported verbally to some selected senior doctors but not to Mrs Savage, although he was apparently dismayed that she had not been informed of the content. As far as we know, Sir Malcolm has not put his report in writing. This catalogue of events suggests that there has been little or no true reform of the division of Obstetrics at the London Hospital. Some might hold that such difficulties are almost inevitable when strong personalities meet head on and that the whole sorry tale merely represents an extreme battle of wills. But it is far more then a domestic tiff. Despite many hours of people's time, considerable sums of (largely public) money, and much heart searching, it is plain that there is still no satisfactory machinery for dealing with professional disagreements. In Mrs Savage's case, a disciplinary enquiry was asked to settle a dispute between professional colleagues; she was totally exonerated of the charge of incompetence yet has been effectively barred from practising as she would wish. Clearly her colleagues in the division of Obstetrics were never prepared to accept a verdict of not guilty; if they had been, presumably they would have made more effort to behave in a manner befitting the corporate ethic of the profession. This lengthy dispute has not benefited any of the participants. The opportunity was there for a much-needed comparison of community-based versus hospital-based obstetrics. Instead, the acrimony that has enveloped the case shows no signs of diminishing.

Mrs Savage, who last month was elected to the General Medical Council, has now been advised to take legal action against the health authority for not honouring her terms of employment, with respect to both the direction of the Beaumont enquiry and the findings of the Munro panel. The recommendations of the Munro panel had been accepted as binding by the health authority and by Mrs Savage; an action will now be started.

I had not decided to take legal action, only considered it, and the *Lancet* published a correction the following week.[7]

Following this editorial, two letters were published. Tony Jewell, who had been active in my defence and now on the DHA as the GP nominee, wrote about the confusion of management functions caused by the number of institutions involved. His letter ends:

> As you point out there is an issue here of professional management that is broader than the specific and difficult Savage saga. We are witnessing a failure of management: consultants and professors, beneath their professional mantles, remain employees, with terms and conditions of service. Managers, whether University or NHS, need to act on that fact.[8]

Peter Diggory, a distinguished obstetrician and gynaecologist who had been active in the campaign to change the law on abortion in 1967, wrote:

> There is an overriding need to protect patients from incompetent doctors and much thought has been given to achieving this goal. When a doctor is wrongly accused of incompetence and is finally cleared of that charge there is a need to ensure that thereafter he or she is treated as fairly as possible. When the accusation has been adjudged by the doctor's

7 *Lancet* (1989c)
8 Jewell (1989)

> employer to be so far justified as to necessitate suspension, before a full enquiry, the reputation of the doctor will have been damaged, even if it is subsequently established that the charge was groundless. There is no provision for redress other than by adequate reporting of the case in the public as well as the professional media. In the rare but especially unfortunate cases in which the accusation comes from the doctor's own professional colleagues, it is manifestly inadequate merely to order reinstatement into a professional atmosphere which must by then be full of recrimination and distrust.

He went on to say the problem was recognised by both the Beaumont and Munro panels and to deplore the secrecy surrounding the report from Professor Sir Malcolm MacNaughton.[9]

The MacNaughton report

I did not start legal action as, on 21 August 1989, after months of delay, we were finally sent the MacNaughton report, a fortnight after the *Lancet* editorial. He confirmed that most of the Munro proposals were not working and could not be implemented. He confirmed that Mr John Hartgill and Professor Gedis Grudzinskas were unhappy for me to look after their patients because of my 'non-interventionist and very conservative' philosophy. He did not feel that Professor Grudzinskas and I would be able to work amicably together in the future, and suggested that:

1. A new consultant be appointed, preferably a woman with an interest in community antenatal care
2. Mr Hartgill, who was shortly due to retire, be replaced by a feto-maternal medicine specialist
3. One of those appointed should be a senior lecturer in the University to support the professor
4. Mrs Savage should stay as senior lecturer in Professor Salkind's department (General Practice) as she relates well to him and can do research there.

He did not favour having two separate units as suggested by the deans (that is, one unit at Mile End and the other at Whitechapel) but said one consultant should work with me. He also suggested that 'the new consultant appointments should be to persons who have previously had nothing to do with the London Hospital. Fresh blood is vital for the Department of Obstetric and Gynaecology'. He ended by saying the department should avoid publicity unless it is of a scientific nature for the next five years, mentioning 'personal antagonisms and statements'.

Professor MacNaughton had been president of the RCOG when I was suspended and I was glad that someone of his experience and standing had recognised the intractable nature of the problem which senior figures at the London had seemed to ignore.

The appointment of two new consultants and the two-firm proposal

Lorne Williamson (LW) had taken over as district general manager after Mr Alway resigned in the summer of 1988. The District Health Authority met in September 1989 and the new Chair Ann Mallinson said the O&G consultants had been given the report

9 Diggory (1989)

but none had replied, so discussion was deferred. In fact, I had replied, and told one of my supporters after the meeting. She raised this in writing and asked the Chair to read her letter out at the October meeting. LW said he did not remember saying that there had been no response! LW then said he needed to investigate how much Munro had been implemented, so delaying any decision for another month.

In medicine, 'firm' is the name given to the team of doctors who work together to look after the patients of one (or more) consultants: the senior house officer (SHO) clerked patients in, and attended outpatient clinics and operating sessions along with the registrar and senior registrar. Students were allocated to firms during their attachments to specialities. Firms did ward rounds together and discussed management of patients, so it was a good basis for the apprenticeship system. I came to the conclusion the best solution to the problems we faced was to have two separate firms so that the juniors were not put in a difficult situation with conflicting loyalties. LW wrote in September rejecting this two-firm proposal as it would 'institutionalize a personality clash which has little if anything to do with how medicine is practised' despite the case made by Professor Salkind and myself to him in the summer of 1989. After I had written to all consultants prior to the Medical Council meeting on 25 October 1989 they agreed to accept the MacNaughton report and the proposal to have two firms. They asked the Special Professional Panel (SPP)[10] to work out the details.

The DGM presented his report to the DHA meeting in November 1989. He had interviewed the O&G consultants and disagreed with some of Professor MacNaughton's findings and recommendations; but it was agreed to accept the report, to let the SPP sort out consultant rotas and that management should decide about a sixth consultant. He admitted that although all consultants would cover for another, this did not mean that they would allow every consultant to cover for their patients. This was my reason for wanting to separate the junior staff into two firms: it did not inspire confidence when juniors knew that my colleagues refused to allow me to cover for them when I was the duty consultant. All of us were on call for our own patients unless out of London, but it was unusual for my colleagues to come in, as they left things to our experienced senior registrars. John Hartgill was due to retire in September 1990. In December the *Lancet* had another editorial confirming the DHA's endorsement of the two-firm proposal and appointment of a sixth consultant.[11]

New consultant appointments

In 1990 agreement was reached with the medical school for a new senior lecturer post. I was asked to write the job description for the NHS consultant with a community interest, and the professor was to write the description for the other post.

If there was to be no gap in service, the replacement for John Hartgill needed to be advertised by March. The job descriptions had to be approved by the department as well as the RCOG, another hurdle I negotiated with the help of some of my expert witnesses. I arrived back in May 1990 after four days' study leave abroad to find the president of the RCOG had intervened to prevent a meeting to discuss them, so it was not until June that the DHA agreed to advertise the two posts.

10 The new name for the 'three wise men', the mechanism previously used in the NHS to resolve problems with and between doctors. Senior consultants were elected by the Medical Council.

11 *Lancet* (1989b)

Fourteen people applied for the consultant post. Five were short-listed, none of them women, and only one, our current senior registrar (SR), was British qualified. One was removed by the RCOG representative and both our SR and another candidate withdrew before the interview. The latter said that despite repeated attempts he had been unable to contact two of my colleagues and could not work without the confidence of all the consultants. So we interviewed just two. At the start Mr Brew, the new Chair of the DHA, asked the Royal College representative if both were suitably qualified and he agreed they were. The members of the appointing panel also agreed that on paper both candidates were suitable. The panel included the Chair of the Governors of the LHMC, Mr Dickinson, Lorne Williamson DGM, a regional consultant representative who was a woman, and Professors Chard and Hudson from Barts, who were the University representatives. Professor Salkind did not have a vote but could comment. David Oram and I represented the district. There is a statutory composition for consultant appointment panels and Mr Brew invoked the provision for an extra district consultant, which worried me in the case of disagreement.[12] In the event, the Chair used his casting vote to appoint Mr V S Pathasundaram, a mature and experienced obstetrician and gynaecologist who had left Sri Lanka for political reasons. The decision was greeted with disbelief by my colleagues, who did all they could behind the scenes to prevent the appointment being ratified by the DHA. However Mr Brew stood firm as he was convinced that Mr Pathasundaram would provide the service needed by the women of Tower Hamlets, which he has conscientiously done. So we had some new blood in the department as Professor MacNaughton had recommended. Mr Pathasundaram was a loyal colleague, worked very hard and remained calm despite all the problems.

The appointments committee for the senior lecturer was held on 27 November 1990. The field was small despite the post being advertised twice, and all three short-listed had worked as trainees in the department. One was our current SR. None was a feto-maternal medicine expert, although this was part of the job description. The person appointed, a Mr Armstrong, was in my opinion the weakest academically of the three. Only two publications by him are listed in Medline in 2006, a letter in 1980 and an article co-authored with Professor Grudzinskas in 1986.

Mr Armstrong was white, while both the other candidates were from ethnic minorities. I felt so strongly that the person I considered the best candidate had been treated unjustly and that we had lost the opportunity to strengthen the academic department that I wrote in confidence to Mr Brew and Mr Dickinson. I said I thought that the two unsuccessful candidates could have a case for racial discrimination and I was disturbed that the successful candidate's application had been received after the closing date. I did not copy the letter to anyone else. Mr Brew replied on 20 December 1990 and dismissed my criticisms of the process. In January I had a letter from the Commission for Racial Equality, to whom a copy of the letter had been sent. I discussed it with the SR concerned but he did not wish to pursue the matter – thinking (probably rightly) it might be detrimental to his career. He obtained a senior lecturer post later in 1991 and was then head-hunted by Harvard University. He had 15 publications at the time of interview and has had another 51 since then.

12 DHSS (1982); and Statutory Instrument No.1,407 (1990)

Progress of the two-firm proposal

With the appointment of someone to work with me, it was possible to implement the two-firm proposal that had been agreed by the SPP in May and endorsed by the DHA in June 1990. The unit general manager (UGM) wrote to all consultants asking them to agree to the proposal for two firms by 1 December 1990. The new system was to start on 1 February 1991 when new SHOs began. All agreed in writing by the deadline although Professor Grudzinskas suggested extra junior staff were needed for firm two. This was unreasonable when one looked at the workload and staff allocation.

The slow and tortuous steps towards the final implementation of a watered-down version of the plan required countless meetings between the SPP and the O&G consultants, as some of my colleagues fought the proposal for the two-firm system at every turn. On 22 February 1991 I wrote again with the help of my solicitor, Brian Raymond, to all consultants before the Medical Council meeting. An extract from the four-page letter is given below:

> For the two-firm proposal to work effectively, however, it is essential that each firm has its own junior staff, separately organised and responsible only to the consultants in that firm. The reason for this is that the implacable hostility of the other consultants towards me inevitably affects the activities of the junior staff, causing confusion over clinical approaches and undermining confidence. A substantial amount of my time is spent counteracting this. I must emphasise that I make no criticism of the junior staff: it is nearly impossible to serve consultant X diligently when consultants W, Y and Z oppose her approach, question her competence and refuse to accord her the most elementary professional courtesy. This was so even in 1984, and vivid examples of the difficulties caused – and the adverse consequences for patient care – were given in evidence to the Beaumont Enquiry. …having agreed last July to the division of junior staff between teams, my colleagues have now reversed their position saying 'times have changed' …the two-firm system now stands in danger of being destroyed unless there is immediate and effective intervention. In this event, the demoralising conditions under which I have been compelled to work since my re-instatement in 1986 will continue for the rest of my working life and many hours of work put in by senior members of the consultant body and senior managers will be thrown away.

I went on to say that I would use any legal remedies open to me. The Medical Council confirmed their support for the SPP and the two-firm proposal, despite two of my colleagues speaking against it.

On 1 April 1991 the London became a first-wave trust and the new Chief Executive, Mike Fairey, took up his post in May. The two-firm agreement had been changed at the last minute by a member of the SPP without discussion with me, and contained an inaccuracy about the rotation of registrars in the region. Mr Fairey was able to impose a solution. A last ditch attempt to de-rail the process in July when there was an RCOG recognition visit (all posts recognised for training by the relevant college were inspected every few years) prompted Brian Raymond to write personally to Mr Fairey. Despite the agreement between the president of the RCOG and the hospital management, and my correspondence about the registrar posts since January, the visitors denied all knowledge of the situation. However, on 1 September 1991 the two-firm system finally started and Mr Pathasundaram and I began a one-in-two rota on call. The department moved to a weekly one-in-six duty consultant schedule for emergencies when he was appointed, having previously had a month on call at a time. Obstetrics had moved from Mile End in July 1991 so all the work was at Whitechapel.

One of the problems for me was the number of people involved and the way that they kept changing, so one had to repeatedly explain the problems, which they came to understand after a few months. At the RCOG there was one person who dealt with registrar timetables, another who dealt with rotations and a third with consultant job descriptions, and, in the hospital, medical staffing dealt with advertisements. Trevor Beedham was district tutor and so related formally to the RCOG, and both Alastair Scotland, regional consultant in public health medicine, and the regional personnel officer got involved because of manpower planning and the initiative to reduce junior doctors' hours.

In addition, there was the problem of legal advice. The system with the medical defence organisations (MDOs) was that if a member's application for assistance was approved, the MDO became the solicitor's client, and could withdraw support at any time. After the Medical Defence Union was forced to pay my legal fees[13] they agreed to let Brian Raymond go on providing legal advice once I returned to work. From then until August 1990 his fees for over 75 hours of work amounted to £13,000. On 1 February 1991 the MDU wrote to say that as things now seemed settled (!) they would no longer continue to pay for his services. This was another anxiety, as Brian was always available or returned a call within a few hours. The first time I contacted the MDU after this, the person allocated to me was away and the help I needed was not there. Fortunately Brian's continued assistance could be paid for by a contingency fund which had been provided by supporters and he remained an immense support to me.

As I read through the large ring binder full of correspondence relating to this battle from 18 October 1990 to 8 October 1991 (one of six following my return to work) in order to write this chapter, I felt physically sick. There were over 150 letters, about half of which were from me, typed by myself at home, and they record the details of the two-firm struggle. On 5 February 1991 when the agreed starting date had passed without implementation, despite the assurances given to new doctors beginning in February, I went to see the Chair of the Medical Council and found he was away for two weeks. The medical director elect was unable to speak to me and I broke down in tears when I went to speak to the member of the SPP who was available. The harrowing story of an anonymous surgeon contained in this book shows that such problems still occur.

Life was certainly better with a colleague to talk to and alternate nights and weekends off and, although the two-firm solution was not ideal, it enabled things to go forward. Trevor Beedham asked me to attend a regional meeting to discuss registrar rotations on his behalf and we exchanged useful letters. He had supported the RCOG proposal that I should be considered for a merit award, so I was hopeful that wounds were healing.

One of the things that kept me going was my weekly visit to antenatal clinics in the community. We discussed problems with the GPs, midwives and health visitors in a friendly and normal professional interaction. The other was the feeling – which I experienced every few weeks – that I had made a difference to the way a woman had given birth.

---

13 Dr Noel Olsen, prompted by his doctor wife, started collecting signatures for an extraordinary general meeting (EGM) of the MDU to ask why they were not paying my legal fees. The MDU Council agreed to do this before the notice of an EGM was sent out, but later the number of signatures needed to call an EGM was increased.

On 22 May 1993, the day my youngest son got married, Brian Raymond died suddenly at the age of 44. This was a huge loss for the legal profession as well as for his family and for me personally. As John Hendy wrote in response to the *Guardian* obituary 'Those of our citizens at risk of being crushed by the big battalions have lost a champion.'[14] Then on 20 June my granddaughter, aged six, was diagnosed with a Wilms' tumour. She was treated by Great Ormond St Hospital and had to have ten weeks of chemotherapy, so the letter sent from the RCOG on 17 May 1993, after the hospital recognition committee visit in March, came at a bad time.

The letter said that unless by 15 June 1993 the on-call accommodation was improved and the registrars and SHOs on firm one changed to a one-in-four rota from the current one-in-three, they would remove recognition from the posts. This would mean that career-minded doctors would not apply for them, as they needed to be in recognised posts to further their professional development. I had devised a timetable which meant, by giving time off after a night on call, they were working – on paper – a 72-hour week (probably 76 in practice). Mr Pathasundaram and I looked after labour ward and gynae emergencies on Wednesday afternoon so that the career SHO and registrars could have an afternoon of teaching (the GP trainees were released that day), so educationally the posts had been improved.

By this time Mr Pathasundaram was Chair of the department and Mr McKelvie was no longer our facilitating Chair, so we had at least two meetings to discuss how we were going to respond to the demands by the RCOG visitors. The usual differences of opinion and intransigence of some of my colleagues showed that nothing had changed. The possibility of getting the DHA to employ another SHO was thought to be unrealistic. I spent hours working out rotas and trying to get people to understand the issues. The proposal by a number of my colleagues that six SHOs were attached to the six consultants and rotated every two months, leaving two to cover for holidays, was educationally inferior to the system we had running and was not appreciated by the junior staff attached to Mr Pathasundaram and myself, even though a reduction in on-call would have been welcome.

Mr Fairey wrote to the RCOG on 15 June 1993 saying that money had been found to improve the staff accommodation and went on to say:

> The Visitors raised as a third matter of immediate concern, the issue of the deficiencies in the rotas in firm one. As you know arrangements for the two-firm system and the work practices associated with it have been in operation for approximately two years. They were arrived at as a result of long, patient, and frequently arduous negotiation, and finally gained agreement, not only with all those involved here at the Royal London Trust, but also from the Royal College itself. You will understand, therefore, that these arrangements, so carefully negotiated, and definitively approved by the Trust Board, are not ones from which the Trust wish lightly to depart. As you would expect, however, the Trust and its consultant staff in obstetrics were concerned to learn of the Royal College's views, and would obviously wish to examine how they might be put into effect, whilst at the same time maintaining the felicitous equilibrium in the affairs of the Department of Obstetrics and Gynaecology which have obtained since the new arrangements came into effect on 1 October 1991. You will, I am sure, be as pleased as I am to learn that there appears to

14 Hendy (1993)

> be the possibility that mutually acceptable arrangements can be made to meet the point the College is making. You will, I am sure, equally understand that, in view of the events of recent years, the Trust Board would wish to assure itself that changes in the arrangements should be for the better, and that they do indeed command the necessary support. The Board will therefore be considering that matter at its meeting on Thursday 24 June, and I will be in touch with you as soon as possible thereafter.

However, we had not reached agreement and on 21 July 1993 I learned that the RCOG Council meeting on 24 July was to remove recognition from the posts. I had faxed SHO duty rotas and timetables to the RCOG on 13 July but had no reply. I had been to see Mark Stephens for legal advice and had sent him about 100 photocopies of correspondence to put him in the picture. I finished my letter to Frank Loeffler, who chaired the Hospital Recognition Committee and who had been on Mr Pathasundaram's appointments panel, with the words 'I would not want to see seven reasonable posts turned into eight awful posts and will resist this in any way possible.' He wrote back the following day agreeing to postpone any decision until October and asking for clarification of the timetables.

At one of the meetings Professor Grudzinskas had said that he had never refused to let me cover for his patients. I wrote to him on 29 May 1993 saying that I considered that if his statement had been dishonest this could amount to serious professional misconduct and said: 'I would like you either to confirm in writing what you said in front of witnesses at the meeting on 27 May 1993 or retract the statement'. He replied on 7 June: 'Further to your letter of 29 May, I would like to make it clear that I have not refused to allow you to cover for my patients since the inception of the two-firm system and this is what it was my intention to say. I do not wish to comment on what my attitude was before that time.' I did not pursue the matter.

Mr Pathasundaram and I, with 18 sessions between us, had been responsible for 55 per cent of the births in 1992 and had booked 65 per cent of the women so far in 1993. We shared one SR, while firm two, with four consultants and 30 sessions, had three: a sub-specialist registrar not paid for by the hospital, an NHS SR and the lecturer. We had two registrars, they had two point five; we had three SHOs, they had four. An eighth SHO covered holidays. So it seemed quite unfair to reduce our SHO allocation further.

In a desperate attempt to get the Board to see sense I went to see the Chairman, Michael Haines, but to no avail. Despite the objections of the GP trainees, the allocation of SHOs was changed and they were rotated every two months spending a third of their time in a peripatetic role covering holidays. We returned to the previous system of having one SHO on for obstetrics and one for gynaecology, thereby reducing the opportunity for continuity of care. A weekly teaching session for all staff in training was introduced on Friday afternoons, which was an improvement. However, the consultant staff did not cover the labour ward as Mr Pathasundaram and I had done. In November 1994 after a further RCOG visit it was agreed to give recognition for another five years to the training posts as long as the registrars rotated between firms after six months. Although I thought this was bad for training (with study leave and holidays for both consultant and registrar it was easy for a poor trainee not to be identified and for a good one not to have time to build up the rapport which is essential for a good apprenticeship system), I did not fight it. In retrospect this was probably a mistake.

In February 1996 gynaecology was moved to Barts and again I was the sole voice in opposition. We were promised enough beds so that cases would not be cancelled as had been happening increasingly at Whitechapel. However we were not told that there would only be nine beds for eight gynaecologists: in fact over 40 beds were mentioned, but in the event over half were for the three gynaecological oncologists and so not available for general gynaecological work. In addition we shared the ward with surgeons. Moreover, some beds were removed. So we had underemployed SHOs at Barts and overstretched SHOs at the London and very poor facilities for teaching the students.

Clinical tutor position

In July of that year I was appointed by a panel at the regional postgraduate dean's office to the advertised post of clinical tutor at the London, starting in September. The clinical tutor had oversight of all the doctors in training and liaised with the district tutors in each specialty. The postgraduate centre was situated in Queen Mary College at Mile End, which was not ideal as the majority of the trainees were at Whitechapel, so my first task was to find some space there. Study leave applications came though the office and the previous clinical tutor had set up an excellent system for logging them so one could see which trainees were not getting their allocation. Feedback was obtained about the training they were receiving and fed back to the district tutors. Advice could be given but it was difficult to persuade some consultants to change unacceptable practices. A lunchtime programme for pre-registration house officers was started.

Anonymous complaint

In 1996 the new Barts and The London (and London Chest) Trust was formed and so the question of the clinical tutor for the combined Trust arose. I was asked to go and see the new medical director, Duncan Empey, a physician from the London Chest, on 8 March 1996. When I arrived Duncan told me that he had received an anonymous complaint about my management of five obstetric cases. It was exactly ten years since the last day of my enquiry, and unbelievably, this seemed like another attempt had been made to get rid of me. It was partly to guard against this nightmare that I had fought so long and hard to have two separate firms: so that I could trust the staff and not fear that they were being poisoned against me. I said he was surely not going to take anonymous allegations seriously, but Duncan felt he had to. Obviously he had not been involved in 1985–6 and knew nothing of the history of the department. He wanted to call in an outside assessor, but I resisted this and said I would get computer data to show that my practice was just as safe as those of my colleagues.

I was due at a meeting at the RCOG that day and as I travelled on the tube I went through the staff in my mind – who could it have been? I hated feeling suspicious and as I looked through the cases I could recall that there had been discussion about the management of some of them. As the Munro panel had suggested, I had always been available to discuss issues on the phone and come in out of hours if my management differed from that of my colleagues, for example if a woman wanted to have an attempt to deliver vaginally after two caesarean sections. This is safe, but most obstetricians did not allow it.[15] Although the risk of dehiscence is doubled, the absolute risk is still low, about 1 in 100. When I got to the College, Gordon Stirrat, one of my expert witnesses,[16] was talking to the new president, Naren Patel. He asked me how I was, and I blurted out

15 Roberts et al (1994)

16 Savage (1986) p.160–1

my shock at the events of the morning. I could feel that tears were not far away, but I managed to control them.

So for the next four months I was writing explanations, getting the computer data out, consulting the MDU and explaining management to a physician, resisting his attempts to bring in an outside person, writing to the president of the RCOG and calling on my supporters for advice and help. Having seen the evidence, most of them thought it was unnecessary to bring in an outsider. John McGarry was willing to come and support me if someone was called in to discuss my management. I expressed the view that rather than another enquiry into my competence, an evaluation of our dysfunctional department would be more appropriate.

After my experience with the Hospital Recognition Committee, and knowing that Trevor Beedham now had a senior position in the RCOG (although I did not think he was behind this latest attempt to get rid of me), I did not agree to the proposed external assessor. Eventually Duncan Empey, who had suggested initially that I took early retirement, seemed satisfied and the matter fizzled out. The support of Pam Hibbs was invaluable.

One of these cases showed how strongly some women feel about being able to deliver vaginally. She had booked to have her baby at the London after two caesareans and got to full dilatation, but the second stage was not progressing well. I came in at about 11.00pm and examined her. The baby was in the occipito-posterior position. There was not enough room in the pelvis to rotate the head and a cautious trial with the forceps was followed by a drop in the heart rate. I could see that it was not going to be an easy delivery so I said we should do a third CS. I stayed until the baby was out and the registrar and SR were stitching the uterus. When I got home the SR called to tell me there had been a small tear in the bladder that she was confident they had been able to suture successfully. The woman went home with a catheter in place and did well. A year later I had a postcard from her telling me that she had successfully delivered her fourth baby at home. I wrote back to congratulate her and asked the weight of the baby and its position. This time the head was in the usual occipito-anterior position, which is more favourable for delivery, and he weighed four ounces less.

This second attempt to question my professional standing left me exhausted. When the joint medical school amalgamated academically with Queen Mary College, I had discovered that their staff were offered a term's sabbatical for every seven years in post. Having been in post for almost 20 years, I thought I could apply for a year's leave, and managed to persuade the Warden, Colin Berry, our first facilitating Chair, to support me – but he said it would be unpaid leave. I was fortunate that an outgoing secretary of the joint school agreed that a sabbatical should be paid. I obtained a place to do an MSc in Public Health at the School of Hygiene and Tropical Medicine in September 1996. I found a very experienced Bengali woman obstetrician to do my locum (over 50 per cent of births were to Bengali women), and of course we had a battle about this as Professor Grudzinskas wanted one of our SRs to do it – a white Anglo-Saxon male, who did not share my philosophy. Fortunately, the managers accepted that the department needed a woman and she was appointed.

Another enquiry

When I returned to work on 1 October 1997 I was asked to meet a panel of two obstetricians from Glasgow who were assessing the Department of Obstetrics and Gynaecology. The new management wished us to go on to a one-in-six consultant rota and for there to be consultant cover on the labour ward during the day. This was agreed. The cover was fragmented and it was sometimes difficult to ensure that my patients had the agreed plan carried out, so paradoxically this required more work from me than when Mr Pathasundaram and I covered for each other. As a seven-session academic, I was already doing more work than the RCOG recommended, so the addition of two sessions on Labour Ward and taking on the post of unit training director would push me way over the limit. Nevertheless I complied with the new system.

Academic work

Soon after I returned to work, Professor Chard (Reproductive Physiology, based at Barts) asked me if I would contribute a chapter on caesarean section (CS) to a book he was editing with Martin Richards on obstetric controversies.[17] I wanted to use data from the London Hospital obstetric database comparing CS rates and thought it only polite to show the draft table which compared our results to my colleagues. Professor Grudzinskas's comment was that the table was 'scientifically meaningless'! Fortunately, Professor Chard was happy to publish it and it followed on from a paper that Colin Francome and Peter Huntingford had published in 1980 comparing interventionist and non-interventionist obstetricians at the London Hospital.[18]

Middlesex University

I had lectured on contraception and abortion on an MA course at Middlesex University and had had students on attachment since 1987. In 1991 I was made an Honorary Professor in the Faculty of Social Science and gave my inaugural lecture on 17 November 1992. Colin Francome and I have continued to work on research on caesarean section and abortion.[19]

Women's Health Care Research Unit

Sam Smith[20] had started a fund to pay my legal fees. When the MDU agreed to pay the fees in 1987 (see footnote 14), the money was no longer needed. Brian and I wrote to all those who had contributed and asked if they would like to have their contributions back. Almost none did. They were happy for the money to be used to fund a research post. We set up a charity called Womanschoice in 1988 and appointed Ruth Cochrane as research fellow. Ruth did a study of women's expectations of and feelings about their antenatal care, for which she was awarded an MD by Cardiff University.

Initially I had hoped to draw a random sample of women booking for antenatal care and compare the outcomes of hospital-based and community-based care. Obtaining my colleagues' permission proved a time consuming and frustrating task so we had to use a consecutive sample of women booking under the care of those consultants who did eventually agree to compare with those being looked after in the community. The results were published in a small pamphlet which was circulated to all Professors of Obstetrics and Gynaecology and offered to midwives free of charge.[21]

---

17 Savage (1992) in Richards and Chard (1992)

18 Francome and Huntingford (1980)

19 Munday et al (1989); Savage and Francome (1989); Francome and Savage (1992); Savage and Francome (1993); Francome and Savage (1993); Francome et al (1993); Churchill et al (2006)

20 Savage (1986)

21 Womanschoice (1992)

In the department of General Practice we set up a Women's Health Care Research Unit in 1989 with the help of Professor Salkind who provided the salary for Julie George, our researcher, after an earlier grant ended. The Unit aimed to improve the care given to women. We ran courses for GPs about home birth and organised two conferences, from one of which came a book about the health care of older women.[22] We also published some work on emergency contraception[23] and were commissioned by Newham Health Authority to conduct a survey of family planning services. After Professor Salkind retired we were unable to find further funding to pay Julie George's salary, so we closed the unit in 1994. Because of the continuing difficulties in my NHS work I did not feel able to apply for a large grant spanning several years, as I was unsure if I would be there to see it through, so the whole sad business had yet more detrimental ramifications.

Return to the Academic Department of Obstetrics and Gynaecology

After I returned from my sabbatical, Ovrang Djahanbakhch the senior lecturer in Newham asked me to return to the academic department of O&G and I agreed. During my sabbatical a two-week Community Obstetric and Gynaecology module had been started in the third clinical year and I was asked to organise it, which was very enjoyable. Professor Chard gave me a room in his department at Barts and with a larger department (there was another senior lecturer at the Homerton) academic unit meetings were bearable. Minor problems occurred over secretarial help and over the organisation and setting of examinations. These caused friction between Professor Grudzinskas, Mr Armstrong and myself but overall things were going reasonably well by this time.

In 1999 the medical school asked for an external review of the Academic Unit of Obstetrics and Gynaecology. This was headed by Lord Winston as the infertility expert and two other academics from outside London in the fields of feto-maternal medicine and gynaecological oncology. The visit took place on 25–6 March 1999 and all members of the academic department were interviewed. I do not have a copy of their final report but the summary e-mailed to us all by Professors Chard and Grudzinskas reported on the oral presentation they were given at the end of the visit as follows:

- Individually, most members of the department make a substantial contribution to the school
- There was a serious lack of cohesion between the individuals – lack of overall leadership and lack of strategic vision as to how the department should advance
- The school should identify a new leader for the department, probably from outside, capable of driving forward a new academic vision for the next 5–10 years
- The teaching offered by the department was described as above average
- The strategic plan for Oncology was highly commended
- Those for Reproductive Medicine and Feto-Maternal medicine were considered to be ill-prepared, impractical and lacking in vision
- There was a notable lack of peer-reviewed external research grants

22 George and Ebrahim (1992)
23 George et al (1994)

- Some individuals were considered to contribute less than would be expected from their HEFCE funding and in some cases their publications were in low-impact journals (I probably fell into this category but was not alone)
- There was a total lack of budgetary information or financial planning
- The Reader (Ovrang Djahanbakhch) received insufficient support from the department and school especially in the light of his considerable academic output and the fact that his funding was almost exclusively by the Newham Trust
- The infrastructure for the management of higher degrees was weak – for example there was no figure available for the number of PhD students in the department.

There was also comment about the position of the division within the academic and trust structures and the difficulty of running a department on four sites several miles apart, and the need for central laboratory facilities.

As a result of this damning report (to which I recall Professor Grudzinskas wrote a forthright rebuttal) the division was moved from the community section headed by Professor Sheila Hillier, a sociologist, an arrangement which Professor Grudzinskas had always thought inappropriate, to Oncology, headed by Professor Adrian Newland. I did not really think that Obstetrics fitted this division either, but it made little difference in practice.

Professor Grudzinskas retired in November 2003 and was made Professor Emeritus. One of the fears of the two deans who had written to the Munro panel was that if all my colleagues resigned, as they had threatened to do, the department would be damaged and the medical school's reputation would suffer. As I write, in September 2006, Barts and the London is without a Professor of Obstetrics and it has been difficult to recruit people to the Academic Unit in those intervening years. Had the nettle been grasped in 1987 things might have been very different, but nobody wanted to be critical of Professor Grudzinskas despite Professor Taylor's evidence[24] and, despite his often unrealistic demands, the academic department limped on for 16 years. It seems that the professoriate feel threatened if one of their number is attacked, however poor the behaviour and performance may be.

I retired on 30 September 2000 and held a scientific colloquium. Many old friends and colleagues came and presented papers. This was followed by a dinner which my children also attended and where Mr Pathasundaram spoke. Of my then colleagues at Barts and the London, only Mr Pathasundaram and a locum consultant came, although some sent their apologies.

In this chapter I have concentrated on my hospital work, but I also lectured all over the country in the years after I was reinstated and have continued to do so after my retirement from clinical practice.

Election to the General Medical Council (GMC) 1989

Jean Robinson had worked for the Patients' Association before being appointed as a lay member of the GMC. As a member of AIMS (the Association for the Improvement of Maternity Services) she had been active in my defence, and it was she who suggested that I should stand for the GMC. I was delighted to be elected with the second-highest number of votes after Michael O'Donnell in May 1989.

24 Savage (1986) pp.162–3

The following year I was elected to the standards committee and sat on that until 1999. It was chaired by Donald Irvine and a subcommittee worked on drawing up a positive statement of what doctors *should* do rather than the 'thou shalt not approach' which had prevailed until then. My contribution to *Good Medical Practice* was a positive experience, and collaborating with Michael O'Donnell amongst others was a welcome relief from the many frustrations of life at work.

I was re-elected in 1994, again in 1999, and to the new, reformed GMC in 2002. I was obliged to resign on grounds of age in 2005. I sat on the Professional Conduct Committee, Professional Performance Committee and Interim Orders Committee over the ten years from 1994. In 2000 I became a medical screener of new complaints against doctors, and gained considerable experience in this role of the way the GMC operates. I stood against Sir Donald Irvine in 1999, the first time a sitting president had been challenged. I felt strongly that he was leading the GMC in the wrong direction. My view is that the members need *more* involvement with the day-to-day working not less. I also stood in 2002. This time each of us presented a personal vision of our leadership of the GMC if successful. This set a precedent for the future presidential elections of Council. At the 2002 ballot, Sir Graeme Catto was elected outright on the first round. Jim Drife, a contributor to this book, came second and I came third of the six candidates.

Gossiping doctors

At a GMC Council meeting in 1994 I was trying to get support for a suspended doctor, Dr Helena Daly. The late Bob Kendall, who was then CMO of Scotland repeated some gossip about her which I found quite shocking. I wrote to him and copied the letter to Lord (John) Walton, as I also referred to some gossip that he had passed on in 1986 which had been overheard by a friend of mine. He had said that the reason I had been suspended was because I was 'a socialist feminist lesbian'. I never received a reply from Dr Kendall, but Lord Walton's answer is reproduced below:

> 8 July 1994
>
> Dear Mrs Savage,
>
> I apologize for not having replied to your earlier correspondence as I had been under the impression that you had merely copied the correspondence with Dr Kendall to me for information. I had also thought, and had indeed hoped that Ian Chalmers would have passed on the apology which I had made to him many years ago relating to the comments based on unsubstantiated gossip.
>
> It was in fact a senior obstetrician at the London, whom I would prefer not to name, who told me that you had said to him that you had been suspended for the reasons mentioned in your letter. I should not have passed on his comment at an unguarded moment during a dinner in Green College when a visiting obstetrician was mentioning your problems. I regretted having done so, and when Ian Chalmers mentioned that this quote had been attributed to me in conversation, I asked him to pass on my apologies to you.
>
> Yours sincerely…

I had never said the words attributed to me by a senior obstetrician at the London, but the gossip was widespread at the time of my case. When I returned to work and told the theatre nurses at Mile End about it they fell about laughing. When told these reasons in a major London teaching hospital, another friend of mine replied 'she does have four children and it was in the days before do-it yourself'. Why any of these descriptions would be a reason for suspension is beyond me, yet this explanation was clearly passed around freely.

One of the difficulties that suspended doctors face is the way that their reputations can be damaged by this kind of tittle-tattle, which is hard to counteract, as normally one does not know what is being said. Gossiping may be part of human nature, but one would hope that highly trained professionals in a caring profession would be above that kind of behaviour.

When I was first back at work I would be contacted at least once a month by a distressed doctor wanting advice. After some time I suggested to Peter Tomlin that he set up a group to support these doctors, which he did with the late Dr Harry Jacobs. He has analysed the histories of those doctors who have contacted him. They are not a random sample of suspended doctors, but in my view have a high proportion of those wrongfully suspended because they are seen as 'different' or 'difficult', often because they are more conscientious than some of their colleagues or act as whistleblowers. His latest analysis shows that women doctors are more likely to have had unjustified suspensions – 94 per cent compared with 84 per cent for male doctors.[25]

From this account you can see how difficult management finds it to deal with a situation where a doctor is excluded by her colleagues from normal professional relationships. The problem is compounded by the attitude of some of the most senior people in medicine and the way that many of those in positions of power in the hospital and Royal College hierarchies appear to allow their loyalty to their colleagues to outweigh fairness and justice. This 'club culture' was condemned by Sir Ian Kennedy in his report about Bristol[26] and may explain why some women doctors have such a difficult time. This is still happening, as is portrayed so vividly in section 4 by a woman surgeon suspended three years ago.

References

Churchill H, Savage W and Francome C (2006) *Caesarean Birth in Britain: A book for health professionals and parents*. Revised and Updated. London: Middlesex University Press.

DHSS (1982) *Appointment of Consultants and Senior Registrars*. London: HMSO.

Diggory P (1989) 'Bitter reinstatement', *Lancet* (ii) 806 © reprinted with permission from Elsevier.

Donald I (1955) *Practical Obstetric Problems*. Lloyd Luke.

Ferriman A and Leigh D (1985) 'Women's rights go on trial in childbirth row', *The Observer*, 16 June 1985.

Francome C and Huntingford P (1980) 'Births by Caesarean section in the United States of America and in Britain', *Journal of Biosocial Science* 12(3):353–62.

25 Tomlin (2003)

26 Kennedy (2001)

Francome C and Savage W (1992) 'Gynaecologists abortion practice', *British Journal of Obstetrics and Gynaecology*, 99:153–7.

Francome C and Savage W (1993) 'Caesarean Section in Britain and the United States 12 per cent or 24 per cent: is either the right rate?' *Social Science and Medicine*, 37: 1,199–218.

Francome C, Savage W, Churchill H and Lewison H (1993) *Caesarean Birth in Britain: A book for health professionals and parents*. London: Middlesex University Press in association with The National Childbirth Trust.

George J and Ebrahim S (eds) (1992) *Health Care of Older Women*. Oxford: Oxford University Press.

George J, Turner J, Cooke E, Hennessy E, Savage W, Julian P and Cochrane R (1994) 'Women's Knowledge of Emergency Contraception', *British Journal of General Practice*, 44:451–4.

Hendy (1993) *The Guardian*, 26 May 1993.

Jewell T (1989) 'Bitter reinstatement', *Lancet* (ii) 744 © reprinted with permission from Elsevier.

Kennedy I (2001) *The report of the enquiry into children's heart surgery at Bristol Royal Infirmary 1964–1995: Learning from Bristol*. Chairman Professor Ian Kennedy Cmnd 5,207. London: The Stationery Office.

Lancet (1986) Editorial 'Attitudes in obstetric care', *Lancet* (ii) 257–8.

Lancet (1989a) Editorial 'Bitter reinstatement', *Lancet* (ii) 308–9 © reprinted with permission from Elsevier.

Lancet (1989b) Editorial 'Looking up whilst going full circle', *Lancet* (ii) 1,492–3.

Lancet (1989c) Correction, 12 August 1989, *Lancet* (ii) 402.

Munday D, Francome C and Savage W (1989) 'Twenty one years of legal abortion', *British Medical Journal*, 298:1,231–4.

Munro, Dame Alison (1986) *Report to the Tower Hamlets Health Authority*. Wendy Savage's papers.

Richards M and Chard T (eds) (1992) *Obstetrics in the 1990s: Current Controversies*. London: MacKeith Press.

Roberts LJ, Beardsworth SA and Trew G (1994) 'Labour following caesarean section: current practice in the United Kingdom', *British Journal of Obstetrics & Gynaecology*, 101(2):153–5.

Saha A, Savage W and George J (1992) *The Tower Hamlets Day care Abortion Service*, Study for Doctors for a Womans' Choice on Abortion, funded principally by the GLC Women's committee. London: WHCRU. (Copies available from Wendy Savage.)

Savage W (1986) *A Savage Enquiry: Who Controls Childbirth?* London: Virago.

Savage W (1992) 'The Rise in Caesarean Section: Anxiety not Science' in Richards and Chard (eds) (1992) pp.167–91.

Savage W and Francome C (1989) 'Gynaecologists' attitudes to abortion', *Lancet*, ii:1,323–4.

Savage W and Francome C (1993) 'British caesarean section rates: have we reached a plateau?' *British Journal of Obstetrics & Gynaecology*, 100:493–6.

Statutory Instrument, No.1,407 (1990).

Tomlin PJ (2003) *Journal of Obstetrics & Gynaecology*, Vol.23, 321–7.

Womanschoice (1992) *Antenatal care in the Community*. London: WHCRU. (Out of print.)

1 2 3 4 5 6

Birth and Power

Birth and Power

Wendy Savage

Birth arouses strong emotions in people and the control of it has for centuries been contested. At one time, female midwives were licensed to practise by the Church, which was more concerned with their morals than their competence. Gradually, male doctors became important in providing care, initially for wealthy women, and over the last 250 years doctors have taken over the provision and organisation of services for pregnant women.[1] The medical model, which is the prevailing one in the Western world today, holds that 'No birth is safe except in retrospect' and many obstetricians sincerely believe that the reduction in the PMR (perinatal mortality rate, the number of stillbirths and deaths in the first week of life per 1,000 births) over the last 50 years is due to their efforts to persuade all women to give birth in hospital. The alternative social model, which takes account of the immense importance of birth as a rite of passage for women, its significance within the family and wider community and its normality as a physiological process, asserts that 'birth is not an illness' and is still widely accepted in Holland and by a minority of doctors and midwives elsewhere.

There are about 600,000 births per year, 30,000 practising midwives and 2,000 obstetricians in England and Wales, yet women have almost no say in how services are organised. If 3,000 women confronted one obstetrician the power of numbers would be apparent, but all too often an older, socially privileged male obstetrician will explain things in such a way that a young, poorly educated and inexperienced woman having her first baby feels overwhelmed. The government committees that have looked into maternity services, Cranbrook in 1959, Peel in 1971and Short in 1982, were dominated by the views of the obstetricians advising the government. Cranbrook[2] recommended that more hospital beds should be made available. With the increased birth rate after the Second World War, some women who wanted to have their babies in hospital, often because of poor housing conditions, were unable to do so, and healthy women were encouraged to give birth at home. Domiciliary midwifery was still accepted and a third of women had their babies outside consultant obstetric units.[3] The next review, led by Sir John Peel, recommended that all women be 'offered the benefits of hospital confinement', without any evidence that this was a good use of government resources or was wanted by women.[4] By 1970, only 11 per cent of women had their babies outside hospital, either at home or in general practitioner units.[5] In both settings the majority of births were supervised by midwives, which was quite different from the USA where midwives had virtually been eliminated from birth care in the early part of the twentieth century and women were looked after by obstetricians.[6]

---

1 Donnison (1977)

2 MoH(1959)

3 Butler and Bonham (1960)

4 DoH, Standing Maternity and Midwifery Advisory Committee (1970)

5 Chamberlain and Chamberlain (1972)

6 Arney (1982)

By 1980, the proportion of women having their babies at home had fallen to 1 per cent. Despite the transfer of healthy women to hospital care, which one would have expected to lower the rate, the caesarean section rate (CSR) continued to rise without a break.

The 1982 Short report made a classic epidemiological mistake and stated that it was now safer to have a baby in hospital rather than at home.[7] The reason for this was revealed by Rona Campbell's study of all home births in England in 1989. She showed that the statistics used by Short had included as home births both unbooked and unplanned births (that is, births for which no antenatal care at all had been provided and births which had been scheduled for hospital delivery but took place at home, usually because of an emergency of some kind). Unbooked births had a staggering perinatal mortality rate of 196 per 1,000 which means that almost a fifth of these babies died. The hospital-booked women had a rate of 67.5 per 1,000: only by including these figures with planned home births had hospital delivery been 'shown' to be safer.[8] Without the skewed statistics, the home birth PMR was 4.1 – less than a third of the figure for England and Wales in 1979.

The 1991–2 Health Committee, chaired by Nicholas Winterton, was the first to take evidence from individual women and from women's groups such as AIMS and the NCT. Their evidence and that from the Royal College of Midwives (RCM) was well-documented, whereas that from the RCOG relied on opinion.[9] The Winterton report is an excellent piece of work and deserves to be read widely by policy makers and politicians. It is just as relevant today as it was when it was written.

The Audit Commission's report in 1997[10] and numerous local surveys throughout the country show that many women are unhappy with the maternity services offered to them. In 2003 the Health Select Committee decided to review maternity services, including data collection, and produced three reports.[11] They expressed concern about the lack of standardisation of the data collected, the variability of information available to pregnant women, the attitude of some GPs to home birth and the illusion of choice. They recommended that the soon-to-be-published National Service Framework for Children should incorporate the principles of *Changing Childbirth*[12] (see also the introduction to section six). They deplored the fact that, two years after the then Secretary of State for Health had put an extra £100 million into maternity services to promote choice, women were still denied the option of having their babies at home. They noted that despite the rhetoric, the Department of Health had taken no steps to promote the minister's promises. They also endorsed the idea of local decisions, whilst recognising that this might lead to inequitable provision of services such as midwifery-led units. However, despite their recommendations, the shortage of midwives continues and, in September 2006, we have the new chief executive of the NHS saying that maternity units will be closed.[13]

The organisation of maternity services within the NHS is the responsibility of the

7 House of Commons Social Services Committee (1980)
8 Campbell et al (1984)
9 Health Committee (1992)
10 Audit Commission (1997)
11 House of Commons Health Committee (2003a, 2003b and 2003c)
12 DoH (1993)
13 Carvel (2006)

boards of hospitals, now influenced also by the commissioning decisions of primary care trusts. Although the number of women on these decision-making bodies has increased, they are not necessarily representative of the population they serve. The way the service is organised is decided by managers whose decisions are heavily influenced by budgetary constraints and government targets. They are advised by professionals. Obstetricians have consistently had louder voices than midwives and the process of becoming a manager often seems to distance senior midwives from the needs and desires of women. Decisions to close units are sometimes made because of the perceived lack of paediatric cover or junior obstetric availability, meaning that women are forced into ever larger units.

Home birth is viewed as a 'luxury' (see Jane Sandall's chapter in this book) and the decision by the Chelsea and Westminster Hospital in 2006 to offer continuity of midwifery care for £2,000 suggests that this important aspect of care is also now becoming a luxury.[14]

Antenatal care

Antenatal care developed from an idea by Ballantyne in 1909, who saw it as a way of preventing difficulties at the time of birth. The present schedule of visits was designed by Dame Janet Campbell, a far-sighted civil servant, in 1928, and has only recently been challenged. A randomised controlled trial to compare the conventional system with a reduced number of visits (suggested by the RCOG and accepted by the Cumberlege report[15] as something to be looked at) showed little difference in outcomes, but women preferred the conventional schedule of visits.[16] The measurement of blood pressure, testing of urine and examination of the abdomen to check fetal growth are accepted by women as reassurance that they are coping with the pregnancy and that the baby is growing normally; but they often do not feel able to express their own fears and anxieties and would like more time to discuss them. This is one reason why continuity of care is appreciated: it allows the woman to get to know the midwife caring for her and voice these fears and other feelings.

The introduction of prenatal screening for fetal anomaly was not pushed for by women or society but by professional obstetricians and public health doctors, who produced a cost-benefit analysis to justify it. If the option of terminating a pregnancy which would result in the birth of a handicapped child is accepted, the benefits to individual women and their families are considerable; but the process has changed the experience of pregnancy for *all* women. It also raises ethical issues which some women find difficult and distressing; and it is all too often assumed that the woman will want to embark on the testing programme, even though she may not fully understand it.[17]

Routine ultrasound scanning was introduced without adequate evaluation of its possible effects. I understand that when its use was beginning to spread, the Medical Research Council was asked to consider a trial but decided against it. Now it is too late to carry out such a trial, and scanning is seen as a positive experience for women, with some departments providing a picture of the fetus. One Swedish study showed an

---

14 Press reports. *The Times* (2006)

15 DoH (1993)

16 Sikorski et al (1996)

17 Marteau (1995); Sandall et al (2003)

increase in left-handedness in army recruits insonated in utero compared with men who had not been exposed – a subtle effect,[18] but worrying to those of us concerned about the widespread adoption of scanning. Another factor which might merit investigation is the profitable nature of the business of supplying more and more sophisticated ultrasound machines, which are now considered essential for every maternity hospital.

Home birth

For many years the RCOG was against home birth, and taught generations of GP trainees that it was unsafe. The official position has now changed[19] and I know personally of two women consultant obstetricians who have had their babies at home. However, many older obstetricians still view home birth as dangerous, despite the evidence that it is a safe option for healthy women attended by midwives.[20] The subject is discussed by Marsden Wagner in his contribution to this section. This issue demonstrates clearly the power of the obstetric profession, but today the actions of midwifery managers and hard-pressed hospital chief executives and PCT commissioners may be just as powerful in denying women the choice of a home birth.

Interventions and caesarean section

Interventions such as routine shaving and enemas, induction and augmentation of labour, routine electronic fetal monitoring and episiotomy are examples of practices that obstetricians introduced, often without good evidence, and imposed on women. In the 1980s, WHO Europe conducted a study of birth practices in the European region and showed how variable they were in the different countries.[21] But are women in European countries so different from each other? The introduction of the concept of evidence-based medicine has improved matters in many places; the involvement of women in drawing up NICE guidelines may be a mixed blessing, as Beverley Beech suggests in her chapter. As professionals have designed the service, the expectations of women have changed and, living in a technological society, some women do not feel safe without machines and hospital backup.

The ultimate intervention is caesarean section (CS). The rates have increased tenfold since I was a medical student doing my midwifery in 1957 to almost 24 per cent in the UK in 2005. I still believe that the 10 per cent figure justified by the evidence gathered in the WHO consensus conference in 1985[22] is the maximum needed in a healthy population of women. For further discussion of this issue see the revised edition of *Caesarean Birth in Britain*.[23]

Despite the national audit of CS in 2001[24] and the NICE guidelines in 2004,[25] which recommend that every woman should be informed that booking for a home birth halves her risk of having a CS, the rate continues to increase without good evidence of benefit to women or babies. The latest analysis from epidemiologists in the USA is that the risk of the

---

18 Kieler et al (2001)
19 RCOG (1993)
20 Macfarlane and Campbell (1994)
21 Bergsjo et al (1983)
22 WHO (1985)
23 Churchill et al (2006)
24 Thomas and Paranjothy (2001)
25 NICE (2004)

baby dying after non-medically indicated CS in a large cohort of healthy women was twice that for vaginal delivery.[26] Will this evidence change the way that obstetricians behave?

Money

Since the NHS was introduced in 1948, money has not been a major factor in the power struggle between midwives and obstetricians for the control of birth. In countries like the USA, Australia and New Zealand, as Joan Donley's chapter shows, it certainly has been. When we surveyed British obstetricians in 1989 and asked why they thought the US CSR had risen from 4.5 per cent in 1970 to 24 per cent in 1988, the three leading reasons they gave were: litigation, money and private practice. In the UK, where the increase had been less, they put litigation first followed by clinical reasons.

So how can women get the births that they want? If they have money and want an elective CS they can pay for that, but if they want a birth at home without intervention they may have to find an independent midwife. This option is not open to all women as it also costs money. Pregnant women are not at a stage in their lives when they want to fight, but what about all the grandmothers, my age and younger, who know that they and most of their friends gave birth normally? Can't they be mobilised?

What needs to change in the UK

Despite taxpayers' money coming to government, neither ministers nor select committees since the 1990s appear to have been able to influence the way that women give birth to their babies. The repeated change of Secretary of State for Health and junior ministers does not help, and allows civil servants to push policy through; but maternity care is not high on their list of priorities. The Royal College of Midwives should be in a powerful position to ensure that midwives provide services in the way women have repeatedly requested. Yet the RCM was subservient for too long to obstetric views and is internally divided as to the way forward – as well as being currently involved in fighting job cuts. The handful of independent midwives have shown that they achieve good results – individual examples of good practice are scattered throughout the country – but will the 'One Mother, One Midwife' campaign succeed?[27]

AIMs and the NCT are now accepted as representing the views of women. In 1992–3, many people were hopeful that the evidence they had put forward to the select committee along with individual women had been accepted, and that the Cumberlege recommendations would transform maternity care. This has not happened.

Now in 2006, with the changes taking place in the NHS, managerial decisions are becoming increasingly important in shaping the way services are provided. John Eversley's chapter discusses the accountability of boards and PCTs.

The high-handed and unaccountable way that the NHS is being 'reformed' by the present government suggests a hidden agenda of privatisation, and the explanation for this can be found in Colin Leys' book *Market Driven Politics*.[28] The prospect of a privatised, US-style health system bodes ill for women, and we must resist it.

We now have a National Service Framework for maternity[29] and a women's 'Tsar'.

26 Macdorman et al (2006)
27 IMA (2006)
28 Leys (2001)
29 DoH (2004)

Let us work together as women – grandmothers, mothers and midwives – to change the way that services are provided in the way that women want.

In Joan Donley's chapter she traces the hard negotiating and tortuous path of change in New Zealand, where women now have much greater choice about the way they give birth – including being cared for by independent midwives contracting with the health service like GPs. Her tough and outspoken style may upset some who feel her views have no place in an academic book, but to me she exemplifies what it takes to fight the establishment and transform the system. The New Zealand midwives worked with women from the start and, whilst it may be easier to achieve change in a smaller population, the sheer persistence and understanding of the political scene are, I think, as applicable here.

Marsden Wagner has given a global perspective on the powerful forces which prevent midwives and doctors from providing the care that women want in the first chapter in this section. The chapters by Beverley Beech and Jane Sandall later in the book, together with what I have outlined here, show that the services provided for women have developed under the guidance of civil servants, themselves advised by obstetricians, and that women have played little or no part in how these services have developed.

References

Arney WR (1982) *Power and the Profession of Obstetrics*. Chicago: University of Chicago Press.

Audit Commission (1997) *First class delivery: Improving maternity services in England and Wales*. London: Audit Commission.

Bergsjo P, Schmidt E and Pusch D (1983) 'Differences in the reported frequencies of some obstetrical interventions in Europe', *BJOG*, 90:629–33.

Butler NR and Bonham DG (1960) *Perinatal Mortality*. Edinburgh & London: E & S Livingstone.

Campbell R, Davies IM, Macfarlane AJ and Beral V (1984) 'Home Births in England and Wales 1979', *British Medical Journal*, 289 721–4.

Carvel J (2006) 'Plan for wave of closures of NHS services', *Guardian*, 13 September 2006.

Chamberlain G and Chamberlain R (eds) (1972) *British Births*, Vol.1. London: Heinemann Medical Books.

Churchill H, Savage W and Francome C (2006) *Caesarean Birth in Britain, Revised and Updated*. London: Middlesex University Press.

Department of Health (DoH), Standing Maternity and Midwifery Advisory Committee (1970) *Domiciliary Midwifery and Maternity Bed Needs: report of a sub-committee* (The Peel report). London: HMSO.

Department of Health (DoH) (1993) *Changing Childbirth, Part 1: Report of the Expert Maternity Group* (The Cumberlege report). London: HMSO.

Department of Health (DoH) (2004) *National Service Framework for Children, Young People and Maternity Services*. London: DoH.

Donnison J (1977) *Midwives and Medical Men*. New York: Shocken Books.

House of Commons Health Committee (1992) *Second Report, 1991–2 Session, 'The Organisation of Maternity Services'* Vol.I–III (The Winterton report). London: HMSO.

House of Commons Health Committee (2003a) *Provision of Maternity Services, Fourth Report of Session 2002–3,* Vol.1. London: The Stationery Office.

House of Commons Health Committee (2003b) *Inequalities in access to Maternity Services, Eighth Report of Session 2002–3,* Vol.1. London: The Stationery Office.

House of Commons Health Committee (2003c) *Choice in Maternity Services, Ninth Report of Session 2002–3,* Vol.1. London: The Stationery Office.

House of Commons Social Services Committee (1980) *Second Report. Perinatal and Neonatal Mortality Session 1979–80* (The Short report). London: HMSO.

Independent Midwives Association (IMA) (2006) *Community Midwifery Model, One mother One Midwife petition*. http://www.independentmidwives.org.uk/article155.html

Kieler H, Cnattingius S, Haglund B, Palmgren J and Axelsson O (2001) 'Sinistrality – a side-effect of prenatal sonography: a comparative study of young men', *Epidemiology*, 12:618–23.

Leys C (2001) *Market Driven Politics*. London: Verso.

Macdorman et al (2006) 'Infant and Neonatal mortality for Primary Cesarean and Vaginal Births to women with "No indicated risk", United States, 1996–2001 Birth Cohorts', *Birth*, 33: 175–82.

Macfarlane A and Campbell R (1994) *Where to be born: the debate and the evidence*. Second edition. Oxford: National Perinatal Epidemiology Unit.

Marteau T (1995) 'Towards informed decisions about prenatal testing: a review', *Prenatal Diagnosis*, 15:1,215.

Ministry of Health (MoH) (1959) *Report of the Maternity Services Committee* (The Cranbrook report). London: HMSO.

National Institute for Clinical Excellence (NICE) (2004) Caesarean Section, *National Collaborating Centre for Women's and Children's Health, Clinical guidelines*. London: RCOG Press.

Royal College of Obstetricians and Gynaecologists (RCOG) (1993) *Recommendations on the Future of Maternity Services*. London: RCOG Press.

Sandall J, Grellier R and Ahmed S (2003) 'Prenatal screening and diagnosis in a multi-cultural, multi-ethnic society', pp.83–97 in Abramsky L and Chapple J (eds) *Prenatal Diagnosis*. London: Chapman and Hall.

Sikorski J, Wilson J, Clement S, Das S and Smeeton N (1996) 'A randomised controlled trial comparing two schedules of antenatal visits: the antenatal care project', *BMJ*, 312:546–53.

The Times (2006) 'Sentenced to Hard Labour?' 13 March 2006. http://www.reform.co.uk/website/pressroom/articles/aspx?o=221 (accessed 3 October 2006).

Thomas J and Paranjothy S (2001) *National Sentinel caesarean section Audit Report*. Royal College of Obstetricians and Gynaecologists Clinical Effectiveness Unit. London: RCOG Press.

World Health Organisation (WHO) (1985) 'Appropriate technology for Birth', *Lancet*.

Birth and Power

Marsden Wagner

This chapter draws heavily on two previous publications by the author: 'Birth and Power' in Perinatal Health Services in Europe *edited by JML Phaff, Groom Helm, London, 1986 and 'A Global Witch-hunt' in the* Lancet *Vol.346, pp.1,020–22, 1995.*

As a male physician, I have personally experienced the power of the medical profession. While practising medicine for many years, I felt the power over life and death. As a teacher in a medical school, I felt the power of control over the dissemination of knowledge. As a medical researcher, I felt the power of control over deciding what new knowledge would be developed. As a health administrator, I felt the power of control over the nature of health services and how money was to be spent. Finally, as a health service researcher and occasional critic of the health care system, I have sometimes felt the power of the medical profession directed against me. Power and control are most important elements in health care and to date have received little attention. This chapter will explore how power relates to birth and birth care, how power is obtained, the impact of power on the care system and counterbalances to medical power.

I must add that not all doctors are interested in power, and many doctors care about their communities and try to provide humane care. By their silence, however, they allow those of their colleagues who are interested in power to control the direction of their profession.

Furthermore, in my own experience in the medical profession, the doctors who seek power do so with good intentions, honestly believing that they know best and, at least in most cases, wanting to help. They should not be blamed for believing and behaving in this fashion: both the society in which they live and the medical training they have received encourage them to fill a role that results in the accumulation of power. Only more recently have we begun to appreciate that doctors' knowledge is only part of the truth and must be combined with the knowledge and reality of the person they seek to help if we are to avoid the disabling help that results in loss of control over one's own body and destiny.

The source of power

Who in our society today has power over birth and birth care? Who controls where birth happens, how it happens, who is present and other conditions? Medical doctors have nearly absolute control over birth and birth care. How has this nearly absolute power been gathered? There are at least eight ways in which the medical profession has gained its power. First was the redefinition of birth. Sociologists have known for some time that whoever defines a problem controls the solutions. Although birth is a normal biosocial process, it has been redefined as a medical problem that is either pathological or potentially pathological. One can frequently hear doctors say that birth is normal only in retrospect. The medical profession has thereby created the necessity of its presence at the centre of birth.

The second method of obtaining power was moving birth to the doctor's territory, in other words, to the hospital where they exerted absolute control already. To accomplish this move to their own territory, inappropriate or false statistics were necessary to attempt to prove that normal birth is safer in hospital. This is still unproved.[1] It was necessary to promise women safer births if they were willing to give up the obvious advantages of remaining in their own homes to come to a strange place filled with strange people and strange machines. We doctors, nevertheless, succeeded in convincing everyone that this was appropriate and so, in nearly every developed country in the world, almost all birth is in hospital. More recently, following pressure from women, doctors have been trying to make the maternity wards in the hospitals more home-like by hanging curtains and bringing in rocking chairs. This reminds me of the sign in the bakery window: 'We sell home-baked bread'. Also because of pressure from women, the chief physician in the hospital may often decide that women may, for example, walk around during labour if they choose. But whatever the chief physician does not explicitly permit is still forbidden. This, of course, is not real choice for the woman but loss of control. The power of the chief doctor in the hospital to set all of the rules on birth produces the extraordinary conditions today in which routine practices for birth care vary widely from hospital to hospital.

Doctors have increased their control of birth by gradually taking control of the education of birth attendants, such as midwives. Obstetricians are the directors of most schools of midwifery today. (Although not in the UK – but it was only in the last decade that obstetricians stopped sitting as examiners for the qualifying examination for midwives.) As a consequence, doctors control what student midwives should be taught and what their attitude to birth should be.

Limiting the distribution of certain drugs to prescription by licensed doctors is another traditional method of control in health care. This operates equally effectively in birth care where doctors have successfully insisted that only they should prescribe medications and use certain machines and procedures. In the UK, however, where midwives retained more power than in the US, for example, they are licensed to give two doses of pethidine and administer a mixture of nitrous oxide and oxygen without recourse to a doctor.

Doctors have controlled the distribution of money for medical research in most countries for many years. Consequently, doctors control the generation of new knowledge about pregnancy and birth, together with what shall be studied, how it should be studied, and how the results should or should not be disseminated.

The doctors in most countries have controlled the official government guidelines for medical services. This has also been true of the guidelines for birth care and, as a result, national patterns of services for birthing remain under the control of the medical profession. Recently in the UK, user representatives have taken part in drawing up national guidelines for the National Institute for Clinical Excellence (NICE) – in particular those regarding induction of labour and caesarean section – but it is debatable how effective their input is. The National Childbirth Trust (NCT) is also part of the guidelines group in the RCOG.

Over many decades doctors have convinced the public and their representatives that they and they alone are capable of evaluation of their own services. Medicine, in fact, is

---

1 Macfarlane and Campbell (1994); Springer and Van Weel (1996); Chamberlain, Wraight and Crowley (1997); Johnson and Daviss (2005)

the only profession that has gained such absolute control over the evaluation of its activities. This is absolute power indeed. This peer review clearly has a built-in conflict of interest. Nowhere in the world, to my knowledge, has peer review been adequate in controlling any excesses of the medical profession.

The medical profession has used this absolute control of the evaluation of its actions as part of a final strategy for the accumulating and maintaining of power in birth – the witch-hunt.

There is a global witch-hunt in progress – the investigation of health professionals in many countries to accuse them of dangerous maternity practices. This witch-hunt is part of a global struggle for control of maternity services, the key underlying issues being money, power, sex, and choice. The investigation often leads to a public court, a medical review board, or a health insurance review board. Over the past 10 years I have been asked to consult, and in some instances testify, in 20 cases in 10 countries – a very small proportion of the actual cases. In the USA alone, 'though no-one knows how many out-of-hospital midwives have actually been charged, we have reports of legal altercations involving more than 145 out-of-hospital midwives in 36 states'.[2]

Whilst the profession of the accused in my 20 cases includes obstetrics (Austria, Italy, UK), general practice (Australia, New Zealand), and midwifery (Canada, France, Germany, Italy, Sweden, UK, USA), the striking thing is that, of the accused, 70 per cent were midwives and 85 per cent were women. In the 20 cases, all of the accused have one thing in common: at least some of their practice is not mainstream. In other words, what they do is not what the local doctors in authority most commonly do.

Irrespective of the country, certain methods are commonly used by the obstetric establishment to accrue evidence against the accused. For example, in most cases the doctors notify the legal authorities only after a perinatal death. One death, even if not preventable and not the result of any mistake, suddenly negates years of impeccable statistics. This is in stark contrast to what happens when an orthodox doctor is involved in a perinatal death in the hospital – there may be a hospital review committee meeting behind closed doors but it will not come to the attention of the public or legal authorities.

Another ploy is to scrutinise all obstetric patients' records connected with the accused looking for possible mistakes. Such a strategy creates fear in all those in that community who might deviate from orthodox practice.

Once the case is brought before a court or review board, other methods are commonly adopted. Threats may be used to pressurise local doctors who are perceived to be sympathetic to the accused so they will be too afraid to testify. Moreover, tribunals, especially if they are medical or insurance review boards, usually try to forbid the public or media from being present. In London in the 1980s, Mrs Wendy Savage, an obstetrician, caused an enormous upheaval when she demanded – ultimately successfully – a public hearing.[3]

The results of these cases have been mixed. The circumstances of the trial affect the chances that the accused will win the case. The accused who comes before a public court with a jury has the greatest chance of winning. The chances are progressively less with a public court with a judge, then a medical review board open to the public and media, and finally a closed medical review board. If the accused is allowed to bring in experts

2 Korte (1995)
3 Savage (1986)

to testify, including those from other countries, the chances of winning are higher. If the case has media coverage and the accused has visible public support, again there is a better chance of winning, as was the case with Mrs Savage.

If the accused loses, that often means losing the possibility at least temporarily, of continuing to practise. Apart from the great personal losses entailed there is an impact on the health professionals. Midwives in that country feel threatened in their independent practice, rightly fearing loss of medical backup and/or hospital privileges. Doctors are afraid to support midwives or to go along with the wishes of their patients when the requests are outside mainstream policy – water births, for example. Women in that community therefore lose the freedom to choose among a broader set of options for giving birth.

Conversely, investigation of independent midwives and unorthodox doctors, with a possible board hearing or court case, can sometimes have the opposite effect, leading to solidarity among midwives and between midwives, unorthodox doctors, and women, irrespective of whether the accused wins or loses.

The witch-hunt is part of a global struggle for control of maternity systems, and there are several key issues, one of which is economic. As birth rates fall, the competition for pregnant patients increases, especially in countries largely reliant on private medical care, and as more and more countries move towards pluralistic health care systems with private practice, maternity care becomes more competitive. However, in the face of increasingly limited economic resources, governments and insurance companies are becoming more and more concerned with the waste associated with high-technology, high-intervention obstetrics. It is much more difficult for obstetricians to defend this expensive type of practice when midwives and a few doctors are meanwhile showing that a much less expensive type of maternity care is equally safe. The witch-hunt is an attempt to display lack of safety among the competitors.

A second issue is the control of maternity services. Until recently, government regulations in most countries have given medical doctors a monopoly in providing health services. Medical licensure represents 'a social tolerance for a monopoly in return for a promise of social benefit in the form of competent and dedicated medical care'. But this monopoly can easily be abused, especially behind closed doors. The issue becomes one of peer control versus accountability to the public. In medical board reviews of professional behaviour, if the medical profession can make secret judgements on the accused, the doctors have absolute control of their monopoly, and there is the possibility of abusing the system for professional gain.

On the other hand, in a public court in which a judge makes the final decision, there is a danger that the judge, as part of the power elite in the community, will be more influenced by another member of the same elite – the local professor – than by a midwife or even by outside scientific opinion. There is a great difference between unorthodox doctors and midwives being judged by orthodox doctors and judges or being judged by the public – and that is why it is so important to have a medical review board open to the public.

Fortunately the pendulum is swinging, at least in some places, with the coming of quality assurance systems that include public accountability of health care and health care professionals. Maternity services are in the forefront of the controversy over peer control and public accountability because birth, like death, is a deeply personal social and family event and does not fit the doctors' disease model. So today the medical monopoly of maternity services is coming into question and the witch-hunt is one means of reasserting the orthodox doctor's control.

Choice and freedom for health care providers are at stake here. There is considerable peer pressure to conform because deviations may threaten the legitimacy or supremacy of practice based on opinion rather than evidence. It is important to distinguish between the quality assurance function and the witch-hunt function so that the courts and boards are not inappropriately used for professional gain. When making this distinction in a particular case, think about who might gain from a successful prosecution – is the evidence brought against the accused scientifically based?

Whilst tribunals may have a declared function to weed out true incompetence and protect the public, in the cases I describe the real function was to punish deviant professional behaviour that could threaten the income, practice style, prestige, and power of mainstream doctors.

Another issue is the two-hundred-year-old struggle of doctors to control midwifery. It is no coincidence that 70 per cent of the accused in my sample are midwives, all in independent practice where they are not under the immediate control of doctors. Fear of being investigated by the authorities is a strong deterrent amongst independent midwives.

The results of power

In these ways, then, the medical profession has gained power over birth and birth care. What are the results of this control by doctors? The main result is the medicalisation of birth and birth care. This medicalisation is described in some detail in my book *Pursuing the Birth Machine: The Search for Appropriate Perinatal Technology*[4] and the main results will only be briefly summarised here. The first result of the power of doctors over birth is the recent uncontrolled proliferation of technology used during pregnancy and birth. The most serious aspect of this proliferation is that a machine or procedure becomes widely used before it is adequately evaluated, so that nobody knows whether it is useful or even if it is safe. Interestingly, obstetrical intervention rates vary greatly among countries and among hospitals in the same country. Some evidence suggests that rates of obstetrical intervention may be inversely correlated with the independence and strength of the midwifery profession in that hospital, region or country. Thus, the United States has some of the highest obstetrical intervention rates in the world, while the European countries, where there is an independent, strong midwifery profession, generally have some of the lowest rates of obstetrical intervention.

Another consequence of the power of doctors over birth is the increasing number of pregnant and birthing women labelled at risk. While the inability to predict pathology has usually resulted in the failure of the various risk systems to accomplish what they were designed for, they nevertheless persist. The reason may be that the risk systems serve a purpose beyond the medical: power. Risk is the bludgeon used to scare not only women but also politicians and health care providers. A doctor tells a mother, 'You would not want to take a risk with your unborn baby, dear. Would you?'

Another consequence of both the power of doctors over birth and its medicalisation is the increasing use of drugs. Studies have shown that a majority of pregnant women in most countries have taken medication during pregnancy and that a majority of this medication was prescribed by physicians. We doctors have convinced women that they

4 Wagner (1995b)

are in real danger when pregnant or giving birth, then given them drugs for these risky situations and prescribed tranquillisers when they get upset. Doctors prescribe so much medication during pregnancy and birth for several reasons. Firstly, a subtle influence in obstetrics absolves a doctor who interferes with a normal pregnancy but exposes his conservative colleagues to censure for inactivity when an infant is born dead. This places a premium on intervention as a form of personal insurance for the doctor, although the consequences of the intervention may be detrimental to some of his patients. A doctor needs more experience, more judgement and more courage to stand back and do nothing.

We doctors also prescribe drugs so often during pregnancy and birth because, despite more and more sophisticated diagnostic procedures, our therapeutic possibilities unfortunately lag far behind. In other words, we are clever at finding out what is wrong but can do little about it. So the temptation to turn to drugs is great. It can be concluded that doctors see pregnancy and birth as dangerous until proved safe but see drugs, which are artificial interventions and in many cases not tested on pregnant women, as safe until proved dangerous. I think we have things upside down.

Another consequence of medical power over birth is the increasing centralisation of birth care. More and more births take place in fewer and fewer, and larger and larger, hospitals. Care during pregnancy is also becoming more centralised. The result is the loss of all of the great benefits of primary health care.

Another result of the medicalisation of birth brought on by the power of doctors is the neglect of the psychological and social aspects of birth and birth care. Good, solid evidence shows that the psychological and social wellbeing of the woman is essential for the best biological outcome for pregnancy and birth; but the medical profession persists in seeing these psychological and social elements as marginal and deserving of attention only when everything else has been done.

The final consequence of medical power over birth is the loss of the woman's right of informed choice about her own pregnancy and childbirth. Half of informed choice is information: the information provided to pregnant and birthing women has been most inadequate and always very carefully monitored by doctors. I've often heard doctors say that we must not 'scare' pregnant women, as an excuse for not sharing information. If sharing the information does elicit concern or fear in women then, rather than withholding this information, doctors must be prepared to work with women to cope with this anxiety – as well as their own. Sharing information also means sharing power.

The other half of informed choice, of course, is choice. To give women choice is to give up power on two levels. Firstly, the doctor loses control over what happens with that particular woman. Secondly, the doctor implicitly acknowledges that the woman also has valid information and should control her own body and life. Such an acknowledgement by the doctors would shift the ultimate power from the doctor to the woman. Rather than choice, the medical literature today is filled with discussions on patient compliance. To comply means to obey and is the opposite of choice.

The results of the power of doctors over birth might well be summarised by saying that the doctor has written the obstetrical drama so that he is the star, rather than the woman.

Counterbalances to power

Are there counterbalances to this nearly absolute power of doctors over birth? The first and clearly most important counterbalance to the power of doctors is the role that pregnant and birthing women themselves can play in taking control of their own births and birth care. Since the ownership of the knowledge about birth and the freedom to choose what will happen during birth are key elements in the power over birth, informed choice for the birthing woman must be considered a central issue here.

As more and more women have begun to demand informed choice, they have devised certain ways to get it. For example, before coming to the hospital for childbirth, the woman may develop a written birth plan that describes in some detail for the hospital staff the type of birth that she wishes to have. Then she discusses this birth plan with the hospital staff and negotiates her choices. Another important aid for this informed choice has been the development of a guide to good birth. In Britain, such a guide,[5] giving detailed information on the practices in all of the maternity units in Britain, has been a highly successful method of choosing the best place for childbirth. It has also indirectly affected hospital staff, as they may wish to improve their standings in the guide by changing some of their routine practices.

An important facet of the expanding role of birthing women in controlling their own birthing is what I call community epidemiology in maternity care. The idea behind this is simple: the community should have all of the information on its own maternity services and the power to monitor and control them. Thus, for example, caesarean section rates per hospital and per doctor would be provided, along with all other obstetrical intervention rates. The community would receive the information necessary to compute such things as its own perinatal mortality rate, and rate of low-birthweight babies and would compare them with those of neighbouring communities. So-called experts would be called into the community to present data and debate both sides of the issues. All of this, of course, would be fed to the local media for reporting and discussion. The community would decide which issues should be researched and receive all research results. Such community epidemiology would redress the imbalance in power, the unreasonable promises of doctors and the secretive, club-like nature of medical practice. Such a solution is for the future, but we are already moving in this direction. In the United States, hospital statistics are now in the public domain. In the United Kingdom, the Community Health Council was a start in this direction. Sadly this has now been disbanded and replaced by PALs based in and managed by hospitals – which are also about to be re-organised again in summer 2006.

A second important counterbalance to the power of doctors over birth is the role of midwifery. As stated earlier, some evidence suggests that the midwifery profession has acted as an important deterrent to the rising obstetrical intervention rates and other instances of the medicalisation of birth. The diminishing power of midwives over the last 50 years is discussed in *Pursuing the Birth Machine*[6] and will not be repeated here. The important thing is that this essential profession appears to be beginning a resurgence. An independent midwifery profession is likely to play a more and more important role in the future in counterbalancing the power of doctors over birth.

Another important counterbalance to the power of doctors over birth is the courts. The courts must be seen as a kind of complaint procedure. When people feel that they have been mistreated by a physician, they must have a source of redress and this cannot be another doctor, whoever that doctor is, because of the obvious conflict of interest and the

5 Kitzinger (1983)
6 Wagner (1995b)

club-like nature of the medical profession. In some countries, numbers of court cases concerning childbirth have risen alarmingly, and doctors have blamed women and lawyers. Perhaps doctors should consider the most important role that they themselves have played in this increasing litigation on birth. For many years now, doctors have been selling hospital birth as the safe alternative. Women give up much in going to the hospital, but for the most part they do so because they have been promised safety there. So when a woman has a hospital birth in which something goes wrong, she feels deceived. Such a sense of betrayal motivates them to turn to the courts, and behind this feeling lie doctors' promises of a risk-free birth. To summarise, if you play God, don't be surprised if you are blamed for natural disasters. The courts are far from ideal but nevertheless remain an essential counterbalance to the nearly absolute power of doctors over birth.

A fourth important counterbalance to the power of doctors over birth is the public health authorities. In most countries, these authorities are responsible for evaluating health care services and controlling health care practices. While in the past the public health authorities have tended to be controlled rather completely by the medical profession, this is becoming less true. In evaluating health care services, the public health authorities usually create a most important balance between the case-by-case clinical approach of doctors and the population-based approach of epidemiologists. Therefore, an evaluation is more likely to be unbiased and scientific. To the extent that the public health authorities carry out such unbiased, scientific evaluations of services and follow them up with recommendations or regulations for practices, they are very likely to come into conflict with clinical practitioners. Such conflict is very easy to see in a number of countries in Europe today over pregnancy and birth services. The important thing here is that the public health authorities in these countries have the courage and foresight to take action, in spite of an inevitable confrontation with some practising doctors. The epidemiologists and other medical scientists who have been carrying out careful, controlled scientific research on pregnancy and birth are essential to this process and the findings of these epidemiologists and scientists, reinforced by the public health authorities, are likely to be more and more important as a counterbalance to the power of practising doctors over birth.

The final counterbalance to be mentioned to the power of doctors over birth is the general public through its representatives in government. As mentioned near the beginning of this chapter, in the past doctors have successfully convinced the general public and their representatives that they and they alone could decide the content of health care. As a consequence, in the past the guidelines for care during pregnancy and birth were nearly always drafted by doctors. This is gradually changing, however, as the general public becomes more and more aware that its health and health care is far too important to leave exclusively in the hands of doctors.

As all of these counterbalances to the power of doctors gradually increase in the future, I believe that birth and birth care can be confidently predicted to become the responsibility of all. When this happens, the obstetrical scenario will be rewritten so that birth ceases to be an obstetrical drama and becomes a human drama.

Update

This chapter was first written ten years ago. Sad to say, it is actually quite up-to-date as there has been little change in the power structure of maternity care in the interim. The intransigent nature of obstetrics is illustrated by recent events surrounding the issue of the safety of home birth. Home birth is an issue vital to obstetrics because the profession can only retain its power by keeping childbirth where it has control: in the hospital. The American College of Obstetricians and Gynaecologists (ACOG) has an official, published opinion that home birth is dangerous, an opinion given in 1975 and reaffirmed in 2002. In both cases, no references from the literature were given to back up this opinion.

Then in 2005 a paper appeared in the *British Medical Journal*[7] reporting on an excellent prospective study of over 5,000 planned home births attended by direct entry (non-nurse) midwives. The study found planned home birth to be as safe as hospital birth for low-risk pregnancies. This study resulted in over 40 letters to the *BMJ* online response page but not a single one was from an obstetrician. It was not possible to shoot down this study as the methodology was too good and the sample size too large; so apparently the strategy of obstetrics is to ignore it and hope it goes away.

But since the publication of this study, ACOG has taken two actions regarding home birth. First, in February 2006 ACOG released a Statement of Policy 'Lay Midwifery' in which it says it 'does not support the provision of care by lay midwives or other midwives who are not certified by the AMCB'. Now, the direct-entry midwives who participated in the study of 5,000 planned home births are not certified by the AMCB but by another certification process which has been documented to be equal to or even superior to the AMCB process. So ACOG's statement completely ignores a fully developed training and certification process involving thousands of American midwives. But ACOG, by calling them by the pejorative 'lay midwives' rather than identifying them as direct-entry midwives and by not supporting these direct-entry midwives, is indirectly trying to shoot down the study. And in May 2006 at the annual ACOG convention, ACOG inserted into the convention package given to all of the thousands of participants, a bumper sticker 'Home delivery is for pizza' – another attempt to indirectly shoot down the study. Obstetrics will use every tactic to maintain its power.

I have documented in detail the continuing power and control which obstetricians have over maternity services in my new book: *Born in the USA: How a broken maternity system must be fixed to put women and children first.*[8] And in another new book, *Creating your Birth Plan,*[9] I help pregnant women to gain control over their own bodies and their maternity care so that they are empowered rather than the obstetricians.

---

7 Johnson and Daviss (2005)

8 Wagner (2006)

9 Wagner and Gunning (2006)

References

Chamberlain G, Wraight A and Crowley P (1997) *Home Birth*. Carnforth (UK) and New York (USA): Parthenon Press.

Johnson KC and Daviss B (2005) 'Outcomes of planned home births with certified professional midwives: large prospective study in North America', *BMJ*, 330: 1,416–1419.

Kitzinger S (1983) *The new good birth guide*. Harmondsworth: Penguin.

Korte D (1995) 'Midwifery on Trial', *Mothering*, fall issue, pp.21–5.

Macfarlane A and Campbell R (1994) *Where to be born: the debate and the evidence*, second edition. Oxford: National Perinatal Epidemiology Unit.

Savage W (1986) *A Savage Enquiry: Who Controls Childbirth?* London: Virago.

Springer NP and Van Weel C (1996) 'Home birth', *BMJ*, 313:1, 276–7.

Wagner M (1986) 'Birth and Power' in Phaff JML (ed.) *Perinatal Health Services in Europe*. London: Groom Helm.

Wagner M (1995a) 'A Global Witch-hunt', *Lancet*, Vol.346, pp.1,020–2.

Wagner M (1995b) *Pursuing the Birth Machine*. Sydney: ACE Graphic.

Wagner M (2006) *Born in the USA*. Berkeley: University of California Press.

Wagner M and Gunning S (2006) *Creating Your Birth Plan*. New York: Penguin.

Behind Every Midwife is a Doctor Trying to Stop Her[1]

Joan Donley

The 1990 amendment to the Nurses Act 1977 restored autonomous practice to New Zealand midwives. They could now 'carry out obstetric nursing' without a medical practitioner 'undertaking responsibility for the care of the patient', which had been a requirement since the Nurses Act 1971.

The two-clause bill was introduced in November 1989, and during its passage through Parliament, amendments to other legislation enlarged the scope for midwives to become autonomous *in practice* as well as in principle. They could order laboratory tests, prescribe relevant prescription medicines, have access to public hospital facilities on the same basis as GPs and claim on the maternity benefit used to pay general practitioners who undertook maternity care.

In addition, the Nursing Council was required to give serious consideration to women entering midwifery directly, rather than through nursing, after years of sustained opposition to direct entry (DE) midwifery education. Remarkably, by 1992, three-year direct entry Bachelor of Midwifery degree programmes were established at Otago Polytech and Auckland Institute of Technology. By 1999, five centres were established, and these had graduated more than 100 midwives. By 2004, 196 of 3,087 midwives on the register had qualified in this way.[2]

These radical changes were the result of a number of factors. The growth of the grass roots home birth movement threatened the position of the midwives in the New Zealand Nurses Association (NZNA) who wished to remain representatives of the profession within the increasingly medicalised maternity hierarchy. The 1987–8 Cartwright enquiry into cervical cancer at the National Women's Hospital questioned doctors' 'clinical freedom'.[3] This undermined the credibility of the Postgraduate School of Obstetrics and Gynaecology (O&G). Finally, there was a supportive Labour government with a visionary and courageous Minister of Health, the Right Honourable Helen Clark, who became Prime Minister in 1999.

The New Zealand Homebirth Association (NZHBA) had a thorough historical and political understanding of New Zealand's maternity services and a cohesive partnership between women and midwives. NZHBA fought the regionalisation and medicalisation of childbirth using international networks. It argued from the strength of WHO's Alma Ata Primary Health Care (PHC) initiative and *Appropriate Technology for Birth* (1985). It used its electoral power, leaked documents and guerrilla tactics to discredit and challenge the bureaucratic status quo.

---

1 Apologies to Katherine Mansfield

2 NZHIS (2006a)

3 Coney (1988)

Background

There was opposition from both nurses and doctors as midwives began to work towards restoring their autonomy as an independent profession in 1980.

Nursing opposition

The NZNA attitude to home birth as shown in their *Policy Statement on Home Confinement* (1980) was negative – the 'reluctant acceptance of a fait accompli'. It recommended 'disciplinary action' against domiciliary midwives who tended other than low-risk women – as defined by obstetricians. (Domiciliary midwifery was subsidised under the Social Security Act 1938. When maternity care was transferred from the Department of Health to hospital boards (1969), the three existing DMs were overlooked.)

In response to the NZNA action eight of the 17 DMs throughout New Zealand met and formed the Domiciliary Midwives Society Incorporated. They boldly advised NZNA and the Department of Health (DOH) that in future *they* would speak for DMs – not the NZNA National Executive 'career midwives' dedicated to maintaining the hierarchical system which legitimised their power.

NZNA wanted 'changes and innovations in the delivery of maternal and infant care'. They suggested establishing a new 'comprehensive' family health nurse who would provide continuity of care from birth to menopause.[4]

A 1983 amendment to the Nurses Act allowed any nurse to carry out 'obstetric nursing' under medical supervision. This blow to the status of all midwives quickly politicised the hospital midwives. They joined the handful of DMs and the NZHBA in the struggle to maintain midwifery as a profession.

DMs with the support of NZHBA established the Domiciliary Midwives Review Committee, outflanking moves by NZNA and the Maternity Services Committee[5] to have DM practice monitored by the Obstetric Standards Review Committees (OSRC) who approved GP access to hospital facilities. Annual review of DM practice by equal numbers of consumers and midwives was later extended to monitor the practice of independent midwives.

When seven local branches formed the national NZHBA, the senior obstetric nurses in the NZNA responded quickly and said that the 'relative independence' of the domiciliary midwives (DMs) was 'a threat to their scope of practice'.[6]

This unity (which included NZNA voting power) forced the NZNA to change its definition of a midwife to the ICM one (1985) and reluctantly accept the concept of a one-year midwifery course to replace the brief midwifery option within the Advanced Diploma of Nursing. A consumer-oriented task force to promote direct entry education contended that midwifery as a postgraduate nursing course was misconceived and should be abolished.

As 80 per cent of the 3,000 midwives worked in hospitals and the NZNA negotiated their work and pay conditions, the possibility that midwives might break away from the more than 20,000 strong NZNA was hardly discussed. The 1987 'market-led' Labour Relations Act, which signalled the end of collective bargaining, reduced the dependence of midwives on the NZNA.

---

4 NZNA (1981)

5 Maternity Services Committee (1983)

6 Department of Health (1985)

Rather than become moas – an extinct species – midwives in 1988 took their destiny into their own hands, accepting the concept of forming the New Zealand College of Midwives (NZCOM), including consumers as members. This became reality in 1989. Karen Guilliland, president of NZNA Midwives Section at the time, became president. A leading obstetrician responded that the 'three greatest threats to obstetrics were feminism, consumerism and midwives'.

Medical opposition[7]

The entrepreneurial doctors in their long-held monopoly position were unable to cope with the reality that fewer than 100 independent midwives (mainly DMs) were accessing what they saw as *their* maternity benefit. This fee-for-service system, developed over a period of 50 years, was based on the medical model and the subsidised but unacknowledged support of the midwife. It now needed adjustment to accommodate midwives as autonomous practitioners.

The Department of Health (DoH) had long considered that doctors over-utilised and abused the fee-for-service maternity benefit. NZCOM now provided the lever – and the heaven-sent scapegoats – to restructure the maternity payment system. The doctors representing the New Zealand Medical Association (NZMA) boycotted three DoH attempts at negotiation. Waving the safety shroud, GPs, in collusion with the Obstetric Standard Review Committees (OSRCs), obstructed midwives' access to hospital board facilities. They questioned the boards' liability for incompetent midwives – although the COM midwives were the only health professionals to have established standards of practice. The managers commissioned a legal opinion only to find that an autonomous midwife is medically and ethically responsible for her practice.

Attracted by the doctors' $285 labour and delivery fee plus $69.80[8] per half-hour for prolonged attendance, increasing numbers of hospital midwives opted for independence. Many, working with specialists, did only hospital intrapartum care – hardly independent midwifery!

With the election of the right-wing National government (October 1990) dedicated to market-led health *de*forms, the doctors mounted a media campaign accusing midwives of 'blowing out the budget' during this period of 'fiscal restraint'. They demanded their legal right to a tribunal to put midwives back on a separate schedule.

Tribunal

A five-member tribunal was set up in November 1992. The NZCOM nominee was President Sally Pairman. NZMA hired a QC for $40,000. With a membership of

---

7 **Wendy Savage adds:** When I went to New Zealand in 1973, the system was that women had antenatal care from their GP, saw the hospital midwives for booking and then arrived in labour. The midwives looked after her and called the GP when she was about to deliver and s/he came and 'caught the baby'. My post was a new one: to provide hospital obstetric care for those women who needed it with one of the two obstetricians who had been employed for gynaecology by the hospital board. They only did private obstetrics and might be called in by the GP if there were problems he could not deal with. The new Medical Superintendent thought this was a bad system so persuaded the board to create this post. I also did a locum in Gisborne in 2001 after I retired. The system had been transformed and the independent midwives worked well with the GPs, most of whom had opted out of maternity care. In 2003, 98.3 per cent of women were booked initially under the care of a midwife – the highest proportion in New Zealand (NZHIS, 2006b).

8 There were about three NZ$ to the £ at the time, so this would be about £95 for the birth and £23 per half hour in attendance.

approximately 1,200, COM had to rely on its own resources. Karen Guilliland, COM National Co-ordinator, and Stephanie Breen (Nurses Union) acted as counsels. Vital evidence was given by a team of four midwives and a consumer/accountant and the economist Prue Hyman, Reader in Economics, Victoria University submitted that the Public Finance Act focuses on outcomes, therefore if outcomes (normal birth) were substantially similar, the work was of equal value and should be paid accordingly. The DoH, noting the 'clear philosophical differences' between the two parties (doctors focused on the risks and midwives viewed birth as a normal life event) confirmed that the fee is for a service of equal value of which responsibility is a factor, so 'two scales is clearly an untenable argument'.

The 1993 Health and Disabilities Services Act based on competitive contracts and capped budgets would corporatise the public health system for eventual privatisation. It replaced the DoH with a ministry to advise, monitor and disburse Crown funds to four competitive Regional Health Authorities (RHAs) as purchasing agencies. The public hospitals became 23 profit-oriented and competitive Crown Health Enterprises (CHEs) each under business management.

This economic retreat from the welfare state in New Zealand was known as 'Rogernomics' after its promoter, Roger Douglas, Labour Minister of Finance. The policies were supported by the Business Roundtable and their Treasury clones, who had been advised by an American, Dr Patricia Danzon. Health care was to become a commodity with 'health a privilege, not a right'.[9]

Section 51

Section 51 of this Act established a maternity negotiating committee comprised of NZMA, NZCOM and the RHAs (the funders). Section 51 replaced Section 106 of the Social Security Act 1964, which guaranteed a fully subsidised maternity service with every woman having the right to select her practitioner(s). However, ministry policy guidelines charged RHAs to use the inequities of the uncapped maternity benefit to bring all demand-driven expenditure under control (to pave the way for budget holding or managed care – a modular system with specified services which can be sold in the private insurance market).

There were approximately 57,000 births a year and the maternity budget was capped at $96 million for primary care. The 1993 maternity benefit per birth was $1,398.[10] It was in this quagmire that COM and NZMA had to negotiate 'a new pay structure, based on fiscal neutrality, agreeable to doctors and midwives'.

NZMA, claiming the 1990 Nurses Amendment Act was the root of all evil in the maternity services,[11] had two basic aims:

- To put midwives back where they belonged – under medical supervision
- To maintain fee-for-service.

Fee-for-service was seen as the basis of the doctor/patient relationship – the 'foundation stone of general practice'. Removal threatened 'clinical freedom' which allowed doctors to avoid 'any limitations on the number or cost of consultations, procedures, prescriptions

9 Williamson (1993)
10 English (1997)
11 NZMA (1993)

and referrals'. It would also give management 'more control over what GPs do and how they do it'. NZMA therefore opposed both the 'modular' payment system (recommended by the tribunal) and 'budget holding'. It claimed budget holding was a 'managed care' tool to shift financial risk to the budget holder, with no chance to recoup losses from either the patient or a third party. Although 50 per cent of New Zealand's approximately 2,300 GPs were already under budget-holding contracts through Independent Practitioner Associations (IPAs), they could still charge the patient. They also got computers and 'management' funding.

A GP action group (the GPA) formed a national S51 body to fight for fee-for-service with 'niche contracting'. Although only the 15 per cent of GPs with a Diploma of Obstetrics (Dip Obs) were directly affected, all GPs took up arms – 'Today maternity care, tomorrow general practice'. To prevent the GPs from forming a power block, ministry plans to reduce the four RHAs to one were put on hold.

Unwilling to be 'sacrificed while NZMA put its vested interests ahead of maternity services for women', COM insisted that the system must be women centred, encouraging continuity of care, equity, choice, quality and accessibility. It must be adequately funded to discourage under-servicing. COM also agreed that as primary care givers, midwives are the only health professionals able to provide a total service and continuity of care.

Lead maternity carer: primary provider of care and budget holder

The lead maternity carer (LMC) concept was basic to the maternity service 'reforms'. At the tribunal, Professors Hutton and Mantell had argued the case for only one labour and delivery fee to be paid to the person having ultimate clinical responsibility and the skills to effect a safe outcome (the doctor). This would eliminate 'duplication of services' – and costs. Prior to 1990 both doctors and domiciliary midwives were paid – albeit at different rates – for attendance at labour and birth. The idea of a capped budget which could be held by a midwife (July 1995) made doctors realise the real threat of competition from just 500 independent midwives. Further, 20 per cent of women were choosing midwife-only care while 60 per cent knew the midwife who attended them in labour. The idea of a midwife as the 'gatekeeper' was unthinkable. Having to negotiate with a midwife LMC for payment of services was anathema. GPs claimed that with fees 'screwed to base level and no fat left', one fee for labour and delivery would drive them out of the market.

Although sharing control with a midwife LMC was seen as demeaning the role of the GP and displacing the 'team' approach (with the doctor as head of the team), 'shared care' as 'women's choice' was now promoted. Despite the Professors' opinion at the tribunal that 'shared care results in poor outcomes', doctors used their well-established media contacts to scaremonger. Using safety as a red herring to keep women medically dependent (and disempowered), NZMA campaigned for 'shared care' with the GP as LMC – not too difficult after 50 years' conditioning to be 'under the doctor'. Even some of the DMs, out of 'loyalty' to home birth GPs continued with shared care.

COM was also concerned about inadequate funding, especially the absence of provision for rural midwifery services and the miserly $380 for the postnatal home-care module (after early discharge from hospital). Closure of rural hospitals and lack of health facilities denied '*equity*' of access to the one-fifth of the population living in rural areas. COM insisted on rural midwifery funding. (GPs are subsidised for rural services.) COM also expressed fears that medical control of the budget would promote medicalisation, undervalue a woman's role in her own experience, reinforce the '*invisibility*' of the midwife and contravene the Nurses Amendment Act. The RHAs agreed to 'have another look'.

Meanwhile, in a leading daily newspaper[12] a GP hysterically warned parents about the dangers associated with midwives who preach 'active inactivity' (midwifery support) at birth. A charge midwife responded and '*awarded the GP "A" for effort as he positioned himself to fire. He presented the flank of his experience, signalled with the bunting of his qualifications, ran up the flag of his appointments and shouted the strength of his convictions before he discharged his gun... Nothing solid passed between himself and his target beyond the smoke of anecdote, the hot air of hearsay and some flashes of allegations. His cannon lacked balls.*'[13]

Despite medical opposition, in May 1996 the RHAs announced that the new maternity benefit schedule (MBS) would become effective as of 1 July 1996, budget capped at $323 million.[14] COM considered that the document formalised autonomous midwifery practice as it existed, so was positive for women and midwives. It therefore agreed to provisionally work with the RHAs to improve postnatal and rural funding. Eventually, the RHAs came back with a $1.4 million rural supplement and an increased home-visiting mileage rate – still not adequate, but an improvement.

NZMA totally rejected the proposal. Threatening boycott, they advised women not to get pregnant until things were 'settled'. Minister of Health Jenny Shipley offered doctors $1.5 million to enable women to consult a GP who was not their LMC. This was refused as inadequate for 'women's choice' of shared care. NZMA used the RHA failure to give the required six months' notice of their decision on the MBS to demand further negotiations to address their 'greatest concern'.

Consumers, who had no official voice in the negotiations, expressed concern that the focus on funding constraints rather than women's needs could deprive women at risk from obtaining primary care – the business model had separated the previous integration of secondary and primary care. The RHAs came up with 'referral criteria' to secondary care. Both NZMA and COM opposed the inappropriate linking of protocols to payment. COM felt 'risk lists' would emphasise birth as pathological and distort clinical judgement. The obstetricians refused to act as 'obstetric police'.

Midwives manoeuvred their way through the minefields of competitive laws relating to marketing and small business practice, survived stressful Health Benefits Ltd[15]

---

12 Sutherland (1995)

13 Lewis (1995)

14 Maternity benefit schedule fees (1996, when approximately 3NZ$ = £1)
Providing options – $10
Registration (booking) – $75
2nd trimester – $165
3rd trimester – $230
Labour & birth:
Primip (a woman's first birth) – $950, multip (subsequent births) – $750
Home birth – extra $180
Birth unit – extra $100
P/N – leaving delivery unit within 12 hours – $380; > 12 hours – $280.
Rural home visit supplements categories A – plus $200, B – plus $350

15 HBL, a company which paid claims on behalf of the RHA

negotiations and fraud squad audit and got on with booking women under the 1996 MBS. In an attempt to retain the GP workforce – and since doctors cannot provide a maternity service without midwives – the RHAs separated the single labour and birth fee, introducing a cheap midwifery 'support' option for doctors only – a return to pre-1990 fragmented care.

RHAs had not negotiated with the competitive debt-ridden CHEs (19 of the 23 Crown Health Enterprises had a combined debt of $1.2 billion in 1997) as to how 'primary' funding could be used to pay doctors or whether this would distort funds available to subsidise secondary services. Doctor LMCs opted for this cheaper service, discouraging (even illegally forbidding) women from choosing their own midwife. This resulted in CHE (hospital) staff shortages and created tension between hospital and independent midwives. It placed hospital midwives under medicalised 'standing orders', prevented them from becoming LMCs (which could have fostered their autonomy, increased CHE funding) and undermined established 'know your midwife' schemes. It also contravened the Commerce Act.

COM considered the $360 midwifery services fee to be 'insulting' to hospital midwives. Midwives would provide 95 per cent of the care, while the doctor would rush in for the birth (or shortly after) and claim an average $590. The tribunal had stated that although it had no authority with regard to hospital midwives' salaries, it felt that an unrealistic conduct of labour fee would increase disparity. This could send signals to consumers and professionals that this work was not valued – negating the intent of the Nurses Amendment Act. Specialists charge $1,800–2,200 as well as collecting the MBS, so can afford to engage an independent midwife.

In their opportunistic lobbying for 'women's choice', the GPA demanded that any GP be able to provide antenatal care to 28 weeks. In order to retain families, an increasing number of IPA GPs (unsuccessfully) pressured midwives to buy into their companies so they could contract to bulk fund for maternity services. Wellington O&Gs complained that, due to so many independent midwife and GP deliveries, Wellington Women's Hospital was running low on 'public babies'. This was undermining its accreditation.

Persuaded by the doctors that 'shared care' was the safer option, during October 1996 the RHAs assisted the NZMA to develop a 'financially transparent' capped 'fee-for-service' proposal that completely destroyed three years of negotiation. The LMC as 'provider' was changed to 'managing provision of care'. Antenatal care was divided into three 'fee-for-service' type modules, opening the door to subcontracting. Women could now 'choose' a GP, who had not done six months of obstetrics after qualifying so as to obtain a diploma, for two-thirds of their antenatal care! As medical students, doctors get only four weeks obstetric hospital 'attachment' in years IV and V, and a six-week 'allocation as apprentice' on an obstetric team in the sixth, trainee intern year. Some choice.

For her MA thesis (1998) Karen Guilliland[16] surveyed 2,212 births of self-employed/independent midwives (December 1995 to March 1996) in relation to Maternity Care Provider and outcomes.[17]

---

16 Guilliland (1997)

17 **Wendy Savage adds**: the obstetricians may have had more women with risk factors; however, the resultant outcomes show that midwifery care has good results with lower intervention rates, in keeping with experience in the Netherlands. (van Alten et al, 1989)

Carer	No.	NVD	Forceps/ ventouse	C/S	PNMR Per 1,000
Midwife only	1,094	88%	5.7%	6.2%	3.8
Midwife/GP	605	82%	9.3%	8.8%	11.1
Midwife/O&G	134	60.4%	18.7%	20.9%	14.9

Women complained about being discharged from hospital within 12 to 24 hours without adequate postnatal care. The proportion of babies fully breast-fed at two weeks declined from 83 per cent in 1993 to 72 per cent in 1997, and at six weeks from 75 per cent to 64 per cent. Postnatal distress and depression increased. The heroic RHA bean counters, with no concern about the needs of pregnant and lactating women, 'laboured' to make NZMA's structure functional. The 'proposed amendments' introducing 39 different funding streams compared to MBS's 16 streams were received by COM on Christmas Eve 1996 with 'despair'!

Karen urged midwives to remain focused on women's needs. 'Women need strong midwives in order to claim their personal autonomy – midwives strong enough to enter into a true informed and negotiated partnership. To deny the right to autonomy indicates a profession's insecurity'.

Midwifery entered 1997 under siege. They faced an unprecedented number of complaints through the Health and Disability Commissioner Act 1994 based on the consumer Code of Rights 1996. Doctors encouraged dissatisfied consumers to use the Commissioner's wide-ranging powers to bring disciplinary action against midwives. The most common complaint was failure to inform of significant risks. Many complaints against doctors were settled by mediation; those against midwives went directly to the Nursing Council, even bypassing the Preliminary Proceedings Committee. Although complaints against midwives accounted for only one per cent of the whole profession, midwives got the publicity! Sensational, misinformed reports from an unfriendly press were disheartening. Our brilliant midwife legal advisor, Jackie Pearse, claimed 'vicious criminals were accorded more protection under the Human Rights Act than a professional being investigated over standards of practice'. Jackie told the NZCOM conference (August 1998) that 'Many wonderful, experienced midwives have walked away because they can no longer practise without fear. Sadly, practising well no longer immunises a midwife against a complaint.'

As midwives were being victimised, the doctors were backing themselves into a corner. No doubt emboldened by earlier RHA support, the Royal New Zealand College of General Practitioners rejected the 'proposed amendments' because they failed to meet seven NZMA-specified conditions! This left NZMA in 'limbo' with no credibility or fallback position. The doctors had defeated themselves. By May 1997, the RHA reverted to the MBS. Although a complicated claiming system, the MBS provided 'an appropriately financed framework to nurture midwives as autonomous practitioners, at their own pace, allowing those unable to accept challenges to practise in their "comfort zone"'. In 1997, self-employed midwives made up 42 per cent of the midwifery workforce. These plus employed midwives provided 60 per cent of New Zealand women with an LMC service up from 53 per cent in 1996. An estimated 50 per cent of women were choosing midwife-only care. By 2003, 78.1 per cent of women registered with a midwife initially. One third of practising midwives were self-employed.[18]

The health services were in chaos. The four expensive, inefficient RHA bureaucracies were reduced to one Transitional Health Authority (THA) to become a Health Funding Authority (HFA) by January 1998.

In September 1997, the THA finally provided COM with $3 million to establish a limited liability Maternity Provider Organisation (MPO) for the Southern Region – effective from 1 March 1998 and subject to negotiation of collective arrangements with IPAs, GPs and obstetricians. This protects midwifery autonomy at a macro economic and social level. COM has also developed a national database which allows the profession to describe the work and outcomes of midwifery practice throughout New Zealand. HBL is working with MPO to adapt the COM-owned database to deal with claims electronically.

An IPA report to the THA claimed payments to LMC doctors ranged from $1,600 to more than $2,000. Doctors were selecting only low-risk women, forcing the high-risk ones into the public hospital system. There was also increased handing over to secondary care to avoid clinical risk. They urged fence mending between IPAs and CHEs as well as with midwives.

Doctors were dissatisfied with the March 1998 Section 51 amendments that deducted hospital midwifery service costs from their MBS – $280 for postnatal care and $450 for a primipara labour and delivery ($350 for subsequent births). CHE midwives were unhappy that they were seen as worth less than independent midwives. NZCOM lodged a complaint with the Commerce Commission about setting the price of one midwifery service against another.

By September 1998, HBL showed that only 451 doctors had registered as LMCs, compared to 845 in 1997. Some GP groups are illegally charging women. One group with specialist affiliations charges a woman $900 entitling her to two specialist consultations – seldom needed in a normal pregnancy.

Individual GPs collect $10–20 'donation' per visit. Another group of seven rostered GPs charge a $100 'administration' fee. The HFA has threatened doctors with HBL audit. Doctors calling themselves GP obstetricians (GPOs) want urgent research to see if a correlation can be shown between the availability of GPOs and infant mortality rates, New Zealand having slipped to 15th in infant mortality among 21 OECD countries.[19] No doubt the government will throw some money at that idea rather than acknowledge that the cause is poverty!

Despite five years of Section 51 negotiation the GPs still want midwives back on a separate, lower pay schedule. As Karen told the conference, the determination of NZCOM to struggle in 'this painful and difficult environment to ensure the transition from dependent to independent has been revolutionary for us as professionals and as women. We have not only changed ourselves, we have also changed our world. The energy involved in change of this magnitude cannot be overestimated.'

Also, COM has substantially delayed the government's resolve to privatise the health services – to make the primary sector limit access to secondary care and transfer financial and political risk to providers and consumers. So now the HFA has to deal with the private maternity contracts subsidised by the CHEs. Another recent plus is that the HFA

18 NZHIS (2006b)
19 OECD (2006)

has given COM one-off funding to set up a breastfeeding committee to establish the Baby Friendly Hospital Initiative in New Zealand. Previously, COM was told by Jenny Shipley, then Minister of Health, to find a sponsor!

HFA claims it is committed to Section 51. It aims for national consistency of all primary care and CHE/secondary care contracts. As a result of ordering GPs to stop illegally charging women, the issue of the 'pitiful' funding has again erupted. The minister has ordered a review in 1999 of the 'fraught' public maternity services.

This review is to be carried out by the National Health Committee (NHC) which advises the Minister of Health on the quality and mix of services that should, in the Committee's opinion, be publicly funded. The terms of reference are to assess:

- The quality of public maternity services and scope for improvement
- Women's satisfaction concerning ability to make informed choices
- Barriers to access of maternity care of the type and quality women need and ways to achieve better use of available resources *within current funding levels*.

The review process is to be 'consumer-centred'. A 'parallel process' will include data collection and analysis to review pregnancy complications, clinical interventions during delivery and outcomes and the interface between primary and secondary care. 'Stakeholders' groups are to be established to discuss working conditions. The final report is due 31 August 1999.

With a national election due by November the review will no doubt be positive for women and midwives!

'Midwives are like cockroaches, you can't stamp 'em out'.

Wendy Savage adds: Joan's chapter was written in March 1999 and ended here, so I have looked at what has happened since then.

The NHC concluded that maternity services were safe but urged more co-operation:

> There is no evidence to suggest any reduction in recent years in the safety of maternity care that women are receiving... Faced with such findings the NHC sees no reason to recommend major changes in the current system of maternity care in New Zealand.[20]

In 2002 the Ministry of Health carried out a survey of women's satisfaction with their care and concluded that:

> The LMC concept with continuity of a primary maternity practitioner is considered important in engendering a relationship of partnership.... The women who were surveyed generally supported the maternity framework and acknowledge the professionalism of the practitioners.

They thought it would be useful to repeat the survey in two to three years' time but this does not seem to have been done.[21] However a consultation was announced in August 2006 about access to maternity services[22] which followed a report by the Health and Disability Commissioner into the unfortunate death of a baby in Nelson from a group B

20 NHC (1999)

21 Department of Health (2003)

22 Department of Health (2006)

streptococcal infection. He considered there was a systems failure although he criticised both the obstetrician and the midwives.[23] The Minister of Health resisted calls for a review of services saying that it would only delay improvements being developed by professionals.[24] This article reports some individual neonatal deaths and there is criticism of midwives, but as Karen Guilliland pointed out, the perinatal mortality rate had continued its slow but steady fall without a break after independent midwifery was introduced.[25] Whilst there may be mistakes in management due to human error there will always be some babies who die around the time of birth and one has to look at the overall results as well as the details of care.

No doubt the battle to control birth will continue but, as the experience in Gisborne shows, where midwives, GPs and obstetricians work together everybody benefits and women get the care that they want.

References

Coney, S (1988) *The Unfortunate Experiment*. Penguin Books (NZ) Limited.

Department of Health (1985) *Study proposal – a qualitative study of Domiciliary midwifery*. Wellington: Department of Health.

Department of Health (2003) 'Maternity Services Consumer Satisfaction Survey 2002'. http://www.moh.govt.nz.moh.nsf/ html

Department of Health (2006) 'Consultation: Access to maternity services'. http://www.noh.govt.nz.moh.nsf/ by+um/ntml (accessed 1 August 2006).

English, B (1997) Minister of Health, Letter, 21 July 1997.

Guilliland, K (1997) *NZCOM Journal*, April 1997.

Guilliland, K (2001) 'Midwifery in New Zealand'. http://www.acegraphics.com.au/articles/guilliland01.html

Health and Disability Commissioner (2006) http://www.hdc.org.nz/files/hdc/opinions/04hdc03530/obstetrican-midwives.dhb.pdf

Lewis, J (1995) *NZ Herald*, 11 January 1995.

Maternity Services Committee (1983) Wellington: Department of Health.

NHC (1999) Media Releases http://www.nhc.govt.nz/media releases/29sept19991/html

NZHIS (2006a) http://www.nzhis.govt.nz/stats/nursestats/html2

NZHIS (2006b) 'Maternity 2003: a snapshot'. http://www.nzhis.govt.nz/stats/maternity stats/html

NZMA (1993) Statement made at first Negotiation Committee meeting.

NZNA (1981) 'Policy Statement on Maternal & Infant Nursing'.

NZPA (2006) 'Hodgson argues against review of Maternity services review'. http://www.nzherald.co.nz/organisation/story (accessed 20 March 2006).

23 Health and Disability Commissioner (2006)

24 NZPA (2006)

25 Guilliland (2001)

OECD (2006) 'OECD in Figures: Statistics on the Member Countries', *OECD Observer*, 2005, Supplement 1.

Sutherland, A (1995) *NZ Herald*, 3 January 1995.

van Alten D, Eskes M and Treffers PE (1989) 'Midwifery in the Netherlands. The Wormerveer Study, selection, mode of delivery, perinatal mortality and infant morbidity', *BJOG*, 96:656–62.

Williamson, M (1993) Associate Minister of Health (National party).

1 2 3 4 5 6

Accountability

Accountability of Doctors and the District Health Authority

Wendy Savage

Accountability appears to me to involve three elements: disclosure, explanation and justification. If people are to be held accountable for their actions then they must be ready to disclose what they have done, to explain why they did it and to justify it as reasonable or appropriate in the circumstances. Explanation and justification may often appear to merge in practice, but I think that they are logically distinct processes.

Accountability of doctors

I fully accept that doctors are accountable to their patients, to their regulatory body and to their employer for their actions whilst carrying out their professional duties. Clearly if a doctor's behaviour or actions, personal or clinical, appear to be affecting patient safety then their colleagues should take action, but their first step must be to speak to the doctor concerned. I first heard of my professor's doubts about my competence when I was told that I was to be suspended.

The cost of my suspension and the enquiry was put, at the time, at £250,000.[1] It seems incredible that a handful of doctors were able to set in motion a process which deprived the NHS of much-needed resources because their obstetric philosophy differed from mine. Yet this kind of outrage is still happening (see section four of this book). The justification offered by my accusers was that there was a danger to patients. Yet we had monthly perinatal mortality meetings where we scrutinised the case of every baby who had died around the time of birth, and we had a computerised obstetric data system which could have shown that my results did not differ significantly from theirs. Moreover, most of them had no first-hand knowledge of my practice because they worked exclusively at the Whitechapel site, while I was based at Mile End.

Four of the five cases cited to justify my suspension concerned caesarean sections. When called to account for my conduct of these cases, I explained that I had worked in Africa, and knew that some cultures viewed a caesarean delivery as a failure on the part of the woman. As long as it was safe to do so, therefore, I was willing to give more time for a natural birth than some of my colleagues might have done. I thought that this was justifiable because doctors have a responsibility to care for the whole patient, and not just to consider the purely physical which might point to an earlier intervention. My colleagues disagreed. I do not believe that either side in this controversy can show that the other is wrong in any objective sense. One can only take people over one's ideas about how matters should be handled, and appeal to them to imagine what it is like for a mother to see the birth of her baby as a failure. Perhaps that leap of imagination is easier for a woman doctor than it is for a man. I certainly believe that I acted reasonably and appropriately, but convincing others can be difficult in a discipline which is rent –

1 Savage (1986) p.178

as obstetrics was and is – by competing paradigms of how birth is to be managed. Regrettably, when the case against me was put to the lay chairman there was no explanation of the wide spectrum of obstetric opinion.

At the time of my suspension, the General Medical Council's (GMC) guidance to doctors *Professional Conduct and Discipline: Fitness to Practise* (colloquially known as 'The Blue Book')[2] contained a section about the depreciation of other doctors:

> The Council also regards as capable of amounting to serious professional misconduct:
> (i) The depreciation by a doctor of the professional skill, knowledge, qualifications or services of another doctor or doctors.

Luke Zander, a general practitioner from Lambeth and senior lecturer at St Thomas', was a great support to me during the case, although we had hardly known each other beforehand. He did home births, and is a very thoughtful doctor with a holistic approach to medical care. He wrote to the chairman of the Standards Committee at the GMC after I was reinstated to enquire whether my colleagues' conduct amounted to serious professional misconduct and whether reporting them to the GMC would be a useful way forward. The response from Donald Irvine was equivocal, and the GMC has been reluctant to intervene in cases where doctors hold different opinions. In any event, I did not feel that I wanted to pursue this course of action. It seemed that the enquiry panel had given my colleagues a face-saving way out of the situation, and a GMC case would have taken years. It would have kept the whole battle running and prevented us working together amicably. Had I known how difficult working with them was going to prove, and how many more doctors were to be suspended for so-called 'genuine concerns', I might have agreed with Luke and pursued the question of whether my colleagues conduct was a breach of professional ethics. However the media coverage in the broadsheets, TV and the medical press made me hopeful in 1986 that managers and doctors would be more careful in the future.

The result was that my colleagues, who believed that their view of how obstetrics should be run justified them in pursuing an expensive, damaging and non-evidence based case in order to remove me from my post, were never held to account for their actions.

Two cases have helped to change doctors' attitudes towards accountability since then: first, that of an anaesthetist who dismissed a locum for poor practice but failed to inform both the GMC and a colleague who had been asked to write a reference for the locum;[3] second, the striking off of the medical director in Bristol for what were judged to be his failures to deal with problems relating to paediatric cardiac surgery at the Bristol Royal Infirmary.[4]

Doctors are much more accountable nowadays than they were when I was suspended, for a number of reasons. There has been an increase in the number of cases referred to the GMC over the last two decades.[5] There has been a growth in litigation. The regular appraisal of doctors has been introduced and revalidation may follow. The system of clinical governance is attempting to make chief executives of hospitals responsible for the standard of care, as well as for the financial stability of the hospital. The Health Care

---

2 GMC (1983) p.16

3 GMC (1994)

4 Privy Council (1999)

5 GMC Annual reports

Commission (HCC) is now responsible for monitoring compliance, and trusts have to produce detailed formal statements which are rigorously monitored each year. Targets are set and indicators of success published on the HCC website.[6] The HCC can mount investigations if standards of care cause concern, so a doctor's practice may be examined in context, as part of this exercise.

However these measures have not stopped inappropriate suspension of doctors (see section four of this book).

As well as being accountable to the GMC and their employer, hospital doctors may also be sued in the civil courts or prosecuted in the criminal courts. If a patient dies they may be charged with manslaughter.[7] GPs are now accountable to 14 different systems.[8] The creation of the Council for Health Regulation of Professionals (CHRP) in 2003, which metamorphosed into CHRE (The Council for Healthcare Regulatory Excellence) adds another layer of accountability. The CHRE can challenge the decisions of the health care regulatory bodies like the GMC and Nurses and Midwives Board. This means that a doctor may go through a long and painful GMC fitness-to-practise hearing, be found not guilty, and then come before the High Court for a further trial.[9]

In July 2006[10] the Chief Medical Officer (CMO) published his response to the Secretary of State's request to examine the weaknesses in the system to protect patients from harm which had been identified by Dame Janet Smith in her fifth report of the enquiry into Dr Harold Shipman.[11] This single-handed GP was found guilty of the murder of 15 patients in 2000 and committed suicide in prison in 2004. The enquiry estimated that he had killed about 250 of his patients between 1972 and 1998.

The CMO has made 44 recommendations on matters ranging from transferring responsibility for undergraduate education from the GMC to the new PMETB (Postgraduate Medical Education and Training Board) to the way appraisals should be conducted and the kind of structures needed for the proposed revalidation system.

The problems with the applications for the first Foundation Year One posts in 2006 – when hundreds of undergraduates in their final year received no offer of an appointment – suggest that putting more power in the hands of the Department of Health may not be altogether wise.[12] On accountability he suggests a new system, with GMC-trained affiliates responsible for the standard of care of doctors in each hospital, assisted by a local lay person. This seems to me to be a step too far, and a slur on the professionalism of the majority of the 100,000 doctors in NHS practice. As Onora O'Neill said in her Reith lectures, 'The efforts to prevent the abuse of trust are gigantic, relentless, and expensive; their results are always less than perfect'.[13] My own experience makes me sceptical about the independence of the proposed affiliate doctors within institutions where they know and are known by everybody. The risk of bias is clearly a difficult issue. There may also be a conflict of interest, with affiliate doctors feeling that their own careers may be jeopardised by a negative report on a colleague.

---

6 Health Care Commission
7 Ferner and McDowell (2006)
8 Holden (2005)
9 Samanta and Samanta (2005)
10 Chief Medical Officer (2006)
11 Smith (2004)
12 McCullum et al (2006)
13 O'Neill (2002)

Accountability of the DHA or successor bodies

In 1985 the DHA was made up of a number of people appointed to represent the views of doctors, nurses and the public via local authority members and independent members appointed by the Regional Health Authority. There was no clear and transparent process for these appointments but names 'emerged', and within the hospital structure, the chair of the Medical Council would suggest names which were usually accepted without debate. The University nominees might well be decided upon locally rather than, for example, in Senate House in London. GP nominees came through the Local Medical Committee to which GPs were elected by their peers. Some of those appointed did feel a strong sense that they were responsible for the delivery of health care in the district. Meetings were held monthly and in public, apart from confidential matters to do with employees which were discussed in private. The DHA was not involved in the decision to suspend me but was presented with a fait accompli and then told that the matter could not be discussed because it was 'sub judice'. Following the enquiry and my re-instatement, the DHA asked two of its members to conduct an internal enquiry as to how this debacle had occurred. The members found that proper procedures had not been followed and were critical of the chair, the late Francis Cumberlege. He declined to resign, but one of the independent members, the Reverend Bourne, resigned in protest.

The 1989 'reforms' introduced by Kenneth Clarke[14] and continued with renewed vigour by New Labour, after a short break when Frank Dobson was Secretary of State for Health in 1997–8, divided the NHS into purchasers (Primary Care Groups then Primary Care Trusts, PCTs) and providers (NHS trust hospitals). A business model was imposed, with a board consisting of senior managers in the organisation and non-executive directors appointed by the Secretary of State. Initially there was no formal appointments procedure, but now posts are advertised and applicants are interviewed. Their prime responsibility and statutory duty is to balance the books, and business people with no knowledge or understanding of the NHS are frequently appointed. They are not accountable to the local community, only to the Secretary of State for Health.

The direct link with the local authority has not been maintained. Instead, health overview and scrutiny committees (HOSCs) have been set up for each local government area. HOSCs can launch local investigations into any aspect of the NHS. They also have to be consulted about service planning, operational matters and the development of proposals for changes in provision as part of the process by which patients and the public are required to be involved in these issues under Section 11 of the Health and Social Care Act 2001.[15] If HOSCs are unhappy about a proposal, they can either seek judicial review on process type grounds or refer the matter to the Independent Reconfiguration Panel via ministers. Very few have become actively involved in this way. However, with the introduction of the Private Finance Initiative (PFI) and contracting with private companies, the concept of 'commercial confidentiality' has been introduced so that even less information is available for local people.

Despite the statutory duties to consult, most people feel disillusioned by the process, which costs a lot of money but rarely seems to result in the views of the community being taken seriously. The recent High Court decision in the case where a local PCT awarded a practice in East Derbyshire to a subsidiary of an American health insurance

---

14 Department of Health (1990)

15 HMSO (2001)

organisation with no experience of British general practice[16] exemplifies the problem. The judge ruled that the local population should have been consulted about the decision, but then refused a judicial review on the grounds that the plaintiff had not used 'an alternative route'. The route which apparently should have been followed was said to be the Patients Advisory and Liaison Service, PALS (set up after Community Health Councils were abolished). The plaintiff did not know that this organisation existed, but had she consulted it, she would have found that it had no power to act. It can only refer matters to the scrutiny committee of the Local Authority, whose only redress is to refer issues to the Secretary of State. It was scarcely to be expected that a cabinet minister would rule against a decision which was so in tune with government policy. In August 2006 Pam Smith won her appeal against the High Court decision: the judges ruled that Section 11 of the Social Care Act (2001) did apply, and that the PCT had failed in its duty to consult the local population.[17] The Department of Health denied that this was a significant victory.

Despite all the talk about 'openness and transparency' and accountability, I believe that the system of management of the NHS today means that there is even less accountability to the public than there was in 1985. Despite the rhetoric of 'patient choice', the recent debacle following the relatively minor deficits in the NHS budget of £76 billion led to the closure of community hospitals, wards and specialist services and to massive job losses. This in turn has sparked demonstrations by local communities throughout the country.[18]

The NHS has been repeatedly reorganised: 14 Regional Health Authorities (RHAs) became nine, and were replaced first by regional outposts of the NHSE, then by 28 Strategic Health Authorities, which were recently merged so that we now have ten. This is virtually the same as the number of RHAs 15 years ago. Apart from the almost constant upheaval, there has been a loss of collective experience as each reorganisation loses key people. Foundation hospitals, established after a considerable battle in Parliament, ostensibly to give hospitals more freedom from central control by the DoH, are supposed to engage with their local communities, but so far there is little sign of this.[19]

In this section, James Drife writes about the accountability of doctors. Professor Drife is a former Vice President of the RCOG and was for several years an elected member of the GMC. A reference for the disgraced gynaecologist Richard Neale (who was erased from the register in 2000), which he had given, in good faith in 1996, was criticised by the Neale enquiry. He was referred via the GMC's solicitors to the GMC and found guilty of 'impaired fitness to practise'. He resigned from the GMC after this judgement.

John Eversley, a lay member of the DHA in Tower Hamlets after my reinstatement, who later became an executive director of the East London and City Health Authority, writes about accountability in DHAs and their successor bodies.

---

16 Dyer (2006)

17 Kelly (2006)

18 O'Dowd (2006); Triggle (2006); BBC News (2006)

19 Kings Fund (2005)

References

BBC News (2006) 'Timeline of health service job cuts'. http://www.bbc.co.uk/health (accessed 26 July 2006).

Chief Medical Officer (2006) *Good doctors: Safer patients. Proposals to strengthen the system to assure and to protect the safety of patients*. London: Department of Health.

Department of Health (1990) *Working for Patients*. London: Department of Health.

Dyer O (2006) 'Councillor loses legal battle over Derbyshire General Practice', *BMJ*, 332:1,469.

Ferner RE and McDowell SE (2006) 'Doctors charged with manslaughter 1795–2005: a literature review', *Journal of Royal Society of Medicine*, 99:309–14.

GMC (1983) *Professional Conduct and Discipline: Fitness to Practise*. London: GMC.

GMC (1994) Professional Conduct Committee. GMC vs Dr Dunn, 14–18 March 1994.

GMC annual reports, http://www.gmc-uk.org

Health Care Commission, http://www.healthcarecommission.nhs.uk

HMSO (2001) *Health and Social Care Act 2001*. London: HMSO.

Holden J (2005) 'British GPs are accountable to 14 systems', BMJ.com (accessed 15 January 2005).

Kelly A (2006) 'Code of practice', *Society Guardian*, 30 August 2006, p.7.

Kings Fund (2005) 'Promised democracy in Foundation hospitals yet to materialise'. http://www.kingsfund.org.uk (accessed 13 October 2005).

McCullum C and 85 others (2006) 'Choose doctors by interview not by computer', Letters, *The Times*, 4 March 2006 p.22.

O'Dowd A (2006) 'NHS deficit doubles to £512 million but true figure may be higher', *BMJ*, 332:1411.

O'Neill O (2002) *A question of Trust*. Cambridge: Cambridge University Press.

Privy Council (1999) 'Dr John Roylance vs the General Medical Council'. Oral judgement upon petition. Privy Council Appeal No.49 of 1998. http://www.privycouncil.org.uk

Samanta A and Samanta J (2005) 'Referring GMC decisions to the High Court', Editorial, *BMJ*, 330:103–4.

Savage W (1986) *A Savage Enquiry: Who Controls Childbirth?* London: Virago.

Smith J (2004) *The Shipman Enquiry: fifth report; safeguarding patients. Lessons from the past – proposals for the future.* Chairman Dame Janet Smith. CMD 6394. London: The Stationery Office.

Triggle N (2006) 'Are NHS managers really to blame?' http://www.bbc.co.uk/health (accessed 10 July 2006).

The Health Authority: Accountable for What, to Whom and How?

John Eversley

Wendy's case was important for public policy at the time because it raised questions about to whom doctors were accountable, for what and how. That in turn raised the question, as Wendy asks at the end of her 1986 book, to whom were the chair and members of district health authorities accountable? This reflects an even wider issue about non-elected public bodies generally.[1] If anything the issues the case raised are even more apparent and unresolved now. Some would say that despite major organisational and cultural changes in the accountability of professionals – and others would say *because* of these – the role of health body members may have become even more important, but not more transparent.

As well as to whom NHS staff, including doctors, are accountable, it is important to ask for what and how they are accountable. This will not be discussed in any depth here because it is complex and extensively debated, whereas the role of NHS bodies is rather neglected. Apart from a rather generally expressed dissatisfaction with a 'democratic deficit', there has been little analysis of the role played by the executive committees, boards and other such bodies that have existed throughout the history of the NHS.[2] The major exception is the work of Klein and Day.[3] This is particularly relevant because their field work was done in the period just before the Savage case and was published just as that case was drawing to a close.

This chapter will argue that there were serious flaws in the arrangements for accountability in the NHS at the time of Wendy's case which in many respects have got worse since then. It argues that these flaws arise from:

1. A misconception about accountability: it is seen as a linear 'chain' – usually going upwards to national government in the classic organogram of a pyramid with the Secretary of State for Health at the top.
2. Requirements for lateral and downward accountabilities being ignored that are sometimes inconsistent and incompatible with upward political accountability.
3. This idea of upward political accountability in the NHS as consistent with downward delegation of responsibility being simplistic and unworkable.
4. The other dimensions being treated as irrelevant or illegitimate, thus reinforcing abuses of position. The winners in this situation are generally privileged – the professional providers of health care (clinicians and managers), national politicians and sometimes patients with the means to articulate their cause – the groups most often represented in the bodies in question. The losers are the people who are not represented and frequently most dependent on the NHS.

---

1 Savage (1986) pp.175, 178

2 Hereafter called 'NHS bodies'

3 Day and Klein (1987)

Even in this brief introduction, it is obvious that the concept of accountability is closely tied up with wider political ideas about democracy and representation, with questions about what the NHS is there to do and how decisions in larger organisations are taken. A framework is needed to incorporate these elements and others.

A conceptual framework

Accountability in the public sector

Lawton and Rose[4] talk about five dimensions of accountability in the public sector:

- Political
- Managerial
- Legal
- Consumer
- Professional

This model is intended to cover individuals, occupations (such as the professions) and bodies. Implicitly it is understood that different individuals, professionals and bodies might give priority to different aspects. It would be expected that a director of finance would give priority to financial management but in this model s/he also needs to take into account, say, the best interests of the patients or the standards of professional accountants. In the case of the health authority in the Savage case, different strands of accountability pulled in different directions. Individual members interpreted their responsibilities in different ways.

The chapter explores the *what* and the *how* of accountability in relation to each of the five constituencies identified by Lawton and Rose. Wendy's case is used to illustrate the issues.

What are individuals and bodies accountable for?

The *Code of Conduct and Code of Accountability* in the NHS says of accountability that 'everything done by those who work in the NHS must be able to stand the test of parliamentary scrutiny, public judgements and professional codes of conduct'.[5]

Political accountability and professional accountability are usually expressed in slightly different language to describe similar distinctions in what individuals and bodies are accountable for.

Political accountability is couched in terms of responsibility for policy – strategy, overall levels of resources and outcomes – usually considered as ministerial responsibilities at the highest level, and responsibility for operations – methods, process, inputs and outputs – for which civil service or NHS staff are responsible.[6]

Studies of professional competence make a distinction between *fitness to practise* which in very simple terms generally means minimum standards of competence and *fitness for purpose* which often reflects best practice. The notion of fitness for purpose comes from manufacturing industry – giving the customer a product that does what they want it to do.[7]

4 Quoted in Pyper (ed.) (1996) p.7

5 NHS Appointments Commission and Department Of Health (2004)

6 Day and Klein (1987)

7 Harvey (2004)

Professional fitness to practise often focuses on loss, danger, the breaking of clear rules. Questions of fitness to practise often focus on behaviour or methods – 'doing the thing right'.[8] Fitness for purpose more often includes explicitly questions of values, questions about the direction of behaviour – doing the right thing – and more explicitly on the outcomes. Here it is argued that strategy/operations and purpose/practice should not be seen as entirely separate categories but rather as on a continuum. When the Home Secretary says the Home Office is not fit for purpose, he is complaining that it is not getting the required results.[9] For NHS bodies, fitness to practise has often not been clearly defined – it is obviously about the methods used but beyond that it is not clear what level of detail they are responsible for. Whether it is to observe, test or question decisions, or to make them is often obscure. Boards of NHS trusts appear to take major decisions on building hospitals, closing services, making and ending contracts with organisations and individuals. The distinction between strategy and operations is often unclear. Members of NHS bodies are told that they should not get involved in day-to-day operations; they are also told that they are there to implement national and regional policies and priorities. This is explored further below.

The Latin roots of *governance* lie in the notion of steering a ship rather than driving cattle, which is the root of the word *management*. Board members are neither navigating nor herding. Aneurin Bevan said in 1945 that NHS bodies would be agents ('though not in a derogatory sense') of his department.[10] He also implicitly compared members of hospital boards to chauffeurs (see below). Members of NHS bodies might like to think of themselves as a shepherd or sports coach, but in reality they are more like a sports commentator – one influence among many. What they are usually doing is giving or withholding confidence in someone else's judgement. They are also frequently making an assessment of things outside their direct control. A decision about building a new hospital (almost invariably now with Private Finance Initiative money) is largely not a local decision.

How are NHS bodies accountable?

Mechanisms of accountability take three broad forms:

- *Executive:* behaviour is mandatory – individuals or bodies must behave or not behave in particular ways. In common with many approaches to planning and performance management it is assumed that having facts available (information, disclosure, transparency and so on) is in itself some form of management. The idea that transparency is in itself a form of accountability is one that has grown in the NHS since the 1980s. In 1981 Patrick Nairne, the Permanent Secretary at the DHSS, told a select committee that the department was 'investigating enhancing efficiency and a sense of local accountability by requiring health authorities to publish information to Community Health Councils and the local press with formal accountability upwards matched by a greater degree of informal accountability downwards'.[11] Information may or may not be a means of control: Day and Klein also reported that district health authority members themselves complained of having too much of the wrong kind and too little of the right kind of information and that they did not trust

8 Argyris and Schön (1974)

9 See for example Walker (2006)

10 Quoted in Day and Klein (1987)

11 Day and Klein (1987)

the district management teams of full time officers.

There are external and internal, explicit and implicit rules for NHS bodies about how often they meet, meeting in public and declaring interests. There are occasional examples of members of an NHS body being removed because they have broken one of these rules. This is most often when an individual dissents from a collective decision and expresses it through 'leaking' or 'whistle blowing'. As will be described below, 'interests' are interpreted in a very narrow way.

- *Education or exhortation:* rather than being told what to do, members of NHS bodies are given advice, information and training. This strategy has been part of the NHS for a long time. In 1950 Bevan wrote, 'We have deliberately come down in favour of maximum decentralisation of local bodies, relying for economy on education rather than a tight and detailed departmental grip'.[12] Sixty years later, board away days, board development programmes and mentoring contracts signed by non-executive members to undertake training are all part of the 'education' armoury.
- *Redress:* a key part of accountability may be putting things right or compensation for the consequences of action. It could also include punishment for errors. NHS bodies do issue apologies and pay compensation for clinical failures for example. Board members are also subject to periodic interviews by the chair about what they have done and s/he is interviewed by someone else in turn. However none of this amounts to redress for personal actions.

Within each of these approaches there are potentially adversarial and supportive, formal and informal, public and private approaches. The practice tends to be supportive and informal. Compared to the mechanisms used in relation to elected politicians (usually adversarial, often public or semi-public) or professions – often formal and adversarial – the position of members of NHS bodies seems highly protected.

To whom are members of NHS bodies accountable and what for?

Political

Before the NHS was born, doctors were arguing about what it would mean for accountability to be part of a state medical service with medical practitioners describing the power of ministers to discipline doctors as 'autocratic and dictatorial… very much like the [Nazi] regime that is coming to its sorry end in Nuremburg'.[13]

Aneurin Bevan struggled with questions of political accountability from the earliest days: in October 1945 he was arguing in cabinet with Herbert Morrison about the role of the Regional Hospital Boards. Morrison said they would 'either be creatures of government [or have] dangerous freedom to pursue policies of their own at the expense of the exchequer'. Bevan replied that there was room for development in the techniques of government.[14] Observers of the debate about Foundation Hospitals will recognise the style of the exchange. He also said 'it is no use giving orders to the chauffeur if the steering column is not connected to the front wheels'[15] and that 'when a maid kicks over

12 Quoted in Day and Klein (1987)
13 Honigsbaum (1989) p.98
14 Campbell (1987) p.170
15 Webster (1991)

a pail on a ward, Whitehall shakes'.[16] Many, perhaps all, health ministers since then have felt these two grievances – the NHS is not responsive enough to their demands but if something goes wrong, ministers are blamed even if it is beyond anything they can or should control – or even know about. Richard Crossman compared relations with hospital boards to that of a Persian satrap to a weak Persian Emperor. 'If the Emperor tried to enforce his authority too far he lost his throne or at least lost his resources or something broke down'.[17]

At the time of Wendy's suspension, health authorities consisted of a chairman [sic] and 16–17 other members – four appointed by the local authority (in inner London, one is also appointed by the Inner London Education Authority), nominees of hospital consultants, GPs, trade unions and nurses and the local medical school, plus up to nine generalists nominated by the regional health authority. The criteria for choosing them were set out in guidance from the department and included:

- Ability to devote sufficient time
- Health and vigour to make an effective contribution
- Experience of management, finance etc
- A balance of age, sex, geographical spread
- 'In appropriate cases' suitable representation of ethnic minorities.[18]

Despite the last two points, the Tower Hamlets DHA was overwhelmingly white in a multiracial area, comprised mainly older people from professional backgrounds and was predominantly male.

The era in which Wendy was suspended has been described by Rudolf Klein as one in which the politics of value for money dominated. It took several forms. One was that central government forced health authorities 'to be efficient' – for example by imposing compulsory competitive tendering. However ministers still wanted to make a distinction between management and politics. They did this at national level initially with a Supervisory Board and a Management Board and locally by tighter control of who sat on health authority boards and what they did.[19]

The chair of the Tower Hamlets authority played a highly controversial role in the Savage case. Rather than seeing *whether* there was a prima facie case to answer, he saw his role as 'to establish' that there was a prima facie case against Wendy.[20] During the case he was reappointed by the Secretary of State – a fact that probably prolonged the case. In the very long, drawn-out period after the enquiry in which Wendy was unable to return to normal clinical and teaching arrangements, the new chairman also played a controversial role. She was a Conservative councillor from Westminster whose only connection with East London was through her husband's business. When she talked about 'going up the hill' to DHA members, it was not immediately understood that this was a reference to grouse shooting in Scotland rather than getting out of the tube at Tower Hill!

Beyond being accountable to an elected national government, there are other kinds

16 Quoted in Foot (1975)
17 Klein (1995)
18 1981 Health Circular quoted by Day and Klein (1987)
19 Klein (1995)
20 Savage (1986) p.53

of political accountability. After the enquiry finished, over 100 MPs signed an early day motion of support for Wendy[21] and two MPs were on the first march in support of her.[22]

Although several members of the authority were nominated by authorities controlled by Labour at the time (London Borough Tower Hamlets and the ILEA) and others worked or had worked for one or other body, there was no question of 'caucusing', bloc voting or 'whipping'. Memorably, when political accountability did become an issue in the Wendy Savage case, the chair of the Health Authority acted in such a way as to undermine it: he called a DHA meeting on the day of the general election when the political party members of the authority were unable to attend – and then used his casting vote in a partisan way, not, as a chair should, to ensure procedural propriety.[23]

Haywood and Ranade and Klein and Day writing in the 1980s adopted a threefold typology of DHA members, based on ancient Rome:

- Tribunes – whose prime loyalty was to the local community
- Prefects – whose loyalty was to government or the Region
- Patriarchs – whose loyalty was to HA staff. [24]

If this typology is applied to Tower Hamlets DHA at the time of Wendy's suspension, a majority of members would probably have said they were Tribunes – the problem was there was little consensus or shared perception of what the interests and wishes of the local community were. There were certainly Prefects – whose loyalty was to the NHS hierarchy or ministers. There were some members who were Patriarchs – supporting the interests of the clinical and management establishment. The three groups made a highly toxic mix from Wendy's point of view.

The current trend is to appoint as chairs and members of NHS bodies people who declare that they have no current political interests. What this means is that they declare that they are either not members of or active in a political party. There is a proper distinction to be made between support for an institution or a group such as a political party and support for policies that may be favoured or opposed by a party. However where an individual has interests or opinions that support or oppose policies that have direct bearing on the work of the NHS body, the distinction is rather artificial. This was evident during the Wendy Savage case. It is still an issue. In the mid 1980s one of the Health Authority members was a very active and traditional member of the Catholic Church. It is hard to imagine he did not act on his beliefs in relation to Wendy's, whose views and practice on abortions would have been unacceptable to him. The District Medical Officer told Wendy that some of the opposition to her stemmed from the day care abortion service that 'had turned Tower Hamlets into the abortion capital of London'.[25] Among medical staff at the London Hospital at the time there was an active Masonic lodge.[26] It was believed that Masonic members played a crucial part in decision-making about the construction of a new children's unit at Whitechapel. Suspicions were rife, but no evidence was found that Masonic networks played a part in the events surrounding

21 Savage (1986) p 178
22 Ibid. p.70
23 Pratten (1990) p.27
24 Cited in Day and Klein (1987)
25 Savage (1986) p.22
26 Knight (1985)

Wendy's case, though there were unexpected interventions or decisions that seemed to have been made elsewhere than the place they were supposed to be.

Since 1994 the 'Code of Conduct' for NHS non-executive directors has said that:

> Chairs and board directors should act impartially and should not be influenced by social or business relationships. No-one should use their public position to further their private interests. …When a conflict of interest is established the board director should withdraw and play no part in the relevant discussion or decision. [27]

Recent (July 2006) appointments to the Strategic Health Authority for London illustrate that the distinction between political, policy and business interests remains an arbitrary one. The chair has a professional background in firms producing confectionery (Mars), over-the-counter medicines (Reckitt) and cigarettes (British American Tobacco), and running pubs (Terra Firma – also potentially bidding to take over Thames Water). He is chairman of a water company (East Surrey) and a former chairman of a food retail chain (Iceland).[28] There are not many decisions that the Strategic Health Authority has to take that are neither influenced by nor have an influence on the companies he has been associated with. One wonders how policies on fluoridation, obesity, availability of new drugs and cancer prevention can be developed with a chair with such a background. One of the members of the new board is a former member of the Prime Minister's Strategy Unit. Only in a very mechanical conception of the state is independence of government only a formal separation of responsibilities – more sophisticated models would see the movement of people between civil service, non-executive and political roles as an indication of a ruling elite or a hegemonic structure. Perhaps the most striking case in point is the present Health Minister, Lord Warner, whose career has included being a civil servant, a local government officer, the non-executive chair of a health authority, the executive chair of the Youth Offending Board and now a minister. [29]

The structure adopted by the NHS is based on the idea that non-executive directors need to be independent of the managers or executive directors. One wonders how much it has changed from the 1980s, when the DHA members reported on by Day and Klein said how dependent they felt on the District Management Team.[30]

Most NHS bodies have executive and non-executive directors, and a system of reporting and controls first proposed in 1992 by the Cadbury committee (set up by the London Stock Exchange and others[31]) for the management of private enterprises. The committee started meeting before the events which gave it prominence and force – the collapse of the bank BCCI and of Robert Maxwell's business empire. The non-executive directors are intended to bring independent judgement to bear on issues of strategy, performance, resources (including key appointments) and standards of conduct. The accountability of non-executive directors in the Cadbury model is simply to shareholders. There are important questions about the (in)efficacy of corporate governance in the private sector: interestingly the American regulatory authorities are investigating the 'independence' of non-executive directors of United Health – the company whose

---

27 NHS Appointments Commission and Department of Health (2004)

28 Gould (2006)

29 Edwards et al (2006)

30 Day and Klein (1987)

31 World Bank (2005)

European arm, headed by a former Downing Street health adviser, is seeking to take over NHS services.[32] That aside, the difficulty in applying the shareholder model in the NHS is apparent. Who are the shareholders? The NHS prefers the language of *stakeholders*.[33] The origins of the term are contested. It could be either in the fight for control of territory in the Wild West or Australia when competing settlers raced to mark out their claim on free land (in fact land often owned by the indigenous communities) or in the role of the person holding stakes during betting. Both derivations underline the difficulty of seeing political accountability as a 'one answer' problem. There are always winners and losers. Foundation trusts have to 'earn autonomy'[34] by achieving government targets before they can be created. They are encouraged to think of local residents as shareholders but not if it means providing services at the expense of financial control by the NHS. They also have structures that clearly distinguish between governors (who may be numerous and broadly representative) and a board that may be very technocratic and focused on government performance targets. Primary care trusts also have two- or three-tier structures. While the board has non-executive members, there are professional executive committees dominated by clinicians of various kinds; and the executive directors play a crucial role in decision making, as do the strategic health authority's performance managers. The shareholder/stakeholder analogy highlights the tensions rather than resolves them.

All non-executives are appointed by the NHS Appointments Commission, which was established in 2001. The Commission has taken over from health ministers the statutory duty of appointing chairs and non-executives to all local NHS boards. The Commission has to ensure that chairs and non-executives have annual performance appraisals, receive proper training and get full support for their board work. It cost £5.0 million to run during 2004–05 and made over 1,250 appointments, an increase of 20 per cent on the previous year. The Commission's analysis of appointments shows that there remain serious issues about how unrepresentative of society appointments are:

- More than half as many men again as women apply to be non-executive directors and the actual number of women appointed has fallen; women make up 46 per cent of appointments.
- The proportion of non-executive directors and chairs from black and minority ethnic communities has remained constant at around 11 per cent.
- The number of people declaring themselves disabled has increased to around 8 per cent; however, the Commission believes this is partly due to more accurate data.
- More than two-thirds of appointments are of people over the age of 50 – even higher in the case of chairs.
- More than two-thirds of appointees claim not to be politically active. However, in the biographies published by the appointments commissioners, this only refers to current political activity, and many were formerly active in party politics. Of those that are currently active, Labour activists outnumber activists from all the other political parties put together and nearly three times as many Labour activists are appointed as the next biggest group – Conservatives.[35]

---

32 Urban and Moore (2006)

33 See for example, the National Audit (2005) p.3

34 *Health Service Journal* (2003)

35 NHS Appointments Commission and Department of Health (2005)

In terms of the framework of this chapter, there are a number of conclusions in relation to political accountability:

- It could certainly be argued that Wendy's conduct was presented by the (un-elected) politicians as an individual issue of fitness to practise when it was in fact a wider question of whether the obstetric practice of an individual consultant – or the profession collectively – was fit for purpose. The rise in caesareans, and concerns about junior obstetricians carrying out caesareans rather than take responsibility for difficult vaginal deliveries, suggests that it would have been much better to discuss the issues in terms of what is the right thing to do (purpose) rather than what is the right way to do it (practice).
- The approach taken by the Health Authority was in contrast to the ways the conduct of its own members would be handled. It behaved in an executive (punitive) way towards Wendy and the case was conducted in an adversarial manner when a collaborative educational approach (learning the lessons) and a strategy of rebuilding relationships between colleagues might have been more appropriate.
- More generally, political accountability was (and still is) narrowly interpreted. Wider questions need to be asked of members about affiliations and identity that may affect their ability to take decisions in the interests of the NHS, including questions of cultural competence.
- It is important to note that having elections to NHS bodies would not in itself solve these problems, though it would make some of the issues more transparent.

Managerial

The Griffiths report in 1983 led to the introduction of general management in the NHS. Quite explicitly, it gave managers (whatever their background) more control over what clinicians did. In the case of Tower Hamlets DHA, although the District Administrator was a long-time NHS administrator, he had a new authority which was starkly evident in Wendy's suspension.

On 24 April 1985 Wendy was 'suspended by the District Health Authority' – except of course that the decision was not taken by the DHA, it was taken by the chair of the DHA on the advice of the District Administrator, another consultant, in his capacity as Regional Assessor for the DHSS, and the District Medical Officer.[36] Members of the Health Authority were not told until two weeks later.[37] This pattern was repeated throughout the whole period of suspension and reinstatement – the Health Authority members generally were not even kept informed, let alone asked to take decisions at crucial moments.

In the event it was the HA that set up the enquiry – when ordered to do so by the High Court. The internal enquiry by the DHA found that the enquiry should never have taken place under the disciplinary procedure but rather it should have been dealt with as a complaint[38] – in other words, it related to accountability to consumers, not professional or managerial accountability. There were probably three reasons why this did not happen:

First, some of the patients concerned did not believe there was reason to complain. This would have contributed to the second reason – that a complaint case would be hard

36 Pratten (1990) p.15; Savage (1986) p.3

37 Pratten (1990) p.58

38 Ibid. pp.26–7

to prove. But the third reason is probably the most significant: sanctions against doctors for complaints are either minimal or very long and drawn out, involving the GMC or the courts.

However, the sequence of events that led up to that point began when the District Medical Officer (the professional lead on public health for the District Health Authority) asked for a report on Wendy's competence initially from the very same members of the department who had raised questions in the first place, although they declined to produce one.[39]

The nexus between managerial and professional lines of accountability is apparent in the roles of the District Medical Officer and the Regional Assessor, who was reported to have opposed Wendy's initial appointment, had appointed the professor criticising her and was a member of the same academic unit.[40] This confusion of roles is even more apparent in the behaviour of the head of the Professorial Unit, who argued that Wendy owed loyalty to the Department, the Academic Unit and himself personally and threatened her with dismissal.[41] Dismissal is significant as a sanction because it is clearly a managerial prerogative not a professional one.

After Wendy's exoneration in July 1986, she was unable to return to work because other consultants in the department threatened to resign if she did.[42] This again illustrates how conflicts between managerial and professional accountability were used as weapons by the other consultants. In a normal industrial relations situation, an order to reinstate an employee which was followed by a refusal to work with him or her would normally be followed by the suspension and dismissal of the protesters. In essence those managerially responsible for the NHS hid behind professional accountability.

The steady increase in the power or responsibility of paid managers is not clearly accompanied by an increase in the managerial accountability *to* or *of* board members.

The 'Code of Accountability' for NHS board members says that the role of an NHS board is to:

- Be collectively responsible for adding value to the organisation, for promoting the success of the organisation by directing and supervising the organisation's affairs;
- Provide active leadership of the organisation within a framework of prudent and effective controls which enable risk to be assessed and managed;
- Set the organisation's strategic aims, ensure that the necessary financial and human resources are in place for the organisation to meet the objectives, and review management performance;
- Set the organisation's values and standards and ensure that its obligations to patients, the local community and the Secretary of State are understood and met.[43]

Board members generally now have job descriptions and these are often accompanied by specific tasks, such as responsibility for audit, remuneration or equalities. They may be set objectives against which they are monitored. This gives the form of managerial accountability without the substance. They have very limited

39 Pratten (1990) p.22
40 Savage (1986) pp.28, 102
41 Pratten (1990) p.24
42 Ibid. p.25
43 NHS Appointments Commission and Department of Health (2004)

resources of their own (a tiny board secretariat) so that their ability to initiate activity, inspect or investigate or even to arrange meetings, is dependent on the goodwill of the executive directors. They have no right to have questions answered. For example if the lead member for equalities wanted to know the profile of applicants or staff in categories not required by the Department of Health, they would probably be told it was not possible to provide the information, either technically or because of resource constraints.

Anyone wanting to enhance the managerial accountability of NHS bodies could learn lessons from local government. In the 20 years since the Savage enquiry, this has undergone many changes. One is that councils increasingly operate through cabinets (rather than the traditional committee structure). Cabinet members generally have a 'support office' with limited dedicated resources, but the executive directors are also more clearly responsible to individual cabinet members. This enhances both the accountability to and of the cabinet member. This is not to say that this is a perfect situation – since the 1980s officers have been given substantial responsibilities in law that they can exercise whether the members agree or not, including budget setting.

Legal

In July 1985, Wendy took her case to the High Court. The principal grounds for her case were in employment law: that she had suffered a breach of contract.[44] In September the court ruled that a professional could best be judged by her peers, a judge could not presume to comment on such a complicated issue – and therefore the case should be heard before an enquiry set up by the Health Authority.[45]

The legal process was invoked by the chair of the Health Authority as a reason for not discussing the case at Health Authority meetings or in public while the enquiry was going on. In fact the chair was wrong about this.[46] However, it is one of the reasons why enquiries are often used – while they are going on they give people who wish to be secretive an opportunity to delay or avoid making information public as in the 'arms to Iraq' or the Hutton enquiries.

Wendy was concerned that her original lawyers were part of the same (medical) establishment which was attacking her, and that they were usually on the side of doctors against patients.[47] The introduction of a solicitor with a human rights background and a barrister with an employment law specialism undoubtedly influenced the way that the professional enquiry was conducted; but this did not alter the fact that it was an enquiry into professional competence. Arguably Wendy's case should have been considered an employment case all along.

The area of law that probably gets the most attention from the NHS is where clinical negligence is alleged. According to the NHS Litigation Authority, at 31 March 2005 there were over 18,600 live claims against the NHS for clinical negligence. Over 5,600 new claims had been made in the previous year. Although surgery accounts for the largest number of claims (over 11,250 since 1995), obstetrics and gynaecology (over 6,200) accounts for the highest cost of potential claims – over £1.66 billion.[48] This compares to the total costs of running maternity services in 2003–4 (the latest year for which figures

44 Savage (1986) p.80

45 Pratten (1990) pp.16–17

46 Ibid. p.59

47 Savage (1986) p.68

48 NHS Litigation Authority (July 2005)

are available) of £2.57 billion.[49] Less than 2 per cent of claims are settled in court in favour of the claimant. Nearly 40 per cent of cases are abandoned by the claimant.

Important though all this is to the service that the NHS provides and its costs, it is probably less of an issue for NHS bodies than judicial reviews, statutory enquiries and employment tribunals:

- There have been a number of high profile judicial reviews when a provider has refused a treatment, such as Herceptin for early stage breast cancer. Although these cases involve individual clinical decisions, NHS bodies are being held responsible for the policy frameworks in which these decisions take place. Judicial reviews are also regularly used when it is planned to change or cease a service, for example the closing of a maternity unit or an A & E department.
- In cases of homicide or suicide while under NHS care, the Secretary of State for Health can, and regularly does, order an enquiry. Sometimes the NHS bodies are among a number of bodies whose conduct and policies are investigated – as in the Laming enquiry into the death of Victoria Climbie. Other enquiries, such as that into the death of David 'Rocky' Bennett, focus only on the NHS. In both these examples, the enquiries found policies as well as practice to be inadequate – policies for which NHS boards could properly be expected to take responsibility.
- Employment Tribunals – particularly for trusts – are also an important focus for legal action against NHS bodies. The NHS is the largest employer in the UK. Many human resource practices are clearly centrally driven by the Department of Health or professional bodies, but responsibility in law generally rests with the local body. Occasional cases, such as that of the finance director at St George's, may involve an executive board member[50] of whom non-executive board members could be expected to have personal knowledge. Many more cases are likely to involve decisions that they were not individually involved in initially but where they are responsible for the policies and supervision of the senior staff, or for conducting appeals. Collective responsibility and responsibility for decisions and events of which an individual has no personal knowledge are often unclear in large organisations. The problem is compounded in NHS bodies. There is no mechanism for the public to express a view – through elections – of what it thinks is reasonable.

Many people would argue that there is an unhealthy trend towards using legal mechanisms to get acknowledgement, redress or prevention of mistakes and to settle policy questions in relation to public services. In relation to clinical negligence, it is clearly a trend and one which the government wishes to curtail. Trends in relation to the other areas of law are less easy to identify. What does seem clear is that members of NHS bodies need to understand that they are legally responsible for policies and that if they want to avoid legal actions they need to use other mechanisms to debate and decide policy questions, to deal with policies with unanticipated or undesirable consequences and to acknowledge and put right mistakes.

Perhaps the major change since the 1980s is that then, as Day and Klein pointed out, judicial review generally focused on whether bodies had exceeded their authority and/or not followed the laws of natural justice (administrative process). Consistency with human

49 Department of Health (2005a)

50 *Observer* (2003)

rights grounds was not clearly defined. The passing of particularly the Human Rights Act in 1998, but also of various equality acts, has clarified and strengthened the grounds for review.

Professional

Despite the label of 'professional committee person' that is applied to some members of NHS bodies, being a member of an NHS body is not a profession. Professions characteristically:[51]

- *Have control over entry to employment through legal limitations and/or the requirement to have formal credentials.* Although, for example, the NHS Appointments Commission is itself drawn from the ranks of committee people and there are now person specifications for most NHS board appointments, the formal entry requirements are very few. You need to be an adult and, for example, asylum seekers (but not refugees with settled status) are excluded.
- *Are defined by activities, knowledge or attitudes. Activities may be processes or outcomes.* There have been various attempts – some initiated or endorsed by government, others not – that have tried to articulate values and standards of conduct for those are in 'public life'. Despite this, it would be difficult to define a canon of knowledge or set of values (other than the very bland and general) to which all or most members of NHS bodies would subscribe. Some of the issues of interests and identities have already been discussed above, such as when a private or personal interest is an impediment and when it's an asset in relation to propriety.
- *Historically have been regulated by themselves and 'professional autonomy' – the right not to be told by outsiders what they must or must not do or know – has been critical.* When the General Medical Council was set up in 1858 it was profoundly opposed to defining what a doctor should or should not do. Between the establishment of the GMC and 1990 it used the so-called 'John Wayne' formula[52] – that doctors duties were to provide 'all necessary and appropriate services of a type usually provided' as the basis for the duties of a doctor. Since 1990, doctors' duties have become more specifically defined and also the General Medical Council has increasing numbers of lay people on it (see James Drife's chapter in this book). Compared to elected politicians, doctors, lawyers or accountants the autonomy of members of NHS bodies is very limited.

However, that does not mean that professional accountability is irrelevant to members of NHS bodies. Two of the crucial and sensitive areas of accountability are how much members have to do as professionals want and how much do they have to do as members want. As was indicated above, in the debates surrounding the establishment of the NHS, a key question was how much non-clinicians (politicians and board members) would be able to direct clinicians. How much clinicians could direct non-clinicians was a more implicit question.

The Savage case was precipitated or activated by the 'concerns' felt by some clinical colleagues about Wendy. She argued that 'no doctor… could direct my clinical decisions

---

51 Witz (1992)

52 'A man's got to do what man's got to do'. What John Wayne actually said was: 'A man ought to do what he thinks is right' (in the film *Hondo*).

as long as they were within the bounds of acceptable medical practice'.[53] The head of her academic unit argued that 'If one holds an academic unit position then the clinical autonomy may have to be modified'. The meaning of this was unclear in his evidence. He said that in that position one should explain one's action more clearly but implied that it might mean taking different clinical decisions.[54] He also argued that he personally was owed loyalty and that disloyalty could result in termination of employment.[55] One of his early complaints was that Wendy was not doing enough research and was doing too much clinical work.[56] University teachers and researchers would also argue that they have professional autonomy. If doctors, teachers and researchers do not like their peers instructing them, their objections to outsiders intervening are usually even stronger. The Health Authority – or some members of it – felt it could and should act on the concerns of colleagues. In the years since the Savage case, the arguments have been increasingly forcefully put that professions should not regulate themselves. This has been argued on a number of grounds:

- A perception that peers fail to prevent, detect, report or act firmly enough when there are problems with colleagues. The cases of Harold Shipman, the Bristol Heart Surgeons, retention of organs at Alder Hey or Rodney Ledward, Richard Neale and Clifford Ayling[57] are often cited as evidence of this in relation to doctors.
- A wider perception that peers in service organisations 'look after their own' at the expense of the public or service users. This is applied to a wide range of public life – politicians, police officers, sports bodies, estate agents or retailers – and has particularly led to the argument, discussed below, that users should have a stronger voice.
- A view that good practice frequently requires inter-professional working and that accountability is owed not simply or preferentially to members of the same profession, let alone the same specialty or one individual as some of Wendy's colleagues argued.
- A view that where public money and services provided under statute are concerned, the government can exercise rights as the funder.

The argument has been taken forward in various ways – more lay people on regulatory bodies, for example – but one of the major initiatives has been the introduction of clinical governance. It was first promoted in the NHS more than ten years after Wendy's reinstatement. The term was derived from corporate governance (see above). Like corporate governance it assumed a great importance because of events that happened before the term was coined, whose implications only became fully apparent afterwards. An elaborate structure has been set up. Probably the area in which it has most relevance to the Savage case is that the 'picking off' of a handful of cases of an individual consultant that occurred in 1984 is less likely now than a general requirement for systematic record-keeping, analysis and reflection on the work of a department. A member of an NHS board is usually appointed as a lead on clinical governance, working with someone with a clinical background.

---

53 Savage (1986) p.30
54 Ibid. p.121
55 Ibid. pp.31–2
56 Ibid. p.32
57 Alden (2005)

Consumers or public participation

Women who had been attended by Wendy played a very small part in the formal proceedings of the case but a much larger role in the public expression of disquiet at her treatment. There were (and are) very few opportunities for service users to express or explore their views about the treatment they receive. Even less was there any role for patients of other consultants to express their views so that a comparison might be made. There was no great expression of the majority of Health Authority members (those in favour of suspension) being champions of service users. The minority members (against suspension, for reinstatement) did sometimes argue that they were representing users. On the detail of the situation the majority would have had a hard case to make: two of the five women (and a sixth peripherally involved) explicitly said that they had no complaint about their treatment.[58] One of the most distressing aspects of the events between 1984 and 1986 was that the Mrs AU and her family did not get an explanation of how their baby had died. This was not because they exercised their right not to have a post mortem (part of the cultural context which practice has to recognise), but because the perinatal mortality discussion which should have taken place was postponed so that the case against Wendy could be made.[59] Accountability to service users repeatedly took second place. The wider question of whether members had a responsibility to represent users or to be held to account by them, since the inception of the NHS, has been discouraged. When Community Health Councils were created (in 1974) they were explicitly compared to school parent–teacher associations,[60] a separate role with only observer status at the open part of DHA meetings – though in fact Wendy's case was mostly considered in private.

Health Authority and Family Practitioner Committee (later FHSA) members had a part to play in hearing complaints – that role has now gone. Community Health Councils have now been abolished. They have been replaced by Patient Advice and Liaison Services (PALS) and Patient and Public Involvement Forums. Neither deals with complaints from patients and carers.[61]

PPI forums are made up of local volunteers and representatives of local voluntary organisations, and they:

- Monitor and review the range and operation of services provided and commissioned by the NHS
- Provide advice, reports and recommendations based on the reviews that they carry out
- Obtain the views of patients and their carers about the range and operation of services
- Make available to patients and their carers advice and information about services.[62]

Although this may sound as though PPI forums might play a role in cases like Wendy's, it is highly unlikely. They have no staff and they are serviced by agencies under contract from an NHS agency that agrees very specific work programmes with them. PPI forums too are now to be abolished.

At the same time that CHCs have been abolished and their replacements made marginal in such cases, another institution has been created which might take up the

58 Savage (1986) pp.52, 93–6
59 Ibid. p.40
60 Webster (1996) p.460
61 Department of Health (2005b)
62 Department of Health (2005c)

kind of issues raised by the Savage case. Local authorities are increasingly moving to a pattern of executive cabinets and monitoring by scrutiny committees. Many local authorities have health scrutiny committees. They can require NHS bodies to provide information about the planning, provision and operation of health services and to make them respond to reports and recommendations of health scrutiny committees but not require them to implement recommendations.[63] They cannot inspect NHS premises, but PPI forums can.

Potentially the Health Service Ombudsman might be involved in some aspects of the conduct of a health authority but the Commissioners (as they are officially called) are explicitly barred from any investigation into decisions 'taken solely in the exercise of clinical judgement'.

Martin Gorsky provides historical evidence that popular participation in managing health care has always been problematic. Certainly, anyone who thinks that paying for health care encourages participation should review the period when patients had to make financial contributions.[64]

Conclusion

Shifting the balance of accountabilities

NHS bodies lack legitimacy, and accountability is upward within the NHS to ministers. The understanding of political interests is formalistic and naïve. Accountability to 'local strategic partners', users or the public is token. Managerial accountability is there in form but not in substance. The relationship to professional accountability is underdeveloped and not yet clearly linked to fitness for purpose. The institutions of political accountability need to be strengthened to include a more direct and powerful role for the public-scrutiny committees are possibly a starting point. Legal mechanisms are being used in the absence of other forms of dialogue, and more for compensation than putting things right.

Aneurin Bevan, having created a structure based on un-elected bodies, argued that if local government were reformed, it could play a more direct role in running the National Health Service. Richard Crossman, who later went on to be Secretary of State for Health and Social Security, pointed out in 1953 that no effort had been made to encourage popular participation in the welfare state. He said Britain was a nation inhibited by an oligarchic tradition, which makes responsibility the privilege of an educated minority. The governors are not accountable to the governed... direct answerability to the people is required.[65] 'Answerability' may not sound like a rallying cry for reform of the NHS but then 'choice' or 'contestability' are hardly inspiring – so perhaps there is hope.

63 Democratic Health Network (2005)

64 Gorsky (2006)

65 Quoted in Day and Klein (1987)

References

Alden C (2005) http://www.chrisalden.co.uk/journalism/medicalscandals.html (accessed 26 October 2005).

Argyris M, Schön D (1974) *Theory in Practice. Increasing professional effectiveness.* San Francisco: Jossey-Bass.

Campbell J (1987) *Nye Bevan – A Biography*. Hodder & Stoughton.

Day P and Klein R (1987) *Accountabilities in five public services*. Tavistock Publications.

Democratic Health Network (2005) http://www.dhn.org.uk/health_improve_facts.taf?_ (accessed 31 October 2005).

Department of Health (2005a) *Departmental Report 2005* http://www.dh.gov.uk/assetRoot/04/11/37/90/04113790.pdf (accessed 29 October 2005).

Department of Health (2005b) http://www.dh.gov.uk/PolicyAndGuidance/OrganisationPolicy/ComplaintsPolicy/ (accessed 31 October 2005).

Department of Health (2005c) http://www.dh.gov.uk/assetRoot/04/07/42/88/04074288.pdf (accessed 31 October 2005).

Edwards N et al (2006) 'Proud to introduce the NHS top table', *Health Service Journal*, 4 September 2006.

Foot M (1975) *Aneurin Bevan*, Vol.2, 1945–1960. Paladin.

Gould M (2006) 'Critics round on London SHA Chief', *Health Service Journal*, 31 August 2006.

Gorsky M (2006) 'Hospital governance and community involvement in Britain: evidence from before the National Health Service History and Policy'. http://www.historyandpolicy.org/archive/policy-paper-40.html (accessed 21 September 2006).

Harvey L (2004) *Analytic Quality Glossary*, Quality Research International. http://www.qualityresearchinternational.com/glossary/ (accessed 14 September 2006).

Health Service Journal (2003) 'PCTs can earn autonomy', *Health Service Journal*, 13 March 2003.

Honigsbaum F (1989) *Health, Happiness and Security – the creation of the National Health Service*. Routledge.

Klein R (1995) *The New Politics of the NHS* (3rd Edition).

Knight S (1985) *The Brotherhood: the secret world of the Freemasons*. Panther.

National Audit Office (2005) *A Safer Place for Patients*. http://www.nao.org.uk/publications/nao_reports/05-06/0506456.pdf (accessed 3 November 2005).

NHS Appointments Commission (2005) http://www.appointments.org.uk/docs/annualreport0405.pdf (accessed 29 October 2005).

NHS Appointments Commission and Department of Health, (2004) *The Code of Conduct and Code of Accountability in the NHS*. NHS Appointments Commission. http://www.appointments.org.uk/docs/code_of_conduct.pdf (accessed 23 September 2006).

NHS Litigation Authority (July 2005) *Factsheet 3: information on claims*. http://www.nhsla.com/home.htm (accessed 29 October 2005).

Observer, 26 January 2003.

Pratten B (1990) *Power, Politics and Pregnancy.*

Pyper R (ed.) (1996) *Aspects of Accountability in the British System of Government*. Tudor.

Savage W (1986) *A Savage Enquiry – Who Controls Childbirth?* London: Virago.

Urban R and Moore D (2006) *United Health's Directors Hold $230 Million in Stock (Update3),* Bloomberg News, 10 August. http://www.bloomberg.com/apps/news?pid=20601170&sid=arcGCC5pTiLk&refer=home (accessed 29 August 2006).

Walker D (2006) 'A performance spotlight falls on Whitehall', *Guardian*, 17 May.

Webster C (1991) *Aneurin Bevan on the National Health Service*. Oxford: Wellcome Unit for the History of Medicine, University of Oxford.

Webster C (1996) *The Health Services since the War*, Vol.II. London: The Stationery Office.

Witz A (1992) *Professions and Patriarchy*. Routledge.

World Bank (2005) http://rru.worldbank.org/Documents/PapersLinks/1253.pdf (accessed 26 October 2005).

The Accountability of Doctors

James Drife

Doctors' accountability has been talked about for many years but as this book goes to press there is a feeling in the air that talk is turning into action. Sir Liam Donaldson, the UK's Chief Medical Officer (CMO), has published his report, *Good Doctors, Safer Patients*, proposing radical reforms to medical regulation in the UK.[1] His ideas have the political wind behind them, following Dame Janet Smith's trenchant observations published in 2004 at the end of the Shipman enquiry.[2] In addition, the medical royal colleges are eager to help turn assessment of doctors into reality, and the Royal College of Obstetricians and Gynaecologists (RCOG) is about to discuss the final draft of a report, *Bridging the gap between appraisal and assessment*, with detailed proposals on how to assess the quality of a specialist's practice.[3]

Nevertheless, perhaps we should not hold our breath. Calls for action have been appearing for the last twenty years. For example:

> It is now clearly unacceptable to society that health professionals qualifying in their 20s should remain registered for 40 or 50 years with no attempt to ensure that they remained competent.[4]

These words from a 2005 article in the *British Medical Journal (BMJ)* echo those of a 1987 *BMJ* editorial entitled 'Consultant accountability':

> After being appointed consultant... a doctor has a secure job and does not appear to be accountable for the quantity or the quality of his work... Consultants should co-operate in developing a more sensitive system of accountability than we have at present.[5]

Sceptics will say the only thing that has changed since 1987 is that we no longer routinely use the word 'his' when referring to doctors, and they will blame this inertia on an unwillingness among the medical profession to be held to account by anyone.

This is not the reason, however, for the slow pace of change. Doctors are deeply interested in the quality of the care they provide, and most doctors will sympathise with the words of Professor David Hatch, quoted in *Good Doctors, Safer Patients*:

> I was appointed as a consultant anaesthetist in 1969. In that 30 years nobody has given me an opportunity to demonstrate that I am fit to practise and up to date. I would welcome the opportunity to try and show that to the parents of the children I anaesthetise and the children themselves in some cases.[6]

---

1 Donaldson (2006)
2 Smith (2004)
3 Royal College of Obstetricians and Gynaecologists (2006a)
4 Walshe and Benson (2005)
5 Drife (1987)
6 Donaldson (2006)

Moreover, a substantial number of doctors, including some still in active practice, are keen to inspect the work of their medical colleagues.

There are two reasons why progress is slow. One is that there is no mechanism for driving change in the medical profession. In the words of the 1987 *BMJ* editorial[7] (written, incidentally, by the present author):

> Most organisations – for example, businesses, the armed services, and even the Church of England – have hierarchical structures with lines of responsibility leading to the person at the top… but the accountability of doctors is not clear.

The General Medical Council (GMC) is perceived as being in charge of the profession but its powers are limited. It has only informal links with the NHS (the major employer of doctors in the UK) and the medical royal colleges, which set the standards of practice for each specialty.

The second reason is that quality of medical practice is not easy to measure. Quantity can be assessed and consultants can now be called to account by their NHS line managers, usually for doing too much work rather than too little. Regarding quality, however, discussion is still continuing over how to define and measure it. Over the last twenty years the profession has in fact travelled a long way on what the *BMJ* has called 'the long march to accountability'.[8] This chapter will attempt to summarise where we are now, and discuss how much further we need to go.

Mechanisms of accountability

George Bernard Shaw's comment in *The Doctor's Dilemma* in 1911, 'All professions are conspiracies against the laity', sums up the view that doctors should be accountable to their patients and to society. The laity, however, lacks expertise so doctors must also be accountable to their professional colleagues. Economic reality requires doctors to be accountable to their employers, though tensions arise when economics conflict with the needs of patients. Ultimately every individual is accountable to his or her own conscience. Thus there are several mechanisms of accountability which can pull a doctor in different directions.

Criminal law

Like any other citizen, a doctor is subject to the criminal law. Doctors who commit crimes such as fraud or assault are treated like anyone else by the law but all convictions are reported to GMC, which then undertakes its own investigation. Drunk driving, for example, routinely triggers a referral to the Health Committee because a doctor's alcoholism may put patients at risk. An offence which does not directly endanger patients may still be seen as bringing the profession into disrepute.

A professional error which causes death can lead to criminal proceedings. The number of doctors charged with manslaughter increased markedly in the 1990s.[9] A mistake caused by excessive tiredness may be treated leniently by the court but a trust which tolerates inadequate supervision of trainees may face a charge of corporate manslaughter.[10] The mechanism for bringing such serious charges against a doctor or a

---

7 Drife (1987)

8 Anonymous (2000)

9 Ferner and McDowell (2006)

10 Samanta and Samanta (2006)

trust is far from transparent. Presumably the police and the Crown Prosecution Service take professional advice, but from whom? In the UK, around 300,000 people die every year in hospital. If an error is suspected someone has to decide whether the police should be informed. The decision may depend on the opinion of a coroner, whose accountability is unclear.

Civil law

All doctors have become used to the threat of litigation but the chances of being sued vary between specialties. Obstetrics is high on the list because people nowadays expect pregnancy to have a good outcome and if something goes wrong they assume someone must have blundered. Being sued, whether the case is won or lost, is very stressful and litigation is cited as one reason why obstetrics has become an unpopular career choice among graduates from UK medical schools.[11] The NHS bears the cost of litigation in the UK but in many countries obstetricians are personally liable and pay large insurance premiums. In parts of the USA it is now impossible to find an obstetrician because doctors have been driven out of the specialty.[12] Audit of pregnancy outcome in the USA is patchy so the effect of this is still unclear but the people who are likely to suffer most are ethnic minorities and the poor, already at higher risk.[13]

Fear of litigation can raise standards – 'defensive medicine' is not necessarily bad medicine – but civil litigation is a hit-and-miss affair. It does not systematically check on practice but depends on patients' perceptions. A good doctor may be sued because of a poor outcome and a bad doctor's mistakes may go unnoticed by patients or relatives.

Employers

The NHS employs over a million people, 100,000 of them doctors. The logistics of dealing with such a large workforce are challenging, the financial pressures imposed by government are well-nigh intolerable, and the NHS is rarely held up as an example of a well-managed organisation. General management was introduced only in 1983[14] but since then there has been progress in improving the accountability of NHS doctors to their employer.

> Management systems in the hospital sector are now mature, with a degree of consistency between NHS organisations. Doctors in secondary care are employees. Directorates, divisions and committees feed up to the NHS Trust board and lines of accountability are clear. The line management of individual consultants is, at least on paper, established through a network of clinical and medical directors.[15]

Line managers are better at setting standards than auditing how doctors measure up to them (see below) but an important step was taken in 2001 when annual appraisal of hospital doctors was introduced. This involves 'meeting with one or more peers to reflect upon prior practice, informed in so far as is possible by evidence and data, in order to identify strengths, weaknesses and areas for improvement'.[16] It has been accepted by

---

11 Royal College of Obstetricians and Gynaecologists (2006b)
12 Elias (2002)
13 Berg et al (2003)
14 Donaldson (2006)
15 Ibid.
16 Ibid.

doctors, who generally gather their own 'evidence and data', since NHS systems for doing so are unreliable.

Professional bodies

Doctors are accountable to the GMC for the standard of their practice. Since its foundation in 1858 the GMC has survived repeated episodes of controversy, succinctly summarised in *Good Doctors, Safer Patients*. During the 1990s the GMC embarked on a programme of reform which began with a new framework for medical education, *Tomorrow's Doctors* (1993), and a first attempt to define the standards expected of a doctor, in *Good Medical Practice* (1995). Until that time the GMC, like the criminal justice system, had focused on what an individual should *not* do. These innovations were well received and remain widely respected. However, just as they appeared, the profession was being overtaken by a series of high-profile scandals, and the reforms appeared to be an inadequate response. Although the GMC was already changing its constitution, increasing its lay representation and streamlining its fitness-to-practise procedures, these changes were not enough to fend off criticism, particularly by the Shipman enquiry.

In the 1990s, the GMC also proposed 'revalidation' of registration, though at the time it was difficult to see how the GMC, without considerable extra resources, could organise regular checks on each doctor's competence. When the NHS introduced annual appraisal it seemed logical to use this as the basis for revalidation. The GMC persuaded the profession to accept this concept, and expected that the process would be refined as systems for collecting 'data and evidence' improved. Dame Janet Smith, however, put an end to this strategy and discussion of the radical changes suggested by the CMO is now starting.

Doctors are not directly accountable to the medical royal colleges, which have no powers to check the practice of individual members or fellows. Colleges have introduced systems of continuing professional development (CPD) but these are voluntary.

Overall accountability

The fact that there are several mechanisms of accountability can lead to problems. Patients find it difficult to know how to complain and doctors worry about multiple jeopardy, with the same complaint being directed to lawyers, the employer, the GMC and the local media. Whatever the mechanism, however, the questions are the same: What are the standards? How is performance audited? What action should be taken if it is substandard? These questions are addressed in the next three sections.

Setting standards

Twenty years ago, standards for medical practice were implicit, not explicit. Medical schools and royal colleges concentrated on producing well-trained entrants to the profession and the specialties, but once in practice doctors were expected to set and maintain their own standards. Most took pride in doing so, but doctors' standards would reflect what they had been taught many years previously. This could lead to older doctors losing touch, not so much with medical progress as with society's expectations.

In the 1990s, once again, another revolution took place with the development of a plethora of guidelines from various bodies. They were introduced tentatively, in the expectation that doctors would object to being told what to do. On the contrary, the profession accepted them with barely a murmur.

GMC

The GMC's move from proscription ('Thou shalt not...') to prescription ('Thou shalt...') began in 1995 with the publication of *Duties of a Doctor*, a list of 14 principles that underpin medical practice. General guidance, *Good Medical Practice*, was published in the same year and has been revised twice, most recently in 2001,[17] with a third revision currently in progress. The second edition, in 1998, warned that 'if serious problems arise which call your registration into question, these are the standards against which you will be judged.' This was felt to be heavy handed and the third edition states that 'serious or persistent failures to meet the standards in this booklet may put your registration at risk' – wording which the CMO now suggests is not tough enough.

All editions of *Good Medical Practice* gave guidance under seven headings such as 'Good clinical care' and 'Probity' but each added more detail. In addition, the GMC has published a further 22 booklets, ranging alphabetically from 'Accountability in Multi-agency and Multi-disciplinary Mental Health Teams' to 'Withholding and withdrawing life-prolonging treatments'. Doctors have welcomed guidance through such ethical and legal minefields but the GMC can offer only generic advice. Detailed clinical guidance on specific conditions comes from elsewhere.

Evidence-based medicine

Fundamental to the development of clinical guidelines was the concept of 'evidence based medicine', a term coined at McMaster Medical School in Canada in the 1980s. It has been defined as 'the process of systematically finding, appraising, and using contemporaneous research findings as the basis for clinical decisions'.[18] Many doctors say this is what they have always tried to do but the key word is 'systematically'. A new specialism developed in which a global network of largely self-appointed experts appraised evidence on behalf of their colleagues. This process began before the advent of computerised search engines and although literature searches are now much easier than they used to be, doctors remain generally content to get their clinical guidance from groups such as the Cochrane Collaboration, whose accountability is again unclear.

NHS standards

In 1999 legislation was introduced requiring the NHS to implement 'clinical governance' programmes, whose underlying principles include 'well-evidenced standards' and 'individual and organisational accountability'. A review in 2003 by the National Audit Office concluded that among the benefits of clinical governance was 'a greater and more explicit accountability for clinical performance'.[19]

Standards for the NHS are set by bodies such as the National Institute for Health and Clinical Excellence (NICE) in England and NHS Quality Improvement Scotland, both originally set up in 1999. NICE guidance covers technology appraisals and interventional procedures as well as clinical guidelines formulated by independent groups which include doctors. The sixteen-strong development group which produced the 2004 NICE guideline on caesarean section included three obstetricians and was chaired by a general practitioner. Also in 2004, guidance on organising maternity services came from the Department of Health's 'National Service Framework for Children, Young People and

---

17 General Medical Council (2001)

18 Rosenberg and Donald (1995)

19 Donaldson (2006)

Maternity Services'. The days when a consultant could decide how to run his or her NHS obstetric practice are long gone.

Specialty bodies

Medical royal colleges and specialist societies began issuing detailed clinical guidelines around ten years ago and those from the RCOG have earned respect from members and fellows. In the late 1990s the RCOG adopted the strapline 'Setting standards to improve women's health'. Since 2002 the College has hosted the National Collaborating Centre for Women's and Children's Health (NCC-WCH), funded by NICE to produce guidelines for the NHS in England and Wales, for example on antenatal and intrapartum care.

The effect of guidelines

Clinicians implement some guidelines and ignore others. The most effective guidelines are local ones, drawn up by interested clinicians and usually informed by national ones. Nevertheless, the mushroom growth of guidance in the last decade has been welcomed by doctors and has changed practice profoundly. Today's well-informed doctor is one who knows the guidelines. Some doctors read and reflect on the original papers, but not many. Although every guideline comes with the caveat that it must not override clinical judgement, it is in reality unlikely to be challenged as doctors like to play safe.

Auditing performance

Once standards are set, the next steps in clinical governance are to measure performance and compare it with the standard. Clinical audit has been encouraged by the NHS for many years and obstetricians have a long record of participating. The Confidential Enquiry into Maternal Deaths, set up fifty years ago, is the longest-running clinical audit in the world.[20] Mortality rates, however, are a sensitive indicator of individual performance only in high-risk specialties, particularly cardiac surgery.[21] In most hospital practice, outcome indicators assess the performance of the multidisciplinary team, not the individual doctor.

The GMC has developed methods of performance assessment but these are labour intensive and costly and are designed to assess doctors whose performance has caused concern. Some royal colleges have been proactive in designing assessment tools and the RCOG has been in the vanguard. Its first report on assessing performance was in 1999 but the college was unwilling to 'go it alone' at that time and in 2006 another working party produced a new report, *Bridging the Gap between Appraisal and Assessment*.[22]

The RCOG report

The 2006 report began by emphasising that the royal colleges are well placed to advise on assessing a specialist workforce. It enumerated five essential criteria for competence:

- That the doctor is adequately qualified for the job he or she is doing
- That he or she is up to date with advances in their area of expertise
- That he or she is a competent diagnostician
- That he or she has appropriate technical ability
- That he or she has good communication and interpersonal skills.

---

20 Lewis (ed.) (2004)

21 Bridgewater et al (2003); Semmens et al (2005); Semmens et al (2006)

22 Royal College of Obstetricians and Gynaecologists (2006a)

It stated that assessment of competence should be a continuous process that builds on the specialty training currently undertaken by UK trainees, and should rely on three pillars:

- Demonstration of CPD
- Directed 360° appraisal
- Assessment of practice by appropriate Objective Structured Assessment of Technical Skills (OSATS) and/or by assessment against national standards.

It recommended that the RCOG CPD programme be widened to include a fifth mandatory category called 'Evidence of Competence'. Directed 360° appraisal should be undertaken on a regular basis and, to keep it simple to administer, should consist of a single questionnaire for use by professional colleagues and patients, though not all questions would apply to both.

Assessment of practice by OSATS and/or by assessment against national standards should be undertaken at less frequent intervals, ranging from annually to five-yearly depending on the skill being assessed. They should be broadly based on those assessments currently undertaken by trainees but with appropriate modification. As with 360° appraisal, some objective assessments may be generic, required by the RCOG, and some more specific, as advised by the specialist societies. Further work on the design of the appropriate OSATS should continue.

The working party recognised that there is a lack of evidence that measures such as these will ensure that all doctors are competent at all times and recognised that the levels of evidence required to signify competence are still unclear. Nevertheless it urged that it is necessary to make a start.

Taking action

If performance is found to be deficient, what action should be taken? Recent NHS innovations include the National Clinical Assessment Authority – now the National Clinical Assessment Service (NCAS) – to help investigate and resolve cases of poor practitioner performance. One lesson learned in the first five years of this service is that doctors can be retrained and rehabilitated if poor practice is detected early, but this is a complex and intensive process which needs expert oversight and control.[23]

The NHS disciplinary framework, which remained largely unchanged for over fifty years, was widely recognised as bureaucratic and unwieldy.[24] Doctors could remain suspended for years and poor performance was often tolerated in preference to disciplinary procedures. In 2003 a new framework was published which provides for an immediate, temporary period of exclusion to allow concern about a doctor's practice to be rapidly investigated and addressed. In 2005 further directions placed the emphasis on local procedures. Doctors are now dealt with under the same disciplinary procedures as any other members of the NHS staff. Re-entry and retraining are encouraged where appropriate and trusts are required to seek the advice of the NCAS.

Summary

The picture painted in this chapter is of the introduction of a 'command and control' structure into UK medicine, a process that is irreversible and almost complete. Time

---

23 Donaldson (2006)
24 Ibid.

may or may not tell whether this has been a good thing. Many medical advances in the past were made by innovative and 'difficult' people who stood against the orthodoxy of the day. Now orthodoxy is being given teeth. State control of doctors is being seen as a good thing as the last century's memories of Nazi Germany and communist Russia fade away. Today's political establishment wants an accountable and docile medical profession and for better or worse this is being delivered.

References

Anonymous (2000) 'Doctors: the long march to accountability', *BMJ*, 321: 0a.

Berg CJ, Chang J, Callaghan WM and Whitehead SJ (2003) 'Pregnancy-related mortality in the United States 1991–1997', *Obstet Gynecol*, 101: 289–96.

Bridgewater B, Grayson AD, Jackson M et al (2003) 'Surgeon specific mortality in adult cardiac surgery: comparison between crude and risk stratified data', *BMJ*, 327: 13–17.

Donaldson L (2006) *Good doctors, safer patients: Proposals to strengthen the system to assure and improve the performance of doctors and to protect the safety of patients*. London: Department of Health.

Drife JO (1987) 'Consultant accountability', *BMJ*, 294: 789–90.

Elias M (2002) 'Obstetricians dwindle amid high malpractice costs', *USA Today*, 5 June 2002.

Ferner RE and McDowell SE (2006) 'Doctors charged with manslaughter in the course of medical practice, 1795–2005: a literature review', *J R Soc Med*, 99: 309–14.

General Medical Council (2001) *Good Medical Practice* (3rd edition). London: GMC.

Lewis G (ed.) (2004) *Why Mothers Die 2000–2002. Report on confidential enquiries into maternal deaths in the United Kingdom*. London: RCOG Press.

Rosenberg W and Donald A (1995) 'Evidence based medicine: an approach to clinical problem solving', *BMJ*, 310: 1122–6.

Royal College of Obstetricians and Gynaecologists (2006a) *Bridging the gap between appraisal and assessment: report of a working party*. London: RCOG.

Royal College of Obstetricians and Gynaecologists (2006b) *A career in obstetrics and gynaecology: recruitment and retention in the specialty*. London: RCOG Press.

Samanta A and Samanta J (2006) 'Charges of corporate manslaughter in the NHS', *BMJ*, 332: 1410–5.

Semmens JB, Aitken RJ, Sanfilippo FM, Mukhtat SA, Haynes NS and Mountain JA (2005) 'The Western Australian Audit of Surgical Mortality: advancing surgical accountability', *Med J Aust*, 183: 504–8.

Semmens JB, Mountain JA, Sanfilippo FM, Barraclough JY, McKenzie A, Haynes NS and Aitken RJ (2006) 'Providers and consumers support the Western Australian audit of surgical mortality', *ANZ J Surg*, 76: 442–7.

Smith J. (2004) *Shipman inquiry fifth report: safeguarding patients: lessons from the past – proposals for the future.* London: The Stationery Office.

Walshe K and Benson L (2005) 'Time for Radical reform', *BMJ*, 330: 1,504–6.

1 2 **3** 4 5 6

Incompetence

Incompetence

Wendy Savage

The *Oxford English Dictionary* defines incompetence in various ways. The one most relevant to medicine is *want of the requisite ability*.[1] It was presumably this meaning which Sir Donald Irvine, a former President of the General Medical Council, had in mind when, in December 2004,[2] he announced that, in his opinion, some three million patients were at risk from eleven thousand incompetent doctors. I believe that an examination of the work of the two bodies charged with upholding standards – the GMC and the National Clinical Assessment Service – shows that Sir Donald's estimate of the extent of incompetence in the medical profession was seriously misleading. However, I also believe that recent changes in professional training have made it likely that more doctors will be found to be incompetent in future. In this introduction, I look first at the new training arrangements, then at the findings of the GMC and the NCAS in cases where incompetence has been alleged.

Although the five-year undergraduate medical course includes the core practical skills of taking a history and examining a patient, the rest of it is mainly theoretical. In 1993, the GMC published a document *Tomorrow's Doctors*[3] which laid more emphasis on developing communication skills and learning about the underlying determinants of health: diet, environment and lifestyle. Sociology was recommended as a core subject along with the traditional anatomy, physiology and pathology. The undergraduate years lay the foundation for the pre-registration year, when doctors (called house officers) acquire basic skills under supervision. Until recently, a second year as a senior house officer was usually undertaken before embarking on either specialist training or the three-year vocational training for general practice. In 2006 a two-year foundation system is being introduced as part of the government-inspired programme 'Modernising Medical Careers' in collaboration with the Postgraduate Medical and Education Training Board (PMETB).[4]

In 1996 a shortened form of specialist training was introduced under the guidance of the Chief Medical Officer, Kenneth Calman. The Calman scheme envisaged that, instead of the 12–13 years that doctors in the medical and surgical specialties spent moving from senior house officer to registrar to senior registrar, there would be five- or six-years' training in the registrar grade. A certificate of completed specialist training (CCST) would be awarded if progress had been satisfactory. The previous apprenticeship arrangement, where a trainee might spend one to two years with a consultant and then work for two to four years in the responsible post of senior registrar in a teaching hospital, was replaced by a more formal system. A dedicated half-day per week of teaching, logbooks and yearly

1 *Shorter Oxford English Dictionary* (1959)

2 Boseley (2004)

3 General Medical Council (1993)

4 The Foundation programme committee of the Academy of Medical Royal Colleges in co-operation with Modern Medical Careers in the Departments of Health (2005)

regional in-service training assessment (RITA) by the Regional Postgraduate Dean's department were all parts of this new scheme. However, the reduction in the hours that trainee doctors worked, whilst welcome in many ways, meant that there was less time for surgery. This, coupled with the European Working Time Directive, has resulted in doctors acquiring considerably less practical experience than they used to. Another problem, which started in the 1990s, was the effect of the quasi-market. Managers reduced beds and cut operating lists if doctors had been too efficient. In my own practice, two in-patient lists a week were reduced to one weekly in-patient and one shorter day-case list per fortnight. When a shift system was imposed on us, and a trainee was on call the night before, they had the day off and missed the list. This meant that in a six-month period a registrar might do 12 hysterectomies whereas in 1985 s/he would have done between 30 and 40.

In the period 1969–71 I was on call for obstetrics on alternate days, and every day when my opposite number was on holiday. This gave me the opportunity to follow women through labour and gain great experience. When my colleagues and I surveyed them in 2005, many consultants thought that the one-in-five rota system and the shorter period of training had led to a decline in operative vaginal skills.[5] These factors were the second most common reason given for the continuing rise in the caesarean section rate.

If there are some justifiable anxieties about the future under the new training regime, an examination of the findings in recent cases of alleged incompetence is more reassuring.

The GMC performance procedures

The experience with the performance procedures of the GMC (now subsumed into generic 'impairment of fitness to practise' procedures) did not confirm the dire predictions of Sir Donald Irvine, who became president at the time they came into operation. He said in council that three to four hundred doctors would be referred at the outset. However, only a handful of doctors were referred in the years 1997–8, and only 105 out of 361 doctors referred by screeners appeared before the Committee on Professional Performance (CPP) between 1998 and October 2004 (when the procedure changed).[6] The screening test is low: 'do the allegations raise a question of seriously deficient performance (SDP)'? The screener does not test the evidence.

The procedures were complex. The Assessment Referral Committee (ARC) saw 82 doctors who questioned the need for an assessment.Twelve accepted voluntary erasure. A CPP assessment panel of council members, including lay people, saw 41 doctors who had not co-operated. Six of these (15 per cent) were thought not to need an assessment. Of the 227 who had an assessment done, almost a third, 72, were not thought to reach the threshold of SDP. The case co-ordinator judged that 39 did not require referral to the Committee on Professional Performance (CPP) and they agreed to a statement of requirements to improve their practice.

The CPP saw 105 doctors in this seven-year period, an average of 15 a year. Sixteen (15 per cent) were not thought to have SDP, 32 were suspended and 52 had conditions applied to their registration. Voluntary erasure was taken by 40 doctors either before or after the performance assessment. The remaining cases were adjourned or had not been

5 Churchill et al (2006) p.155
6 GMC (2001–5)

completed at the end of the year. Assuming that those who took voluntary erasure were incompetent and those who had conditions imposed on their registration were not, that at most would suggest that 72 were actually incompetent and posed a danger to patients: about ten a year, assuming the judgements were correct. Given this remarkably low figure, it is scarcely surprising that Sir Donald's figure of 11,000 incompetent doctors was attacked by several correspondents in the *Guardian*.[7]

The National Clinical Assessment Service (NCAS)

About 10 per cent of cases referred to this service undergo a full assessment using a model developed in Canada[8] and similar to that used by the GMC. Both models involve visits to the workplace, interviews with both medical and non-medical colleagues, objective tests of knowledge and skills, a case-note review and case-based orals using tested instruments. An analysis of the first 50 assessments done by the NCAS (which may not be typical as many of these were long-standing problems) showed clinical performance problems were present in 94 per cent of the group, poor communication with colleagues in 76 per cent, insufficient training or engagement with continuing professional development in 48 per cent and poor mental or physical health in 28 per cent. One can see that there was a multi-factorial problem in this group, which comprised 25 GPs and 25 hospital doctors.[9] The Quebec model looks at the workplace factors which may have affected a doctor's performance. In cases referred to the GMC under the tri-partite system, health concerns and conduct issues were five times more common than performance issues.

An analysis of 50 early cases seen by the CPP showed that, judged against the criteria in *Good Medical Practice*,[10] the issues most commonly identified as problems were: record keeping, working with colleagues, investigations and treatment, provision of a good standard of care, treatment in an emergency and relationships with patients. Of the 25 GPs, 11 were not thought to have seriously deficient performance.[11] Simulated surgeries and objective structured clinical examinations are validated tools for assessing general practitioners, but it is more difficult to assess the technical competence of surgeons. Amongst hospital doctors, substandard treatment was found in 13 of the 25 cases, and practising beyond skills or knowledge in 10. Seven cases were not found to be seriously deficient.[12] The performance criteria used in these cases cover a wider range of considerations than competence, narrowly defined, so once again the figures show that incompetence in the medical profession is rare. This confirms a view which I had personally come to on the basis of 40 years of medical practice in five countries and on four continents.

Incompetence in obstetrics and gynaecology

Two high-profile gynaecological cases – those of Richard Neale and the late Rodney Ledward – came before the GMC's Professional Conduct Committee, not before its Committee on Professional Performance. This reflected the fact that these were not

---

7 *Guardian* (2004)
8 Dauphinee (1999)
9 Berrow (2005)
10 General Medical Council (1995)
11 Vincent and Woloshynowych (2002a)
12 Vincent and Woloshynowych (2002b)

purely matters of competence. Both had their names erased from the register. In Richard Neale's case (on which I sat) it appeared that most of the time his surgery was technically competent but his judgement was questionable and he could not cope if anything went wrong.[13]

The recent enquiry into the high number of maternal deaths at Northwick Park Hospital in 2002–4 decided that poor risk management, inadequate training and supervision of clinical staff, shortages of staff coupled with poor management of temporary employees, and a poor environment with services isolated geographically or clinically, led to the tragic deaths. Only one of those deaths, it was judged, could not have been prevented.[14]

Medical training in the future

The CMO's report[15] has suggested that the GMC should be stripped of its responsibility for overseeing undergraduate education; and changes are being pushed through in the Modernising Medical Careers programme, despite some professional concerns. Whether these will lead to fewer incompetent doctors is unknown. The government response to the consultation has left the supervision of undergraduate education as the responsibility of the GMC[16] but the fiasco over the new Medical Training Application Scheme has serious implications for postgraduate training.[17] The changes in postgraduate education will take several years to come into effect and be evaluated.

In this section Emeritus Professor Ron Taylor, who was Professor of Obstetrics and Gynaecology at St Thomas' Hospital and has done a great deal of medico-legal work since his retirement, will discuss the definition of incompetence.

---

13 Dyer (1998); Dyer (2000)

14 Health Care Commission (2006)

15 Chief Medical Officer (2006) p.96

16 HM Government (2007)

17 Coombes R (2007)

References

Berrow D et al (2005) Anal*ysis of the 50 first NCAS assessment cases*. London: National Clinical Assessment Service. http://www.ncas.npsa.nhs.uk/site/media/documents

Boseley S (2004) *Guardian*, 18 Dec 2004.

Chief Medical Officer (2006) *Good doctors, safer patients*. London: DoH publications.

Churchill H, Savage W and Francome C (2006) *Caesarean Birth in Britain*. London: Middlesex University Press.

Coombes R (2007) 'How specialist training reform sparked crisis of confidence', *BMJ*, 334:508–9.

Dauphinee D (1999) 'Revalidation of doctors in Canada', *BMJ*, 319:1,188–90.

Dyer C (1998) 'Gynaecologist showed lack of care and judgement', *BMJ*, 317:965.

Dyer C (2000) 'Gynaecologist struck off the medical register', *BMJ*, 321:258.

The Foundation programme committee of the Academy of Medical Royal Colleges in co-operation with Modern Medical Careers in the Departments of Health (2005) *Modernising Medical Careers: the new curriculum for the Foundation years in postgraduate training and education*. London: DoH publications.
http://www.dh.gov.uk/AboutUs/MinistersAndDepartmentLeaders/ChiefMedicalOfficer/CMO/GeneralArticle/

General Medical Council (1993) *Tomorrow's Doctors*. London: GMC.

General Medical Council (1995) *Good Medical Practice*. London: GMC.

General Medical Council (2001–5) Council papers 2001–5: Reports of the Fitness to Practise Commitee.

Guardian (2004) letters section of 'Society', *Guardian*, 20 December 2004.

Health Care Commission (2006) 'Healthcare Watchdog renews calls for robust safety checks in maternity units as investigation describes the deaths of 10 women'. Press release, 23 August 2006. http://www.healthcarecommission.org.uk/press reports

HM Government (2007) *Learning from Tragedy, keeping patients safe. Overview of the Government's action programme in response to the recommendations of the Shipman Inquiry.* CM 2014. London: The Stationery Office.

Shorter Oxford English Dictionary (1959, reprint with corrections on 1933). Oxford: Clarendon Press.

Vincent C and Woloshynowych M (2002a) 'The Assessment of Performance: An analysis of general practitioner cases referred to the General Medical Council following the introduction of the Performance Procedures'. Annex A to item 4c of Council papers, 5–6 November.

Vincent C and Woloshynowych M (2002b) 'The Assessment of Performance of Hospital Doctors. An analysis of hospital doctors referred to the General Medical Council following the introduction of the Performance Procedures'. Annex B to item 4c of Council papers, 5–6 November.

Ensuring the Competence of Doctors

Ron Taylor

In his history of medicine, *The Greatest Benefit to Mankind*, Roy Strong commented:

> In myriad ways, medicine continues to advance, new treatments appear, surgery works marvels, and (partly as a result) people live longer. Yet few people today feel confident, either about their personal health or about doctors, health care delivery and the medical profession in general.[1]

In my experience, this is, unfortunately, correct. There are probably many things that contribute to this seeming paradox but I think that one is public concern about the competence of doctors. This is not simply the questioning of a better-educated laity. There is genuine concern, with some basis, that doctors sometimes fail to reach, or perhaps more frequently, slip below an acceptable standard of practice. In compiling this chapter my concern has been to try to determine what we need to do to assuage this concern.

Competence in relation to medical practice is difficult to define satisfactorily. This is in part because the work of doctors is complex and influenced by the character of the patient. I always taught that it was frequently more important to know which patient had the disease than which disease the patient had. This means that individuals have different ideas of what they want from a doctor and, as times change, what we ask of our doctor also changes. A patient's judgement of competence will be to some extent subjective and might be incorrect when judged by objective, professional criteria.

The editor suggests that the term competence should be defined as 'having the requisite ability' and this is the definition that I have had in mind in writing this section.

We can consider someone competent if they are properly qualified for specific tasks. In most technical spheres, qualifications are obtained by undertaking a formal course of instruction and showing by means of an examination that a core of knowledge has been acquired. In some instances, there is a requirement to put that knowledge to use under supervision.

In many occupations and professions, such acquired competence is fairly easy to define and in any event falling below an accepted standard of practice, while it might prove to be expensive, does not usually have grievous consequences.

This can be true in some areas of medicine but there are obviously situations in which incompetence can result in serious injury and even avoidable death. For this reason, competence as defined by the acquisition of a body of knowledge is not always adequate in medicine. It has to be judged additionally by the manner and the consistency with which the knowledge is applied.

A hundred years ago, the body of knowledge acquired during the training of doctors in the United Kingdom was generally expected to fit them for a lifetime in practice.

---

1 Porter (1997)

However, such has been the speed of increase in our knowledge of the body and of disease and in the development of therapeutic techniques, that this is no longer the case. In some branches of medical practice the knowledge that a doctor has on qualification will suffice for only a few years. There is therefore a need for continuous updating and assessment that did not exist previously. The more effective remedies that are available to us today often carry commensurate risks and these are greatest when the therapy is incorrectly applied.[2]

How is the core of knowledge required for the basic medical qualifications determined?

The medical course has evolved over many years with changes decided from time to time – often belatedly – in response to what are the perceived needs of the age. Those who headed academic departments in individual medical schools often made these changes quite arbitrarily in the past. In theory they were acting in concert but in practice it was often difficult to gain universal acceptance of particular changes and medical schools were frequently out of step. In more recent years, a great effort has been made to try to avoid this by regular meetings of senior academics and modern means of communication have facilitated the process.

Problems in accommodating the rapid advances in knowledge and therapeutic techniques are, and will inevitably remain, significant. The time that students have available to complete the course is limited. Now, when most students are expected to bear a considerable part of the cost of their training, they are reasonably reluctant to extend this non-remunerative period in their lives. There must be a serious risk that we will discourage potentially good doctors from taking up training if we make the course too long and therefore too expensive.

The number of topics with which medical students have at least to acquaint themselves has increased and is increasing still. Heads of department often resist any attempt to reduce the proportion of time devoted to teaching their subject, not least because this is likely to reduce the size of their budget and staffing levels, which in turn affect their status and their ability to carry out research, on the results of which some future funding may depend.

In spite of these difficulties, there have been substantial changes in the undergraduate curriculum during the last 50 years. There is, for example, a much-reduced emphasis on memorising human anatomy and greater concern for understanding the normal working of the mind and body and the disturbance of both by disease. Acquiring practical skills and mastering the details of therapeutics have largely been transferred to the postgraduate sphere without apparent detriment. There has been greater emphasis on encouraging students to learn skills that are necessary to relate to patients and, in many schools, they have contact with patients much earlier in the curriculum than they did in the past.

The establishment of new medical schools has facilitated change. They offered opportunities for innovation and some excellent changes have been introduced in this way. The spirit of change does not necessarily persist however, and some of our most recently established schools now appear to be as resistant to change as older institutions.

Interestingly, there is no clear evidence that what appeared to be radical changes in

2 Chantler (1999)

the way that the medical course is organised have made a significant difference to the quality or the attitudes of graduates. This is determined to a considerable extent by the qualities and the motivation that the student had initially. Choosing the right students is notoriously difficult, especially as we usually have to do this when individuals are relatively immature and inevitably have a limited experience of life.

In my experience, the person who has completed a prescribed medical course in the UK, has satisfied the examiners and been awarded a degree, is competent to operate at a junior level and under close supervision. This should be provided during the pre-registration year spent in hospital. Not all prove able to cope with the stress that independent practice can entail and great care must be taken to try to assess their fitness to proceed. At least they might well require detailed help in their choice of a speciality.

Postgraduate training – specialisation

The way in which the basic knowledge acquired during the undergraduate years is applied depends on postgraduate training. No branch of medical practice in the UK is now open without some such training.

The training of specialists in the UK has traditionally been very practical and also prolonged in comparison to other Western countries. This was in part because, somewhat cynically, we used 'specialists in training' to provide cheap residential cover in the hospitals of the National Health Service. Initially this was a haphazard arrangement with priority given to the establishment of posts to fulfil service requirements. Inevitably, the numbers 'in training' for consultant posts were out of proportion to the number of specialist posts available. This was both wasteful and frustrating to many who failed to obtain such posts. During the first 40 years after the establishment of the NHS many who were well qualified by training for consultant posts became general practitioners by second choice. This was possible because at that time there was no special vocational training system for general practice.

This system undoubtedly produced many consultants with sound practical experience but it is no longer possible to defend or impose such a system. Instead, an attempt has been made to match those in training to the specialist posts available and a system of training for general practice has been introduced. A very significant reduction in the hours worked by junior doctors has been accepted as a consequence of the UK's membership of the European Union and this is forcing changes in our approach to postgraduate training.

However, this reduction in time worked each week and time spent on emergency call is undoubtedly reducing the level of expertise of those appointed to consultant posts, in spite of a greater and much to be welcomed emphasis on formal postgraduate instruction. This means that a newly appointed consultant has a greater need than ever before to accept the requirement for ongoing professional development.

One consequence of this more formal teaching has been the establishment of recommended standards for the investigation of symptoms and the treatment of diagnosed disease. The Royal Colleges have taken the lead in formalising these. The wider publication of the results of research, better audit of results and a greater reliance on scientifically validated evidence has made greater standardisation possible and the greater cost of treatments has made its desirability clearer. This is more generally accepted when the cost of expensive therapies falls upon the public purse to which we all contribute.

The establishment of a body to examine new forms of treatment, the National Institute for Health and Clinical Excellence (NICE), was intended to formalise the method of establishing acceptable standards. However, its work has proved more difficult than many politicians and administrators expected. It has not been funded as generously as many think was necessary and as a consequence, its advice often appears to be unreasonably delayed. Furthermore, there is a belief, for which there is some sound evidence, that those who control the purse strings of front line services see these delays as a means of minimising the immediate cost of new forms of treatment.

The effectiveness of any treatment must be properly assessed but those who have tried to do this are aware of how difficult it can be. This is particularly so when we are attempting to assess improvement in a clinical condition, rather than a complete cure. Even when we have a reasonably objective assessment of the value of some intervention, making judgements about cost effectiveness, as politicians and administrators of health care have to do, does not sit easily with a doctor's reasonable belief that s/he should be able to do or prescribe what is best for an individual patient. It will probably prove impossible to eradicate this tension completely.

The establishment of generally accepted standards of practice should help to ensure that good care is more widely available. Those who recall the very uneven standards of care that were available prior to the establishment of the NHS will be particularly aware of the benefits that this will bring.

Recognition of what is an acceptable standard also makes it easier to judge the standard of practice of individual doctors.

It should go without saying that the outcome of an intervention in any individual case is not necessarily an indication of good or bad medical practice. I have had the dubious privilege of assessing, for medico-legal purposes, the standard of practice of medical staff in several thousand cases when the outcome of treatment has been sub-optimal. Although I have often been able to show to the satisfaction of a court that damage could and should have been avoided by proper care, this has not been so in a majority of cases.

An acceptance of standard forms of treatment also makes it easier to set 'targets' for standards of care. These are much favoured by those who think that they will provide a relatively easy means of judging whether the public is getting good value for money spent. However, this is not necessarily the case. One first has to seek the reasons why set targets are not met in individual circumstances. This can take time, and politicians who frequently appear to see no further than the next election are not always prepared to wait to ensure that we get the correct answers before changing systems. Poorly thought out reorganisation has become one curse of the modern NHS.

There is a danger that established standards could act to the detriment of individual patients in some circumstances. Not all diseases present in a standard way and neither individual patients nor diseases always behave in a predictable fashion. Responses to therapy are not always what we expect.

It must therefore be open to a doctor to advise a form of management which deviates from the recommended standard. Good practice will dictate that the reasons for such deviation are set out in the clinical records and explained to the patient in advance. Good practice in this regard is a possible safeguard against vexatious litigation if the results of treatment do not match expectations.

Ranking doctors in terms of skill and effectiveness

Quite reasonably, the starting point here is the result of the management that a doctor recommends; but judging this is not a simple matter like assessing how well a piece of furniture has been made.

Patients and diseases vary in ways that inanimate materials do not. The extent of the disease will vary at the time of diagnosis and its rate of progress can be both variable and difficult to predict. It is therefore difficult to be sure that we are comparing like with like when we compare the results of two doctors, two hospitals or even two different forms of treatment.

Results have to be judged in the knowledge that the ideal desired by those seeking help cannot always be achieved. However high the standard of knowledge brought to bear and however conscientiously it is applied, many of our patients' problems will not be alleviated. Some symptoms will inevitably become worse and some patients will die.

Satisfaction with treatment has to be judged against rising levels of expectation. Some expectations prove to be unreasonable when looked at closely and in many instances, the lay public has been misled by injudicious or premature claims of 'spectacular advances' in the diagnosis and treatment of disease which are made by doctors themselves. To some extent the fault for this lies with medical personnel, anxious to be in the limelight or perhaps to attract funding for further research. The media are always anxious for a good story and often fail to point out the need for caution in interpreting early results.

With advances in medicine, the cost of treatment has risen so that in many areas this can be afforded only through a pooling of resources, with those fortunate enough to enjoy good health providing for those who do not. This can in theory be achieved through some private insurance scheme or a state organised system such as the National Health Service, financed through taxation. Neither system provides a bottomless pool of resources and inevitably disputes will arise about the provision of treatment. Given that some forms of management have marginal benefit and in some cases the results are difficult to predict in advance, there will inevitably be conflict when some decisions are made. This is particularly likely when the provision of services is fragmented, giving rise to what is popularly known as the 'postcode lottery'.

Politicians control the level of funding and set it at the level which they conclude that their electorate will bear. They have singularly failed to stimulate the necessary debate about which of the many treatments that a doctor can provide can reasonably be financed from the taxes of others.

To this extent, politicians determine the level of conflict about the provision of services. However, doctors are commonly the face of the National Health Service as far as the public is concerned and this can determine perceptions of the doctor's competence.

Determining competence in those who have had specialist training

Deciding when a doctor has achieved an appropriate standard of knowledge and skill to justify the designation of 'specialist' is contentious. Qualifying examinations are reasonable ways to test knowledge and it is possible to specify what procedures candidates for this designation should have carried out under supervision. However, levels of performance can only be assessed over a period by senior members of the relevant speciality. By its nature, this system of assessment and certification is subjective.

It is open to error and sometimes abuse.

In my experience it is uncommon for a doctor to be appointed to a specialist role without having achieved a level of skill agreed to be satisfactory by his/her peers.

This does not necessarily mean that the candidate best qualified for a particular post is always appointed. The system for the appointment of specialists in particular is open to abuse because the constitution of appointment committees has a predominance of 'local' representatives. It is reasonable to believe that such people are more likely to appreciate the needs of their local community than outsiders but they can also be self-serving. Most of us who have been members of committees charged with appointing consultants can recall examples of mediocre candidates being appointed to positions because they were seemingly judged unlikely to threaten the established consultants. 'Mediocrity appointing mediocrity!' This is not a way to ensure the best standard of care for any group of patients.

It is possible to point to individual cases where the person appointed has been shown subsequently to be below an accepted standard. It is fortunate that these instances are uncommon because the problem is usually highlighted only when patients have suffered culpable damage. Rectifying such mistakes can be very difficult and almost certainly very costly.

All appointment committees have independent members appointed by the relevant colleges and universities. In practice their opinions can be, and are, ignored in some instances. The system for the appointment of consultants would be more equitable if it were necessary to consider minority reports of the external assessors before Health Authorities accepted recommendations.

It is fashionable to talk of patients as 'consumers' but in practice they do not have the freedom of most consumers because they do not always have the requisite knowledge to judge standards of care adequately. It is the responsibility of the professionals to represent them honestly.

Determining incompetence

Judging when a doctor's level of performance falls far short of that usually achieved by his/her peers – so that it is either incompetent or practice of an unacceptable standard – is subject to the same difficulties experienced when we try to rank doctors in order of performance.

A sub-optimal result might stem from a 'once off failure', an accident, which in other circumstances would probably have been avoided. I have likened this in court to the experienced carpenter who occasionally hits his/her thumb with a hammer when driving a nail. This might be due to some momentary lapse of concentration, or perhaps to a defective nail which breaks. This does not mean that the carpenter is generally a poor craftsman. Similarly, an occasional error by a doctor which results in a sub-optimal result might demand compensation for damage but the doctor does not thereby necessarily show himself/herself to be unfit for practice.

The carpenter who regularly misses the intended target might need further training or an eyesight test. Similarly, a doctor who consistently has poor results requires assessment. It is possible that his/her performance will be found to indicate a lack of adequate training, but more commonly we find that individual's standard of performance has slipped from one that was previously acceptable.

If such failure is to be noted before too much damage has been done, regular audit is essential. In some specialities, notably in obstetrics, auditing of the performance of departments has been practised to some degree for more than half a century. However, regular auditing of individuals in medicine and surgery is a more recent concept and it is not at present common.

There is resistance to such personal scrutiny within the profession. This is partly because of the difficulties in comparing like with like already discussed, partly because a failure to obtain an optimum result is frequently a result of systemic failure and therefore involves more than one individual. There are also justifiable fears that a superficial assessment of the results of an individual doctor will lead to the practice of excluding patients from treatment if assessment suggests that there is a greater than average risk of a poor outcome. Such selection is already practised, quite reasonably at times, in the interests of an individual patient. It is currently being suggested in the interests of economy, which is more difficult to justify.

When an individual doctor's results are consistently and significantly less satisfactory than those of his/her peers, the fact will usually become clear in time. During this time, the number of patients who suffer the effects of poor management will increase. It is therefore important that when a doctor's results are consistently below an accepted standard this fact should be observed and action taken to limit further damage.

As commented, the appointment of sub-standard specialists is uncommon. In practice, we more frequently see instances where individuals who were once competent have fallen below their own standards.

In some instances the problem is one of declining ability with age, a problem that is more likely to affect those in the practical branches of the profession such as surgery and obstetrics. Those in the more contemplative specialities might well see their effectiveness increase with age and experience. Unfortunately, little practical provision is made for such changes in performance in the bureaucratic health service of the UK. This is a problem, which the politicians – medical and lay – are reluctant to address, but for the sake of patients as well as for doctors themselves, it needs attention.

Doctors who develop personal problems, which affect their competence, are a problem which, in theory, should be easier to manage than those who are basically incompetent. Drug and alcohol addiction commonly have their origin in such problems and can aggravate the risk to patients. Not surprisingly it is uncommon for a doctor to admit readily to such problems and there is a natural discomfort felt by colleagues in reporting their concerns. My own experience is that such problems are dealt with quietly and effectively more frequently by the profession than the public realise. When doctors are 'moved sideways' taking them out of situations where patients may be put at risk, the matter is rarely publicised. Nevertheless, when such internal self-regulation fails for whatever reason, the damage to patients and to the reputation of the profession as a whole can be spectacular.

Doctors have considerable ability to hide their mistakes. One gynaecologist, who was at one time a very competent surgeon, had a series of disasters when he tied off the ureter in what should have been a straightforward hysterectomy. I was asked to report on the case by the woman's solicitor and she eventually received compensation through an out of court settlement. However, the publicity that this case received led to a further four, almost identical cases coming to light. The gynaecologist had managed to keep the issue quiet by sending each woman to a urologist in a different hospital for reparative surgery. These women were also subsequently compensated and the gynaecologist struck off the Medical Register by the General Medical Council.

When a doctor has malign intent, he/she can hide this too. The grim facts of Dr Harold Shipman's later career were concealed for a long time and, while some of the changes now suggested in the supervision of doctors will probably reduce the risks of such massive malpractice, I think it would be quite incorrect to think that doctors, and nurses too in some instances, can always be prevented from killing their patients. Other, less extreme forms of poor practice can also be deliberately concealed for some time. It would be foolish to underestimate a doctor's ability in this regard.

Clearly there is need for scrutiny, but this must be the responsibility of the profession: only doctors have the knowledge to uncover devious attempts to cover up errors. Regrettably we do not always manage to do so in time to prevent injury to the public.

I think it would be wrong to suggest that many doctors deliberately protect their colleagues whose practice does fall below an accepted standard. However, it would in my experience be correct to say that in the past we have not been sufficiently vigilant in our scrutiny of friends and colleagues. There has been a reluctance to appear to be acting as 'my brother's keeper'. Hopefully we now understand that this is a duty the profession has to shoulder.

The difficulties of detecting and exposing sub-standard practice are increased when the problem lies not so much in technical incompetence but in personality differences which render teams dysfunctional. This is a problem that is most likely to affect hospital departments where complex teamwork makes harmonious relations essential and problems of contract make solutions more difficult. Again, these problems are best managed by the profession, providing there is the will to deal with them.

In most instances this will need the imposition of a solution devised by someone outside the relevant unit. The professionals involved have an absolute duty to co-operate in such investigations and facilitate solutions that are in the interest of the patients. Only if the profession is seen clearly to be doing this honestly will the public have confidence that they need to be happy with the service we give.

References

Chantler C (1999) 'The role and education of doctors in the delivery of health care', *Lancet*, 353:1,178–81.

Porter R (1997) *The Greatest Benefit to Mankind: A medical history of humanity from antiquity to the present*. London: Harper Collins Publishers.

1 2 3 4 5 6

Disciplining Doctors

Disciplinary Procedure for Doctors and Dentists in the NHS

Wendy Savage

The procedure which was used by the Chair of the DHA to suspend me from practice was set out in HM(61)112,[1] based on the first guidance issued three years after the NHS began in 1948. If the result of the enquiry was dismissal there was the possibility of an appeal (paragraph 190) to the Secretary of State for Health.[2] There were three grounds for suspension: personal misconduct, professional misconduct and professional incompetence.

Personal misconduct is behaviour unrelated to clinical issues including violence towards or sexual harassment of colleagues or staff in the hospital, fraud or theft, or being drunk on duty. Professional misconduct is unacceptable behaviour arising during a doctor's clinical work such as rudeness towards patients, sexual impropriety with a patient, breaches of patient confidentiality or seriously disruptive or unco-operative behaviour towards colleagues. Professional incompetence arises when there is persistent failure to examine or investigate patients properly, to perform surgery adequately or to organise record keeping or one's practice efficiently. In the early years of the NHS it was widely assumed that doctors would be suspended from practice only in exceptional circumstances. These would include when patients were at risk because a doctor was mentally ill, addicted to alcohol or drugs, or arrested for a criminal offence.

It is not known how often this procedure was used, as the whole process was usually shrouded in secrecy. Often if a problem arose which might cause harm to patients it was referred to the 'three wise men'.[3] Concerned doctors or administrators asked a group of three people nominated by the senior doctors in a hospital to discuss the matter with the doctor involved.

At this time the contracts of the senior staff in most hospitals were held by the 14 Regional Health Authorities in the UK. For District General Hospitals the suspension procedure was invoked by the Regional Medical Officers (RMOs) after concerns had been brought to their attention by doctors, managers or the chairperson of a Health Authority.

Donaldson,[4] who published an analysis of all the referrals during five years in the Northern Region, states that 'Action was never taken precipitately because of the concerns of one person, who may have had antipathy towards the doctor concerned'. The RMOs met regularly and shared their experience. Donaldson says that in his region ill health matters were not dealt with using HM(61)112 but by supportive care and by retirement if appropriate. He found that over the five-year period beginning June 1986

1 Ministry of Health (1961a)

2 Ministry of Health (1961b)

3 Department of Health and Social Security (1982)

4 Donaldson (1994)

concerns were raised about 46 consultants and three associate specialists – a total of 49 (6 per cent) out of 850 senior medical staff. More than one issue must have arisen in the case of some doctors, as there was a total of 96 different problems. A third (32) were attitudinal problems, 21 lack of commitment to duties, 19 poor skills and inadequate knowledge, 11 dishonesty, seven sexual matters, five disorganised practice and poor communication with colleagues and one other unspecified.

Half the doctors either retired or resigned and the rest, after counselling, continued to work, some under supervision. Most specialties were represented, with psychiatry (11) having the greatest number; but since the figures for doctors employed by specialty are not given, one cannot tell if this is disproportionate.

Teaching hospitals were treated differently under the old system, so my honorary NHS contract was held by the District Health Authority (DHA) whose members had limited experience of dealing with such problems. It is interesting to speculate that my suspension might not have occurred if the London had been a District General Hospital (DGH). Paul Walker, the RMO of the North East Thames Region (which included the London), suspended a number of doctors over a relatively short period, including the paediatrician Dr Bridget O'Connell, who was unjustly suspended for a record 11 years.[5] By contrast, the late Rosemary Rue, RMO of the Oxford Region, suspended only one doctor throughout her career, and he was later jailed for child sexual offences.[6]

Following my suspension and the subsequent HM(61)112 enquiry (held in public for the first and only time), Norman Fowler, Secretary of State for Health, ordered a review in March 1987 of the procedure for disciplining doctors. This was carried out by a joint working party with six members from the four Departments of Health, four from the British Medical Association, four from the Royal Colleges and two from the NHS. Oddly, their numbers did not include an employment lawyer.

The working party asked RMOs for the number of doctors in their regions currently suspended and found that most were unable to produce a reliable figure. From 1981 there had been 37 appeals against dismissal. Assuming that all of those dismissed decided to appeal, and using the National Audit Office[7] finding that 24 per cent of doctors 'excluded' were dismissed, this suggests about 24 suspensions a year. However the threshold for suspension in the 1980s could have been higher than in the 1990s, so this estimated figure may be too high. I was asked to submit suggestions to the working party and did so, hoping for improvements in the system. My submission is printed as an appendix to this publication. The working party reported eighteen months later[8] and the new procedure was laid down in health circular HC(90)9.[9]

In 1990 the NHS and Community Care Act was passed as part of Kenneth Clarke's reforms of the NHS, *Working for Patients*.[10] This meant that the 270 newly created trust hospitals became the employers of consultants and associate specialists[11] and were responsible for applying the new disciplinary procedure.[12]

5 Public Accounts Committee (1995)
6 Personal communication
7 National Audit Office (2003) paragraph 1.18, p.18 and Figure11, p.19
8 Department of Health and Social Security (1988)
9 Department of Health (1990a)
10 Department of Health (1990b)
11 National Audit Office (2003) paragraph 2.3, p.23
12 Department of Health (1990b)

Donaldson points out that this change led to a loss of collective experience in dealing with these problems, and may well have given rise to an increase in the number of doctors being suspended. Such an increase was reported by a working group of the Society of Clinical Psychiatrists by Dr Harry Jacobs and Dr Peter Tomlin in the 1990s.[13]

Other significant changes were introduced at the same time. There was no longer an option of an enquiry when personal misconduct was alleged, and employers were given powers to deal with doctors as with any other employees of the trust, including the power to order instant dismissal for gross personal misconduct.

All but two of the working party's recommendations were accepted and were incorporated in the new arrangements:

- The right of appeal to the Secretary of State if dismissed for personal misconduct after an enquiry under the HM(61)112 procedure (paragraph 190 appeal)[14] was abolished (recommendation 8, p.10).[15] The possibility of having the case heard in public was also removed.
- A professional review was established to deal with doctors who did not fulfil their contractual commitments (recommendation 1, p.9). This had been suggested by the Joint Consultants Committee (JCC) of the BMA to the Chief Medical Officer (CMO) at the end of 1986. It was seen as an informal mechanism whereby peer pressure could be exerted to deal with the problem. It was proposed that all Health Authorities should set up such a mechanism outside the formal disciplinary procedures.
- An intermediate procedure (recommendation 3) was introduced where a matter was too serious to be resolved by informal discussion with the RMO but not serious enough to warrant dismissal if proved after a full enquiry. The RMO would contact the Joint Consultants Committee of the BMA. They would then nominate impartial assessors from another region to visit the District and assess the situation. When their report had been received and commented on by the doctor concerned, the RMO would decide whether a warning or further disciplinary action was required. It was hoped that this would be used at an earlier stage and prevent cases proceeding to an HM(61)112 enquiry. Consultation with the parties involved was suggested before implementation.
- An indicative timetable recommended that from prima facie case to delivery of the enquiry report to the Health Authority no more than 32 weeks should elapse. My case was unusual in that it had taken only 14 months from suspension to the DHA decision to reinstate me. However many doctors had been suspended for years before decisions were reached. This was both damaging to the doctors and expensive for the NHS. Paragraph 190 appeals were to be used only for full-time doctors and were also to have an indicative time scale (recommendations 6, 11 and 12). It was suggested that a lawyer should assist the professional panel (recommendation 9).
- The new procedures should be monitored and a review should be instituted after three years (recommendation 14).

The two recommendations rejected were the offer of the option of voluntary early retirement (recommendation 13), and the employment of solicitors rather than barristers

---

13 Tomlin (2003)

14 Ministry of Health (1961b)

15 Department of Health and Social Security (1988)

(recommendation 5). Perhaps this last was not accepted because the Secretary of State for Health in 1990 was himself a barrister.

During 1986 Brian Sedgemore posted an early day motion and in an adjournment debate[16] he raised my case and that of Pauline Bousquet, an obstetrician and gynaecologist in the neighbouring district of City and Hackney, who had not been suspended but had had her job whittled away after a whispering campaign about her competence. Mr Sedgemore was supported by Dr John Marek on the shadow health team. The government spokesman refused to comment as 'tribunals were in progress'.

In 1990 Miss Bousquet won her industrial tribunal case against unfair dismissal and the DHA stated that 'any allegations casting doubt on Miss Bousquet's competence were completely unfounded and that her professional competence has never been questioned by the Respondent'.[17] However the women of Hackney lost a dedicated non-interventionist obstetrician and Miss Bousquet's career was ruined.

Bridget O'Connell, a paediatrician in East London, had raised concerns about poor standards of nursing care in the children's wards and inadequate care of newborn babies soon after her appointment in 1977. She was suspended in 1982 for professional misconduct on the grounds of 'her inability to relate effectively to her clinical colleagues'. She received considerable publicity in 1988,[18] but her case dragged on for another six years.

In 1989 the Study Group of the Society of Clinical Psychiatrists published their first report[19] which gave examples of inhumane treatment of doctors and raised the question of whether the disciplinary procedures were an abuse of human rights. There was considerable publicity about the cases of Dr Royce Darnell, a Trent pathologist suspended because of a dispute about the management of the laboratory, and Dr Roy Chaudhury in North East Thames, who had initially refused to sheath needles when collecting blood in the Blood Transfusion Service.[20] Soon after his dismissal, the procedure that Dr Chaudhury had used became official policy.

Diana Brahams, a lawyer, in an article in the *Lancet*[21] discussed the inappropriate use of the disciplinary procedures where there was professional disharmony or intolerance of difference. She suggested referral to the General Medical Council (GMC), which oversees the regulation of doctors, when there is genuine cause for concern, and that the GMC should consider an extension of its powers to deal with incompetence.

In 1992 there was further publicity about Dr Darnell and in 1993 Dr O'Connell finally persuaded the Medical Defence Union with the help of Bindman and Partners (the firm of solicitors who had acted for me) to sue the NETRHA for breach of contract.[22] They had never held an HM(61)112 enquiry but had continued to pay her salary. She accepted a settlement in 1994 – more than eleven years after her suspension. In 1993 the case of Helena Daly, a haematologist loved by her patients, was headline news as marches took place in Cornwall.[23] The following year a last-minute settlement was made

16 Hansard (1986)
17 Public Affairs Division, BMA (1990)
18 Laurance (1988)
19 Tomlin (2003)
20 Greaves (1990)
21 Brahams (1990)
22 Dyer (1993)
23 Crail (1994)

at her paragraph 190 appeal.[24]

In 1994 following concern in Parliament, the Public Accounts Committee held an enquiry into Bridget O'Connell's case and was highly critical of the way that NETRHA had dealt with the case.[25] The responses of the NHSE are reprinted in the NAO report.[26] They declared that they were 'confident that the new guidance will prompt employers to resolve these suspensions quickly', but resisted the suggestion that they should monitor compliance at individual trust level. They did agree to provide a report in 12 months time of the number of suspensions lasting over six months.

The new guidance referred to by the NHSE, HSG(94)49,[27] probably emerged from a joint working party reviewing how HC(90)9 had operated; but the report of this body has not been published. The main changes were that there was to be a nominated officer, normally the Medical Director, who had the power to suspend, and that the Chairman or a nominated non-executive member of the board was be informed immediately. The situation was to be reviewed every two weeks, and the board was to be notified if the investigation had not been completed after three months. Not surprisingly, these modest suggestions, which were not binding on trusts, made little difference to the situation of doctors. The number of suspensions rose from eight in the last half of 1995 (the first available statistics five years after HC(90)9 had ordered their collection) to a peak of 130 in 2002.[28] However the reliability of the statistics before 2000 was unsatisfactory.[29]

One problem that the procedures often did not seem able to deal with was that of doctors whose performance was poor. This was analysed by Rosenthal[30] who interviewed a number of medical managers and recorded their frustrations in 1995. In 1995 the GMC published *Good Medical Practice*[31] in an attempt to state positively what doctors should do rather than what they should not do. In 1997 the General Medical Council launched its performance procedures, which included an assessment of a doctor's knowledge and skills as well as interviews with colleagues at the workplace.[32] This enabled managers to refer doctors whom they had suspended to the GMC, even if their behaviour had not reached the threshold of serious professional misconduct. This has often increased the time that a doctor has been off work. The second report from the Clinical Psychiatrists Study group in 1999[33] showed that they knew of 201 suspended consultants over a 12-year period. Of 154 cases in which the outcome was known at the time of writing, three had died, 25 had been dismissed, 71 had been reinstated and in 55 a settlement had been made.

Liam Donaldson became CMO for England in 1999 and set up the National Clinical Assessment Authority (NCAA) in 2001. Its purpose was to assess consultants whose performance was giving cause for concern but was not so serious as to warrant a referral to the GMC.

---

24 Dyer (1995)
25 Public Accounts Committee (1995)
26 National Audit Office (2003)
27 NHSE (1994)
28 National Audit Office (2003) Figure 5, p.14
29 Carruthers (2006)
30 Rosenthal (1995)
31 General Medical Council (1995)
32 General Medical Council (1997)
33 Tomlin (2003)

In 2002 the National Audit Office[34] issued a comprehensive report after surveying all hospital and ambulance trusts in England by questionnaire. Only seven did not reply, giving a 96 per cent response rate. They visited a number of trusts and also looked into long-term suspensions. They assessed the number and cost of suspended clinicians about most of whom there was no information in the public domain. They used exclusion not suspension to avoid confusion with the GMC's power to suspend from the register.

They found that in England 1,083 clinicians, of whom a fifth were consultants, were excluded during the 15 months they analysed, and that doctors were excluded on average twice as long as other staff. Almost half never returned to work. The cost to the NHS was at least £40 million per year and, extrapolating the costs of the trusts that had recorded them to those trusts that had not, might be as high as £57 million a year.

Some case studies were given. The most expensive was that of consultant breast surgeon Briony Ackroyd, who had been suspended for alleged incompetence. She was referred to the GMC, who did not find her performance seriously deficient and recommended that she should resume work under supervision for a limited period. There was managerial obstruction when she found a suitable hospital to work in, and she eventually gave up and accepted a settlement. She has since retrained as a GP. The cost to the NHS was £825,000.[35] The personal cost to Briony Ackroyd was enormous and that to women patients in the Coventry area incalculable.

Dame Jill Knight, who has pursued the question of suspended doctors first in the Commons and then in the Lords, was highly critical of the NCAA (now the NCAS, part of the National Patient Safety Agency, NPSA). In a debate in 2003 she stated that it had cost £9.5 million since it was set up and had assessed only 16 of the 300 cases referred to it.[36] The government response was to say that many proposed suspensions had been prevented, and that it was too early to judge its cost effectiveness, but that 80 per cent of those using the service in the first 18 months had rated it positively. The current budget is £7 million a year.

Following the NAO report, Liam Donaldson issued new guidance for disciplinary procedures in December 2003.[37] This was classed as a directive, so trusts now had to comply. Hospitals and primary care trusts, which could suspend GPs, were instructed to ring and discuss the case with the NCAS before taking the drastic step of suspension unless there was an immediate threat to patients.

In February 2005 the guidance was strengthened and trusts were instructed to implement it by 1 June 2005,[38] though foundation trusts are excluded from this directive. By 18 July 2005, 85 per cent of trusts had used the NCAS, 1,700 cases where suspension was considered or performance was an issue had been reported and alternatives to exclusion had been found in 85 per cent of cases. Long-term exclusions had been reduced by a half and 25 per cent of cases were being closed every quarter, but no figures were given.[39] A report of the first four years (to March 2005) has been published[40] and 1,772 doctors or dentists were referred. Ten per cent underwent assessment. Suspensions over

34 National Audit Office (2003)

35 Ibid. p.28

36 Hansard (2003)

37 Department of Health (2003); National Audit Office (2003) case 3, p.28

38 Department of Health (2005a)

39 Department of Health (2005b)

40 National Clinical Assessment Service (2006)

six months fell from an average of 29 per quarter in 2000 to 20 in 2005.

On 30 September 2005, 68 GPs, 20 surgeons, 43 other hospital doctors and 12 dentists were currently suspended by the NHS: a total of 143.[41] In 2002 figures were collected for the first time for so called 'gardening leave' – used by some managers to avoid the stigma of formal suspension but seen by some doctors as a managerial device for avoiding the timetable imposed by the regulations. There were 36 found in three months in 2002 but this practice has now been stopped.[42]

Another sanction was introduced in 1997 after anxiety about the time between a concern being raised and action being taken on a doctor's registration. The NHS decided on an 'Alert Letter' issued by the Regional Director of Public Health after a request from senior staff locally. About 70 a year are now issued and circulated throughout the NHS. An analysis by the NW region showed that half of the doctors were considered fit to practise after investigation.[43] I have first-hand knowledge of one of these who was referred to the GMC's performance procedures, and it took almost three years for him to be cleared. There can be devastating consequences if a doctor is unaware of the referral and then finds he loses his job.[44]

In 2000,[45] after the Shipman case, the GMC was enabled to set up the Interim Orders Committee, now Panel. This committee has the power to suspend or impose conditions on a doctor's registration on the basis of a prima facie case. In the first five months 68 per cent of the 187 doctors referred had had their registration affected, over half of which were suspended. The following two years saw a fall in numbers and in 40 per cent no order was made, but in 2005 80 per cent had orders imposed, and the numbers have almost doubled to 274 in 2005.[46] Are more doctors putting patients at risk or has the threshold for referral and action been lowered? This power does raise questions about civil liberties. The criteria for action has been changed from 'cogent and credible prima facie evidence' that the doctor's behaviour required an order to suspend or put conditions on his registration, either to protect the public or the doctor himself, or if it was in the public interest. Now action may be taken if committee is 'satisfied that the fitness to practise *may* be impaired'. The allegations must be credible and backed up by 'corroborative evidence *where possible*' [my emphasis]. This change followed Councel's advice as to how Section 41A of the Medical Act 1983 (as amended) should be interpreted.[47]

One important problem which persists up to the present, is that colleagues and managers may collude to use the disciplinary procedures unjustly to remove a doctor whose 'face does not fit'. As one personnel manager who did not wish to be named said in 1994 'I have been involved at a lot of sites where consultants have been dismissed and I don't know of a single case where the decision on dismissal had not already been taken in advance of proceedings'.[48] I find it depressing that, over 20 years after my case brought the attention of the public and the profession to such inappropriate actions, there are still so many doctors being suspended unjustly. The changes in the NHS, with more

41 National Clinical Assessment Service (2005)
42 Stone (2006)
43 Chief Medical Officer (2006) pp.89–93
44 Personal communication
45 Statutory Instrument (2000)
46 General Medical Council (2001–5)
47 General Medical Council (2006)
48 Glasman (1994)

decentralisation planned and multiple providers and competition, make it likely that the situation will not improve unless increased public and parliamentary pressure is applied. I believe that until managers are subject to regulation by their professional body the unhealthy alliance between doctors and managers will continue to the detriment of hardworking, caring doctors and their patients.

In this section, John Hendy QC, an employment lawyer who was my barrister for the enquiry, reports on his experience of subsequent NHS disciplinary procedures in which he has been involved and suggests how the system could be improved. A woman surgeon suspended in 2003, writes about her experience – anonymously, on legal advice. Professor Michael Goodyear, an oncologist from Canada, also writes about his experience and how the procedure might be improved.

References

Brahams D (1990) 'Suspended doctors, HC(90)9 or the GMC?' *Lancet*, 385:1,089.

Carruthers, Sir Ian (2006) (Acting Chief Executive of the NHSE) letter in reply to query from Wendy Savage, 21 August 2006.

Chief Medical Officer (2006) *Good doctors safer patients*. London: Department of Health.

Crail M (1994) 'Jibe talking', *Health Service Journal*, p.14.

Department of Health (1990a) *Disciplinary procedures for Hospital and Community Medical and Dental Staff.* HC(90)9. London: Department of Health.

Department of Health (1990b) *Working for Patients*. London: Department of Health.

Department of Health (2003) HSC 2003/012 *Maintaining high professional standards in the modern NHS – a framework for the initial handling of concerns about doctors and dentists in the NHS*. London: Department of Health.

Department of Health (2005a) *Maintaining high professional standards in the modern NHS Doctors and dentists disciplinary framework*. http://www.dh.gov.uk (accessed 17 February 2005).

Department of Health (2005b) *Progress on policy. Suspension of doctors*. http://www.dh.gov.uk (accessed 18 July 2006).

Department of Health and Social Security (1982) *Prevention of harm arising from physical or mental disability of hospital or community dental staff.* HC(82)13. London: DHSS.

Department of Health and Social Security (1988) *Disciplinary procedures for Hospital Doctors and Dentists*, Report of the Joint Working Party. London: HMSO.

Donaldson L (1994) 'Doctors with problems in an NHS workforce', *BMJ*, 308:1,277–82.

Dyer C (1993) 'Paediatrician fights 11 year suspension', *BMJ*, 307:1,444.

Dyer O (1995) 'Trust withdraws allegations against consultant', *BMJ*, 310:1,486–7.

General Medical Council (1995) *Good Medical Practice*. London: GMC.

General Medical Council (1997) *Guide to performance procedures*. London: GMC.

General Medical Council (2001–5) Council Papers, Reports on the work of the Interim Orders Committee and, after November 2004, the Interim Orders Panel.

General Medical Council (2006) e-mail reply from Fitness to Practise Directorate, 21 September 2006.

Glasman D (1994) 'The trial', *Health Service Journal*, 7 April 1994, p.9.

Greaves W (1990) 'Guilty until proven innocent', *The Times*, 25 June 1990.

Hansard (1986) '*Women Doctors in Obstetrics and Gynaecology*', 15 March 1986, Vol.93 No.78 pp.1,274–82.

Hansard (2003) House of Lords, 19 March 2003, '*Doctors: Suspension*', p.235.

Laurance J (1988) 'Doctor paid £150,000 to do nothing', *The Sunday Times*, 23 October 1988.

Ministry of Health (1961a) *Disciplinary procedures in cases relating to hospital medical and dental staff.* HM(61)112. London: MoH.

Ministry of Health (1961b) (then DHSS then Department of Health) *Terms and Conditions of Service for Hospital Medical and Dental Staff, for Doctors in Community Medicine and the Community Health Service and for Administrative Dental Officers and Community Clinical dental Officers*. (Paragraph 190 appeal procedure.)

National Audit Office (2003) *The Management of Suspension of Clinical Staff in NHS Hospital and Ambulance Trusts in England*. Norwich: The Stationery Office. http://www.tso.co.uk

National Clinical Assessment Service (2005) *Casework activity – midyear report to the Board in November 2005.* London: NCAS.

National Clinical Assessment Service (2006) *Analysis of the first four years referral data. London*: NCAS. http://www.ncas.npsa.nhs.uk

NHSE (1994) HSG(94)49 'Disciplinary Procedures for hospital and community medical and dental staff'. BAPS, Heywood Lancs.

Public Accounts Committee (1995) '*Suspension of Dr O'Connell' The 40th report of the Committee of Public Accounts*, session 1994–5.

Public Affairs Division, BMA (1990) Press release, 15 June 1990. London: BMA.

Rosenthal MM (1995) *Incompetent Doctor: Behind closed doors*. Open University Press.

Statutory Instrument (2000) No.2,054, Interim Orders Committee amendment to Medical Act (1983). Norwich: The Stationery Office.

Stone I (2006) personal communication. Ian Stone is an advisor to CMO (England) and an HR advisor to NCAS, Market Towers, 1 Nine Elms Lane SW6 5NQ.

Tomlin PJ (2003) 'The suspensions scandal', *Journal of Obstetrics & Gynaecology*, 23(3):221–7.

Employers' Discipline of Doctors in the NHS

....

John Hendy QC[1]

As a consultant obstetrician and gynaecologist at the (then) London Hospital, Wendy Savage was suspended by, and her disciplinary hearing was conducted by, her employing health authority in accordance with the procedure set out in the NHS circular HM(61)112 to which (as I recall) her contract referred. The hearing was conducted with all the formality, intensity, length and expense of a civil trial. However, without such a rigorous quasi-judicial process, there can be little doubt that the spurious and unfounded nature of the bulk of the charges against her would not have been revealed and she would not have been reinstated.

This chapter offers some reflections on the disciplinary procedures of trusts employing hospital doctors in relation to allegations of misconduct. Space does not permit consideration of capability issues nor of the other means by which doctors' behaviour is regulated (such as the GMC).

As Professor Savage sets out in her introduction to this section of the book, the HM(61)112 procedure originated from ministerial guidance first given in 1951, three years after the founding of the NHS. It was superseded in 1990 by HC(90)9 which made relatively modest adjustments to the process. Now this important procedural framework providing vital protections for senior medical and dental staff against false allegations is in the course of being swept away and replaced by whatever disciplinary procedure for alleged misconduct the particular NHS trust adopts for the rest of its staff.[2] This chapter is intended to draw attention to the significance of the loss of some of the characteristics of the old regime under HC(90)9 and the protection it gave to senior medical staff and, thus indirectly, to patients.

The legal basis of HC(90)9

Whilst the NHS was a highly centralised organisation, circulars from the DoH were regarded as binding and there is little doubt that health authorities regarded themselves as bound by them. The NHS standard terms and conditions of employment for consultants of the 1960s, 70s and 80s specifically referred to HM(61)112 as the disciplinary procedure and hence it was incorporated into the contract of employment between the doctor and the employing authority by reason of the application of trite employment contract law.[3] This was fortified by a statutory instrument so that employing

1 Head of Old Square Chambers; Chair of the Institute of Employment Rights; Visiting Professor in the School of Law, King's College London; immediate past chair, Employment Law Bar Association; FRSM.

2 Since 1996, GPs (not being employees) who breach their service conditions have been dealt with by NHS disciplinary committees and the NHS Tribunal, pursuant to the National Health Service (Service Committees and Tribunal) Amendment Regulations 1996 (SI 703/1996). These procedures have changed and are beyond the scope of this chapter.

3 *National Coal Board v Galley* [1958] 1 All ER 91, CA; *Gascol Conversions Ltd v Mercer* [1974] ICR

authorities had no option but to be bound by HC(90)9.[4]

From the late 1990s and in keeping with devolution in the NHS, trusts were encouraged to adapt HC(90)9 and adopt the adapted version as their own procedure, rather than simply making a reference to HC(90)9 in the paragraph dealing with disciplinary matters in the terms and conditions statement they issued to their consultants. Typically, the trust's adapted version was referred to in the contractual document so that it was thereby incorporated into the contract of employment. In my experience the trust variations from the original were not great, as the reported cases (below) show.

HC(90)9 procedures

The procedural characteristics of the HC(90)9 and paragraph 190 procedures are full and, in some respects, complex. The principal features were described by Lord Steyn in the leading decision of the Judicial Committee of the House of Lords in *Skidmore v Dartford & Gravesham NHS Trust* [2003] ICR 721 HL:

2. This appeal raises important issues in respect of hospital disciplinary proceedings. The context is a contractual disciplinary code. Specifically, the issues arise because of the incorporation of Department of Health Circular HC(90)9 dated March 1990 in most hospital doctors' contracts. This Circular governed the hospital sector of the National Health Service before the creation of autonomous trusts under the National Health Service and Community Care Act 1990. It is still in use by autonomous NHS trusts. The disciplinary code provides for a difference in procedure depending on whether the case involves allegations of 'professional conduct' or 'personal conduct.' The former is governed by a judicialised procedure under Circular HC(90)9. The latter is governed by less formal disciplinary procedures without, amongst other things, the right of legal representation. Inevitably this relatively complex structure gives rise to issues of demarcation concerning the category in which a particular case falls...

12. The Circular is a lengthy document. For present purposes it is only necessary to set out a few extracts from it. The Circular draws a distinction between 'personal conduct', 'professional conduct' and 'professional competence'. Those categories of allegations of misconduct are defined in paragraph 3 of the Circular as follows:

    '*Personal conduct*. Performance or behaviour of practitioners due to factors other than those associated with the exercise of medical or dental skills.

    '*Professional Conduct*. Performance or behaviour of practitioners arising from the exercise of medical or dental skills.

    '*Professional Competence*. Adequacy of performance of practitioners related to the exercise of their medical or dental skills and professional judgement.'

    . . .

420, CA; *Keir and Williams v County Council of Hereford and Worcester* [1985] IRLR 505, CA; *Marley v Forward Trust Group Ltd* [1986] ICR 891, CA; *Morris v C H Bailey Ltd* [1969] 2 Lloyd's Rep 215, CA; *Petrie v Mac Fisheries Ltd* [1940] 1 KB 258. Whilst in the past mere 'policies' have not been regarded as incorporated into the contract (*Dryden v Greater Glasgow Health Board* [1992] IRLR 469, EAT; *Wandsworth London Borough Council v D'Silva* [1998] IRLR 193, CA; *Grant v South-West Trains Ltd* [1998] IRLR 188, QBD), with the advent of the implied term of trust and confidence employees are now likely to be able to rely on the latter in order to enforce compliance with a disciplinary 'policy'.

4 Reg. 3 of the National Health Service (Remuneration and Conditions of Service) Regulations 1991 (SI 1991/ 481).

In cases involving personal conduct Annex B provides that 'the position of a doctor or dentist is no different from that of other health service staff'. With regard to cases involving professional misconduct and professional incompetence, Annex B of the Circular provides in paragraph 8 that the panel (consisting usually of three members) should have a legally qualified chairman. Moreover in such cases Annex B of the Circular provides, inter alia, in paragraph 12 for the following further procedural rights:

> 'The practitioner should have the right to appear personally before the investigating panel and to be represented (either by a lawyer... or otherwise), and to hear all the evidence presented to the panel. He should have the right to cross-examine all witnesses and to produce his own witnesses, and they and he may also be subjected to cross-examination'.

By contrast the internal procedure applicable to cases of personal conduct contains no such safeguards and is generally more informal.

13. ...While the distinction between professional and personal conduct goes back to 1956, the disciplinary arrangements presently reflected in HC(90)9 were the result of the deliberations of a Joint Working Party which published a report in August 1988 entitled 'Disciplinary Procedures for Hospital and Community Doctors and Dentists'. The Joint Working Party was made up of representatives of the Health Departments, the NHS and the professions. It was set up to 'review disciplinary procedures for hospital and community doctors and dentists' and specifically to 'consider the scope, operation and effectiveness of the disciplinary procedures' in Circular HM(61)112. Paragraph 3 of the report reads:

> 'The Working Party recognised the professions' concerns that disciplinary procedures for senior doctors and dentists must ensure that the grounds for dismissal have been fully justified, since a specialist who has been dismissed from an NHS post on professional grounds would be unlikely to find alternative employment elsewhere. The professions felt that the procedures used should be sufficiently weighty to reflect both the long periods of training and competitive selection processes which doctors have undergone before appointment to senior posts, and also the potential gravity of the outcome of such procedures'.

The recommendations of the Working Party were accepted and gave rise to HC(90)9 which was published by the Department of Health in March 1990. The terms contained in HC(90)9 were imposed upon doctors by regulation 3 of the National Health Service (Remuneration and Conditions of Service) Regulations 1991 (SI 1991/481). It is now part of the employment contract of Mr Skidmore and of the employment contracts of almost all NHS hospital doctors.

19. ...The line drawn between professional conduct and personal conduct is conduct 'arising from the exercise of medical or dental skills' and 'other' conduct. ...The structure of the disciplinary code set out in HC(90)9 is a classic case requiring a broad and purposive interpretation enabling sensible procedural decisions to be taken.

HC(90)9, Annex B thus provides procedural steps protecting consultants faced with discipline by their employers over matters of professional conduct or professional competence. These steps are notably more extensive than those which applied to allegations of personal misconduct which were left to be dealt with by the employer's ordinary disciplinary procedure applicable to other categories of staff.[5]

The new disciplinary procedure

On 17 February 2005, the Secretary of State for Health[6] issued *Directions on Disciplinary Procedures 2005* which required the Trust (and all other NHS bodies) by 1 June 2005 to implement the guidance contained in the document annexed to the said directions, entitled *Maintaining High Professional Standards in the Modern NHS 2005.*

---

5 In summary the HC(90)9 Annex B procedure required the following steps to be taken:

(i) Following an incident or complaint being made involving the professional conduct or competence of a medical or dental practitioner, the chairman of the NHS body must determine whether there is a *prima facie* case which, if well founded, could result in serious disciplinary action (such as dismissal).

(ii) The prior enquiries to establish whether or not a *prima facie* case exists is undertaken by the Director of Public Health.

(iii) The *'doctor should be warned in writing immediately of the nature of the incident which has been alleged, or of the complaint which has been made, and that the question of an inquiry, which might lead to serious disciplinary action, is under consideration'. Copies of 'all relevant correspondence'* should be sent to the practitioner who is entitled to make comments in response.

(iv) The practitioner should be given '*reasonable time*' to make representations and to seek advice before any final decision is taken (by the chairman) as to whether an enquiry is necessary.

(v) If the chairman decides that a *prima facie* case exists, the NHS body should proceed to an enquiry.

(vi) '*No member of the [enquiry] Panel should be associated with the [organisation(s)] in which [the practitioner] works.'* The panel should be small, normally three persons and chaired by an independent legally qualified chairman nominated by the Secretary of State from a panel appointed by the Lord Chancellor (in practice this is usually a QC). At least one member should be professionally qualified and in competence cases all should be so qualified and at least one of the same specialty as the practitioner in the same grade. Before the professional members are chosen there should be consultation with the Joint Consultants Committee (usually interpreted as a veto exercised by the JCC).

(vii) Terms of reference of the panel should be drafted and given to the practitioner. The practitioner should be provided '*as soon as possible*' with copies of correspondence and witness statements.

(viii) The hearing is held in private (unless the parties agree otherwise). The practitioner has the right to be represented (including legal representation), to be present throughout and to cross-examine witnesses and produce his own. The rules of procedure are determined by the chairman who usually applies, so far as he or she can, the rules of procedure of the civil courts (including as to the standard of proof – often the subject of submissions).

(ix) At the conclusion of the enquiry, the panel is required to prepare a report consisting of two parts. The first part contains the panel's findings. The second part should contain a conclusion as to whether the practitioner is at fault, and may also contain a recommendation as to disciplinary action.

(x) The panel has no power to impose disciplinary sanctions of itself and the penalty is determined by the NHS body (usually the Chief Executive) in a further hearing at which legal representation is not permitted. The Chief Executive is not bound by the recommendation of the panel but must not seek to take into account any aggravating factor and must take into account any mitigation from the practitioner (see *Barros D'Sa v University Hospital Coventry and Warwickshire NHS Trust* [2001] IRLR 691 CA; *Mattu v University Hospitals Coventry and Warwickshire NHS Trusts* [2006] EWHC Civ 1774).

(xi) The practitioner should be given a copy of the first part of the panel report and afforded time to respond with any corrections of fact and other observations. The practitioner should be furnished with a copy of the second part of the enquiry panel's report in good time before any disciplinary hearing called by the NHS body.

(xii) Time limits are set out for each stage and the total up to the disciplinary hearing '*should not exceed 32 weeks*'. In reality, the time limits have been more honoured in the breach than in the observance.

(xiii) There is no provision for appeal save by the Paragraph 190 route, though since NHS bodies have been adapting HC(90)9 to make it their own, they have often included an appeal machinery to members of their board (this is in keeping with section 40 of the General Whitley Council Terms and Conditions of Service which provided such an internal appeal where Paragraph 190 did not apply). Paragraph 190 appeals lay to the Secretary of State where a practitioner felt his or her dismissal was unfair – the reference was to paragraph 190 of the standard NHS Terms and Conditions of Service for Hospital Medical and Dental Staffs. Paragraph 190 provides a right to appeal where the doctor

This document should not be confused with a document of the same name issued[7] in 2003 by the Secretary of State as an annex to HSC 2003/012 which was in itself an annex to the *Restriction of Practice and Exclusion from Work Directions 2003* which required Trusts by 1 April 2004 to implement the 2003 version of *Maintaining High Professional Standards in the Modern NHS*. The 2003 version contained only two parts, the second of which made some very helpful improvements to the regime for suspending doctors and so was to be welcomed. There is no doubt that some consultants have agreed to incorporation into their contracts of the 2005 version thinking that they were getting the benefit only of the new suspension provisions. If so, they have been misled. For the 2005 version, though reproducing the two parts of the 2003 version, contains further parts, amongst which is the new regime for discipline.

The 2005 version of *Maintaining High Professional Standards* (to which the rest of this chapter refers) covers both matters of conduct – both professional and non-professional – and competence (in the latter case involving the performance procedures of the National Clinical Assessment Service, formerly the NCAA, a body established by statutory instrument).

The essential features of the proposed disciplinary procedure were presaged in the Department of Health publication, *Assuring Quality of Medical Practice: Implementing 'Supporting Doctors, Protecting Patients'* (January 2001). Both that and *Maintaining High Professional Standards in the Modern NHS* are lengthy documents but the striking features of the new disciplinary procedure so far as allegations of professional misconduct are concerned are:

- HC(90)9 is abolished with the intention that the HC(90)9 type procedures protecting consultants and senior medical staff in relation to professional misconduct charges are swept away and replaced by the same disciplinary procedures as for all other staff employed by the employer:

> Misconduct matters for doctors and dentists, as for all other staff groups, are matters for local employers and must be resolved locally. All issues regarding the misconduct

---

considers his or her 'appointment is being unfairly terminated'. The right applies only to limited classes of doctor, in particular to consultants. The right is of diminishing significance since trusts and Hospital Authorities were told, and have heeded the advice, not to employ consultants after 1st April 1991 on terms which included paragraph 190. Trusts have excluded a paragraph 190 right of appeal in new contracts, leaving only those employed before 1991 with residual rights. Paragraph 190 cases will soon be of historic interest only. There was no right of appeal under paragraph 190 where the dismissal is on grounds of 'personal misconduct'. This has proved a fraught point in some cases. If a paragraph 190 appeal is lodged the dismissal may not be put into effect (save where the dismissal is summary). The appeal is to a panel which advises the Secretary of State and is chaired by the Chief Medical Officer or his or her deputy sitting with representatives of the profession. The doctor is usually legally represented and the proceedings are formal. The Secretary of State could, on the recommendation of the panel, confirm the dismissal, or direct it to continue, or (the 'third solution') 'arrange some other solution agreeable to the practitioner and the employer'. Before the break up of the NHS into trusts, the third solution was relatively easy to operate by the expedient of moving the doctor to another hospital, near or far. Nowadays the degree of autonomy of trusts means that this option is very difficult and a recommendation of the third solution may be frustrated and end ultimately in unemployment if no employer will take the doctor.

6 Pursuant to powers conferred upon her by section 17 of, and paragraph 10(1) of Schedule 5 and paragraph 8(3) of Schedule 5A to, the National Health Service Act 1977 and paragraph 16(5) of Schedule 2 to the National Health Service and Community Care Act 1990.

7 Also pursuant to the same powers.

of doctors and dentists should be dealt with under the employers' procedures covering other staff charged with similar matters.

- The NCAS is to be involved in all serious cases, for example where exclusion is being considered.
- The 'Paragraph 190' right of appeal is said to be abolished.[8]
- The document contains new capability procedures always involving NCAS and new suspension ('exclusion') procedures.

In the usual conduct case the investigation is to be carried out by a 'case investigator' under the oversight of the Medical Director as 'case manager'. The case investigator must give the opportunity of interview to the doctor under investigation who may be accompanied but, if the companion is legally qualified, 'he or she will not be acting in a legal capacity'. The case manager will decide if there is a case of misconduct which should be put to a 'conduct panel'. Regrettably the document is silent as to the composition of, the procedure before, and any appeal from a 'conduct panel'.[9] These matters are left to the tender mercy of the NHS body's disciplinary procedure for other staff,[10] save (see below) for the provision that the conduct panel must include a medically qualified member if the case involves professional conduct.[11] This contrasts with the detailed provisions for capability cases which go to a 'capability panel', the composition of which, the procedure for which, and the appeal mechanism from which are all set out.[12] In short, where misconduct – professional or otherwise – is alleged, the safeguards provided by the document are virtually non-existent.

The first (of only two) particular protections for the senior clinician under the new procedure is that where the allegation is in relation to professional conduct 'the case investigator must obtain appropriate independent advice' (paragraph 2). It is, of course, common for the trust to obtain an independent medical report or opinion from an expert selected by it, often without the practitioner's knowledge or agreement and with no consultation with him or her. Such reports are, in my experience, not written with the detachment required of medical reports written for the courts where there are explicit duties of independence and where the reporter knows that he or she may well be subjected to probing cross-examination. Under the conduct procedure adopted by trusts it may be unlikely that the reporting doctor will be called to give evidence and certain that he or she will not be subjected to the cross-examination of a professional advocate.

The second protection is that the panel hearing a case of alleged professional misconduct must include a member who is medically qualified and who is not currently employed by the NHS body. There is no requirement of agreement by or even consultation with the accused doctor in the selection of this panel member, no requirement that he or she is of the same specialty, and no requirement of non-association with the NHS employer (nor any requirement that he or she be on an approved list

---

8 Though whether a contractual right to a Paragraph 190 appeal can be abolished in so cavalier a manner may be doubted – see the *Gryf-Lowczowski* case considered below – though since the right of appeal is to a third party, the point is more complex.

9 I, para.17.

10 And the minimal statutory requirements in relation to discipline.

11 III, para.2.

12 IV, paras.13–51 together with Appendix A.

maintained by, for example, the appropriate Royal College).

Without doubt *Maintaining High Professional Standards in the Modern NHS*, in relation to allegations of professional misconduct, constitutes a downgrading of consultants' protection which appears to have met surprisingly little resistance and was agreed by the BMA (and the BDA). The most striking features are the abolition of the independent and legally chaired panel to hear serious disciplinary allegations,[13] and the removal of the right of legal representation. The disciplinary procedures of most NHS bodies applicable to non-senior medical staff put the hearing of disciplinary allegations into the hands of a manager (after 2005 it will presumably be a 'panel' composed of a manager and one other).

Implementation of *Maintaining High Professional Standards in the Modern NHS* 2005

Though all NHS bodies were directed by *Maintaining High Professional Standards in the Modern NHS* 'to implement the framework within their local procedures by 1 June 2005', it was left to them as to how this was to be achieved.[14] The ineptitude of many trusts meant that they failed, in accordance with the well-established principles of contract law, to effect variations to the contracts of employment of their consultants by the due date and consequently found that the HC(90)9 type disciplinary procedures in the existing contracts continue to bind them after June 2005.[15] Thus in ***Gryf-Lowczowski v Hinchingbrooke Healthcare NHS Trust***,[16] Gray J held:

> 12. [The Chief Executive] was asked by Mr Hendy for Mr Gryf-Lowczowski what steps, if any, had been taken by the trust to incorporate the NCAA procedures as part of its contractual relationship with Mr Gryf-Lowczowski. In answer Mr Pattison said that the framework document had been 'adopted at board level within the trust'. He suggested that that amounted to introducing the procedures laid down in the document as terms of Mr Gryf-Lowczowski's contract. Mr Pattison further told me that the framework had been discussed with the relevant professional bodies and that it was widely known. He did, however, concede that the trust had not written to every consultant to seek his or her agreement to the adoption of the new procedures in the contract of employment. No such letter had been written to Mr Gryf-Lowczowski.
>
> ...
>
> 56. The evidence is that the version of the contract of employment which is in the trial bundle was signed by Mr Gryf-Lowczowski on 2 October 2004... It is for the trust to satisfy me that the contract was thereafter varied so as to incorporate the procedure set out in Part IV of the framework document. As stated... above, the DoH directions

---

13 Or, as the press release of 17 February 2006, puts it: 'The employing trust is squarely responsible for the disciplining of its medical and dental staff not outsiders.'

14 Para.3 of *Directions on Disciplinary Procedures* 2005 issued by the Secretary of State for Health under the National Health Service Act 1977 and the National Health Service and Community Care Act 1990.

15 In circumstances where a trust seeks to rely on contractual terms less favourable to the consultant than those found in *Maintaining High Professional Standards* (for example, those in Part II in relation to suspension), then there may be scope for arguing that the trust is bound by the implied duty to maintain trust and confidence to apply terms no less beneficial than those it was obliged to implement by the Secretary of State through his Directions: see *Mezey v South West London and St Georges NHS Trust*, 20 December 2006, transcript awaited.

16 [2006] IRLR 100.

required all NHS bodies to implement the framework by June 2005. In the ordinary way one would expect the trust as employer to draw up a revised contract for affected staff and to submit it to them for signature. That did not happen. [The Chief Executive]'s evidence as to the steps which were taken within the trust are set out at paragraph 12 above. In my judgement they fall well short of what would be required to establish that Mr Gryf-Lowczowski agreed to the variation of his contract for which the trust contends. I should add that I reject the submission of Mr Havers that the reference in clause 7 of the contract of employment (see paragraph 5 above) to 'our disciplinary or capability procedures' is to be construed as meaning 'such disciplinary or capability procedures as the trust may from time to time adopt'. The reference used in my view meant and was understood to mean that the procedures set out in the Disciplinary policy and procedures, based on Health Circular (90)9, were to apply.

Removal of protection

A glance at the new disciplinary procedures in comparison to the old brings vividly to mind words written nearly 160 years ago describing the effect of modern changes to employment relations. They wrote that:

> [capitalism] stripped of its halo every occupation hitherto honoured and looked up to with reverent awe. It has converted the physician, …the man of science, into its paid wage-labourers.[17]

Certainly, the protection of the professional reputation and career of the hospital consultant is now no greater than that of any other NHS employee. Whilst one might not argue that a labourer deserves less protection than a hospital consultant, the Working Party which drafted HC(90)9 was right to emphasise that dismissal from the NHS for a consultant on grounds of professional misconduct almost inevitably means the end of his or her career and vocation. In contrast dismissal of an unskilled worker may be a bitter blow but does not generally mean that he or she is blacklisted by every employer in the fields in which he or she has chosen to work. Furthermore, notwithstanding the Government's controversial impositions of fees on students, the cost to the public of training the consultant runs into hundreds of thousands of pounds, the benefits to the public of which are wholly lost if the consultant is dismissed and rendered unemployable as a doctor.

The removal of protections against disciplining of hospital consultants in relation to professional conduct represents unambiguously an assertion by the NHS towards their senior medical staff of the subservience inherent in the concept of the contract of employment.[18] It is ironic that this development should have coincided temporally with

17 K. Marx and F. Engels, *Manifesto of the Communist Party*, 1st ed., 1848. For a modern and brilliant analysis of the historical development of the employment relationship see S. Deakin and F. Wilkinson, *The Law of the Labour Market*, OUP, 2005, esp. chap.2.

18 As the founder of academic employment law, Professor Sir Otto Kahn-Freund wrote: 'the main object of labour law has always been, and I venture to say will always be, to be a countervailing force to counteract the inequality of bargaining power which is inherent and must be inherent in the employment relationship.' (*Labour and the Law*, 2nd edn, 1977, Chap. 1 at p.6) Also see K. Klare, 'Countervailing Workers' Power as a Regulatory Strategy', and R. Welch, 'Into the Twenty First Century – the continuing Indispensability of Collective Bargaining as a Regulator of the Employment Relation', both in H. Collins, P. Davies, R. Rideout, *Legal Regulation of the Employment Relation*, 2000.

the court's development of a doctrine of fundamental mutuality in the employment relationship both in relation to the essential qualities necessary to create a contract of employment[19] and in the form of implied reciprocal duties to maintain trust and confidence – see below.

No-one can doubt that not only are there incompetent doctors, there are also some who behave so badly that they should be dismissed from employment.[20] The imperative to protect the public is recognised by all. Patient safety must have a higher priority than justice for doctors. But the two are not incompatible. And dismissal of competent doctors falsely accused does nothing to protect patients.

It is a principle of disciplinary practice that the aim should not be to punish but to improve. *The ACAS Code of Practice on Disciplinary and Grievance Procedures* states:

> Disciplinary procedures should not be seen primarily as a means of imposing sanctions but rather as a way of encouraging improvement amongst employees whose conduct or performance is unsatisfactory.[21]

The NHS recognises that 'People with skills are expensive to replace. It makes sense to try to rebuild a career rather than scrapping probably still useful experience, skills and knowledge.'[22]

The fact is, however, that NHS disciplinary procedures are sometimes abused by those with ulterior motives. In his excellent report on the regulation of the medical profession, *Good doctors, safer patients: Proposals to strengthen the system to assure and improve the performance of doctors and to protect the safety of patients*,[23] Sir Liam Donaldson, Chief Medical Officer, Department of Health, found:

> …that there was something of a climate of fear and retribution, so that any lapse in performance or simple human error was seen as punishable by suspension, disciplinary action and referral to the General Medical Council. This remains the case today.[24]

'Today' is the summer of 2006, one year after the 2005 procedures were to be implemented. He pointed out that:

> A culture of blame and retribution has dominated the approach to this whole field so that it has been difficult to draw a distinction between genuine misconduct, individual failure, human error provoked by weak systems, and untoward outcomes which were not the result of any specific failure. An 'off with their heads' approach to every problem will ultimately make healthcare and medical practice more dangerous, since no-one will admit their own mistakes, nor will they want to condemn a colleague's career to ruin.[25]

---

19 *Dacas v Brook Street Bureau* [2004] IRLR 358 CA, para.49; *Cable & Wireless v Muscat* [2006] EWCA Civ 220 CA, para.35, both relying on *Carmichael v National Power* [2000] IRLR 43 HL, para.20 (Lord Irvine) and para.36 (Lord Hoffman) and *Montgomery v Johnson Underwood Ltd* [2001] IRLR 269 CA, paras. 21, 23, 46, and 47.

20 Sufficient to cite Harold Shipman the general practitioner who killed about 250 of his patients between 1972 and 1998, usually with narcotic drugs that he had stockpiled illicitly.

21 Published under statutory powers, September 2004. The first 'core principle of reasonable behaviour' set out in the ACAS Handbook states: 'Use procedures primarily to help and encourage employees to improve rather than just as a way of imposing a punishment.'

22 http://www.ncas.nhs.uk/toolkit/rebuilding.

23 14 July 2006 (part revised 31 August 2006).

24 Introduction at para.9.

25 Summary at para.28.

It follows that whatever modern techniques are used to avoid the blame culture and to enhance performance, senior medical staff who have committed so much of their own lives to their careers and who represent such a high investment by the nation in their careers continue to warrant proper protection against the abuse of discipline.

The reasons for the particular protections intended by the working party which drew up HC(90)9 (cited by Lord Steyn – see above) thus remain unchanged today. *Maintaining High Professional Standards in the Modern NHS* offers no explanation for the need to sweep away the disciplinary protection of consultants. It simply states that 'changes to NHS disciplinary procedures are necessary.'[26] A purported justification for the removal of these rights was asserted by a minister, John Hutton, in the accompanying press release:

> The existing procedures are unjustifiably prolonged and are not fair to NHS staff, taxpayers or patients. The new process ensures resources are not diverted away from patient care into the pockets of lawyers.

There is, as far as I am aware, no evidence that the HC(90)9 procedure was unfair to NHS staff – the usual complaint has been the fact of and the length of suspension prior to hearing. Exclusion and delay were not, however, inherent in the HC(90)9 process but more in the suspension process and the fact that suspension removed the imperative on management to act quickly. The suspension procedure is revised extensively by *Maintaining High Professional Standards in the Modern NHS* (though whether in reality it will improve matters for accused doctors remains to be seen). There can be little doubt that a procedure that gives the decision on whether to dismiss a consultant to management will certainly speed up the disciplinary process; but whether NHS staff would regard that as a price worth paying for avoiding the delays so common under HC(90)9 is dubious.

Mr. Hutton is obviously correct in pointing out that the exclusion of lawyers saves money. What is lost with the demise of HC(90)9 however, is the independence and impartiality of the process – independence which is essential to prevent senior medical staff being dismissed on trumped-up charges generated by personal malice or professional jealousy (in relation to private practice), or intended to neutralise an outspoken defender of patient services from the economic imperatives of management. I regret to say that many (though, of course, not all) of the cases which come across my desk in chambers appear to me to be darkened by the malevolent shadows cast by such (almost inevitably unprovable) factors.

The real reason for the deprivation of the special employment protections of hospital consultants is not obvious. It might well be thought that the current turmoil in the NHS, and in particular the restrictions on funding and their clinical consequences,[27] was a

26 As a result, it states (para.1, explanatory note), of the introduction of *Shifting the Balance of Power*, the Employment Act 2002 and the Follett report *(A Review of Appraisal, Disciplinary and Reporting arrangements for Senior NHS and University Staff with Academic and Clinical Duties)*. I could find nothing in those documents which purported to suggest that there were any reasons for the abolition of HC(90)9 type protections for senior medical staff.

27 For example: 'NHS told: put money before medicine', *Guardian*, 23 January 2006 – Health Secretary said to require trusts to put financial management ahead of clinical objectives; 'Over 6000 jobs lost in the NHS in 2006', *LRD Fact Service*, 13 April 2006, Vol.68, issue 15; 'Poor areas hardest hit by NHS cuts in London', *Guardian*, 7 August 2006; 'NHS becoming a brand like Nike, warns departing health director', *Guardian*, 1 September 2006 – John Ashton resigned as Regional Director of Public Health for the North

factor tending towards measures that might assist in the neutering of opposition from within.[28] Some may consider it to be part of a longer term measure in the NHS whereby administration has been progressively removed from clinicians and placed in the hands of managers in a fast-growing culture which gives primacy not so much to patient care but to the economic performance of the organisation. Perhaps there are other imperatives.

Whether these explanations have any credibility or not, the cases speak for themselves. In case after case heard by the High Court, NHS employers have sought to evade the procedural requirements of the disciplinary procedure of HC(90)9 – and before it HM(61)112. When the power of discipline is transferred from an independent panel chaired judicially to internal management and the consultant deprived of legal representation, it may be assumed that the attempts to evade due process will diminish in proportion to the ease of dismissing the 'difficult' consultant.

Unfair dismissal

It is of course true that a dismissed consultant, like other employees, has a right to make a claim to an employment tribunal for unfair dismissal under the Employment Rights Act 1996. However, the maximum compensation is limited to £58,400 for dismissals after 1 February 2006 and the latest statistics show that the median award actually awarded by tribunals was a mere £3,476 (average award: £7,303).[29] Though reinstatement is ostensibly the primary statutory remedy, in fact it was ordered in only 0.02 percent (14 out of 7,544) cases which went to a hearing.[30] In consequence, the remedy of unfair dismissal is of little value to consultants. If he or she can show that race, sex, religion, whistle-blowing or, now, age discrimination were reasons, awards can be significantly higher. But proving an illegitimate reason for dismissal is much harder than proving, in front of an independent specialist panel, that allegations of professional misconduct or incompetence are not justified.

The courts' protection

I shall conclude this chapter by illustrating what a valuable protection senior NHS medical staff have lost with the demise of HC(90)9 type procedures.[31] For the latter were enforceable as a matter of contract law and NHS employers could be injuncted from evading them.[32]

West and said that there was a danger of two-tier health provision – he resigned because he could not face the fifth reorganisation of his department; 'DHL signs £1.6bn health supply deal', *Financial Times*, 5 September 2006 – this was the outsourcing contract of NHS Logistics, its purchasing arm. UNISON have called strike action (*Financial Times* 11 September 2006); 'Nurses to leave NHS and sell services back through limited company', *Financial Times*, 14 September 2006 – 700 nurses and therapists leave the NHS and set up private company to sell their services back to it; 'Hewitt advisers deny political targeting of hospital closures', *Guardian*, 16 September 2006 – Secretary of State confirms she has a 'heat map' showing where strong opposition is likely to be to government plans to close A&E departments but denies that map is to be used to avoid closures in sensitive marginal seats. See also *R (on appn of Rogers) v Swindon PCT and S of S for Health* [2006] EWHC 171 (QB) – a failed challenge to refusal to fund herceptin for breast cancer patient.

28 It is to be noted that the device of discretionary awards – which are very valuable, measured in tens of thousands of pounds a year – appears sometimes to be the carrot against which the stick of disciplinary charges is juxtaposed to obtain the acquiescence of consultants.

29 Employment Tribunal Service Annual Statistics 2004–2005.

30 Ibid.

31 Regrettably, space does not permit me consideration of the thorny issue of suspension – now given the dismissive and derogatory title of 'exclusion' – though the chapter by Michael Goodyear refers to much of

Before discussing the enforceability of HC(90)9 procedures it is as well to observe that there are a number of legal issues which are beyond the scope of this book but which must be considered when contemplating what appears to be a breach of a contractual procedure such as HC(90)9. One such is the coexistent implied (and often express) term requiring each party to maintain trust and confidence[33] and the unrelated, though similarly named, rule that injunctions will not be granted where the employer has no trust and confidence in the employee.[34] Likewise the possibility of judicial review[35] and the restricted scope of the Human Rights Act are factors to be considered.[36] Though the received wisdom in legal textbooks was for many years that injunctions could not be

---

the extensive literature on the subject. This too was the subject of further guidance in *Maintaining High Professional Standards in the Modern NHS*, superseding HSC 2003/112 which in its turn superseded HSG(94)49. It is said that these developments have diminished the number of doctors on long-term suspension and it may be so. But the suspension procedural requirements are still breached as the recent judgement in Palmer (see footnote below) shows. It is often thought that wrongful suspension is not challengeable but, though difficult, it is possible: see *Palmer; Gogay v Hertfordshire CC* [2000] IRLR 703 CA (damages granted for stress brought on by unjustified suspension); and *Malik v Waltham Forest PCT* and *S of S for Health* [2006] EWHC 487 (Admin).

32 In some cases a declaration of right may be more easily available than an injunction and achieve the same result; see *Gunton v Richmond-upon-Thames London Borough Council* [1980] ICR 755, CA.

33 See *Malik v Bank of Credit and Commerce International SA* [1997] HL the implied term is 'a portmanteau term. Its specific operation in a particular case depends on the circumstances:' *R (Arthurworrey) v. Haringey LBC* [2002] ICR 279 (at 286, para 44). The term does not operate 'on termination', the so-called Johnson exclusion zone (after *Johnson v Unisys Ltd* [2001] IRLR 279 HL), see *Eastwood v Magnox Electric Plc* [2002] IRLR 447 CA, though in *King v University Court of St. Andrews* [2002] IRLR 252 (OH) it was held that the implied duty of trust and confidence subsisted through a disciplinary process which led to the decision to dismissal. See also *McCabe v Cornwall CC* [2005] 1 AC 503 HL and the discussion in Mattu (see footnotes below) at para.89 ff.

34 The employer may not have lost confidence in the doctor's work, for example *Bliss v S.E. Thames RHA* [1987] ICR 700 (breach of contractual term by seeking to impose psychological examination in response to breakdown of personal relationship; no loss of confidence in the doctor's work – injunction granted). Or it may be that the immediate superior is supportive of the worker even if senior management doubts it: *Powell v LB Brent* (see footnotes below). The presence or absence of sufficient mutual trust and confidence is irrelevant if what is sought is preservation of the employment relationship (but not to compel resumption of duties) whilst a contractual disciplinary procedure is adhered to: *Robb v London Borough of Hammersmith and Fulham* [1991] ICR 514, QBD; followed in *Gryf-Lowczowski* and in *Kircher* (see footnotes below); see also *Peace v City and Edinburgh Council* [1999] IRLR 417, Ct of Sess (OH).

35 It is theoretically possible that the procedure was enforceable as a matter of public law. There is limited scope for an 'office holder' to utilise the mechanism of judicial review to restrain dismissal in breach of the rules of natural justice (*Ridge v Baldwin* [1964] AC 40, HL). Judicial review is available to compel the fulfilment of a public duty or to restrain an irrational decision by a public body. But an office holder's claim will not permit judicial review merely because 'his entitlement to a subsisting right in private law... incidentally [involved] the examination of a public law issue' per Lord Bridge in *Roy v Kensington and Chelsea and Westminster Family Practitioner Committee* [1992] IRLR 233, HL (see also McLaren v Home Office [1990] ICR 824, CA and see *R v Secretary of State for Foreign and Commonwealth Affairs, ex p. Council of Civil Service Unions* [1985] ICR 14, HL). But an 'ordinary' employee never could proceed by way of judicial review unless some 'public' element was involved in the decision being challenged, for example where an employer's right to dismiss was restricted or regulated by statute (*Malloch v Aberdeen Corpn* [1971] 1 WLR 158, HL; and *R v Civil Service Appeal Board, ex p Bruce* [1988] ICR 649, DC). In fact, judicial review has been unlikely to be of value to doctors after *R v East Berkshire Health Authority, ex p Walsh* [1984] ICR 743, CA made clear that (notwithstanding *R v British Broadcasting Corpn, ex p Lavelle* [1983] ICR 99, Woolf J), employees' terms of employment are purely matters of private law save to the extent that the employer has failed to incorporate statutory terms and conditions as opposed to failing to implement them properly where they have been incorporated (at p.752EF). See also *R (Arthurworrey) v. Haringey LBC* [2002] ICR 279. For medical personnel this was confirmed in *R v Trent RHA ex p. Jones The Times*, 19 June 1986; and *R v South Glamorgan Health Authority ex p. Phillips* H Ct, 20 November 1986. Since the reported cases are concerned with a failure to follow HC(90)9 rather than a failure to incorporate it or any part of it, judicial review is an unlikely tool against a consultant's employer in this context. Though

granted to enforce a contract of employment,[37] in fact injunctions to restrain dismissals by employers in breach of the contractual disciplinary procedures have long-established antecedents going back nearly a century.[38] There have been many cases since, often involving doctors successfully enforcing NHS disciplinary procedures such as HC(90)9 including, most recently, a quartet of cases reported this year in which I had the honour to be instructed.[39]

---

note the court's acceptance (without discussion of the aforementioned cases) that judicial review was available to a GP suspended by a PCT in breach of statutory regulations: *Malik v Waltham Forest PCT and S of S for Health* [2006] EWHC 487 (Admin), at para.23.

36 The Human Rights Act 1998 incorporating the European Convention, Art.6 of which requires a fair trial, seems to add little to the express provisions of HC(90)9. However reliance on it might be sought under the 2005 procedures. The obligation on public bodies under s.6 HRA means that employment matters in the public sector are not excluded from the Convention: for example, *Halford v UK* [1997] IRLR 471 (art.8); *Ahmed v UK* [1982] 4 EHRR 126 (art.11, art.14). Though private bodies have no direct obligation to apply the Convention under s.6(1) this does not exempt private bodies to which the state has delegated functions: *Castelloe-Roberts v UK* [1982] 4 EHRR 38. Art.6 lays down procedural principles which are an elaboration of the English common law principles of natural justice but go further including, for example, a right to a public hearing. However, 'disputes relating to the recruitment, employment and retirement of public servants are, as a general rule, outside the scope of art.6(1)': *Massa v Italy* (1993) 18 EHRR 266. This includes a claim for unfair dismissal: *Balfour v UK* (Comm. Decn. No. 30976/96) and a reprimand: *X v UK* (1984) 6 EHRR 583. But the category of 'public servants' is limited and may not extend beyond civil servants: *Neigel v France* [1997] EHRLR 424, so that in *Darnell v UK* (1991) 69 DR 306 a doctor employed by a regional health authority under a contract of employment was held not excluded from the protection of Art.6. However, whilst consultants employed by NHS bodies are not within the category of employee denied the protection of Art.6, the circumstances in which they can pray it in aid are limited because Art.6 will not bite unless the dispute involves the *determination of a civil right or obligation*. The general rule is that disciplinary proceedings do not ordinarily involve disputes over civil rights or obligations: *Albert and Le Compte v Belgium* (1983) 5 EHRR 533, para.25. On the other hand, the right to continue in professional practice is a civil right and Art.6 of the Convention will apply to a disciplinary body which is capable of deciding whether or not a consultant can continue in practice, notwithstanding that the body is, in form, private. Thus the GMC is bound: *Wickramsinghe v UK* [1998] EHRLR 338, and analogous medical regulatory bodies in Europe: *Gautrin v France* (1999) 28 EHRR 196; *Albert and Le Compte* (above). There must be doubt whether the consequence of dismissal by an NHS body of being unemployable within or without the NHS neo-monopoly is sufficient to engage Art.6. However, in *Malik v Waltham Forest PCT and S of S for Health* [2006] EWHC 487 (Admin) the English Administrative Court held that Art.6 would have been engaged in relation to a decision by a PCT to suspend a GP in breach of statutory regulations had the penalty been final rather than interim.

37 Relying particularly on *Hill v CA Parsons & Co* [1972] 1 Ch. D. 305.

38 *Crisp v Holden* (1910) Sol. J & Wkly. Rep. 784; *Smith v McNally* [1912] 1 Ch.D. 816.

39 See for example: *Barber v Manchester Regional Hospital Board* [1958] 1 WLR 181 (damages granted for a refusal to permit a paragraph 190 appeal); *Jones v Lee and Guilding* [1980] ICR 310 CA; *Irani v Southampton etc HA* [1985] ICR 590 (injunction to restrain implementation of proposed dismissal unless contractual disputes procedure exhausted – otherwise employer would be 'entitled to snap its fingers at the rights of its employees' at 604F); *Hughes v LB Southwark* [1988] IRLR 55; *Powell v Brent LBC* [1988] ICR176 CA; *Wadcock v LB Brent* [1990] IRLR 223; *Robb v Hammersmith* [1991] ICR 514; *Jones v Gwent CC* [1992] IRLR 521 [tab 13] (final declaration that letter giving notice of dismissal was invalid together with final injunction to restrain dismissal); *Anderson v Pringle of Scotland Ltd* [1998] IRLR 64 Ct of Session (interim injunction to restrain dismissal in breach of a contractually incorporated redundancy procedure); *Peace v City and Edinburgh Council* [1999] IRLR 417, Ct of Sess (OH) (injunction granted to restrain employer from applying unagreed disciplinary procedure in place of contractual procedure; employee suspended; body of authorities recognised in which contractual procedures enforced by injunction: paras.11–12). In *Barros D'Sa v University Hospital Coventry and Warwickshire NHS Trust* [2001] IRLR 691 CA the employer sought to rely on a breakdown in trust and confidence to justify dismissal after HC(90)9 enquiry in which the panel had found minor misconduct which did not justify dismissal; it was held that the trust could not introduce matters of aggravation on which no charge had been put before or investigated by the panel. The quartet in which I was instructed included *Mattu v University Hospitals Coventry and Warwickshire NHS Trust* [2006] EWHC 1774 (QB) against the same

Conclusion

With the replacement of HC(90)9 procedures by 'ordinary' disciplinary procedures applicable to all trust employees, hospital consultants have lost valuable protections in relation to allegations of professional misconduct. The profession should consider carefully whether the restoration of some more formal procedure with an independent, legally chaired panel and a proper opportunity to challenge the charges through a professional advocate is not a necessary step towards the maintenance of the proper role of doctors in the NHS.

---

employer where a similar injunction would have been granted (but for an offered undertaking) to restrain the introduction of similarly aggravating material. The other three cases were: *Gryf-Lowczowski v Hinchingbrook Healthcare NHS Trust* [2006] IRLR 100 (purported termination by frustration was held to be ineffective and an injunction would have been granted to continue the employment, but for undertaking in same terms); *Kircher v Hillingdon PCT* [2006] Lloyds Rep Med 215 (injunction granted to reinstate the employment after a purported dismissal had taken effect, the employer having failed to comply with HC(90)9 procedure); *Palmer v East & North Hertfordshire NHS Trust* [2006] EWHC 1997 (injunction granted to continue employment said to have been terminated by frustration).

Disciplinary Procedures in Health Care: Use and Abuse

Michael Goodyear

The true liberty of the professional man was freedom to exercise his knowledge and skill according to his conscience and his ability, without fear or favour.

Alfred Ernest Brown (1881–1962), Minister of Health (1941–3)[1]

Despite such exalted claims as those of the Minister of Health, most people have accepted that the freedom to practice has been constrained by necessity since the origins of recorded clinical practice. Even in 2200 BC, Babylonian statutes set limitations on clinical practice and prescribed penalties for their violation.[2]

It can be argued that a service that consumes so much of the economy and has such a profound effect on our expectations of life and social function should be accountable.[3,4] Hoffenberg, in his 1986 Carling Lecture *Clinical Freedom*, traces the history of the regulation of the profession for a variety of reasons: technical, moral, ethical, legal and financial. Today there is a general acceptance that professions are accountable through a variety of mechanisms including judicial admonition, peer review, regulations, and formal and informal processes for dealing with performance and conduct problems. As Hoffenberg argues, 'Would our professional freedom not be better preserved if we relied less on the courts and more on our own efforts to monitor and improve our standards?'[5]

Self-regulation and assessment

There has evolved a general tendency to assume that professionals know best how to regulate themselves, even though this remains to be tested empirically.

> A profession… thus carries with it the notion of a standard of performance… a fiduciary trust to maintain certain standards. These are partly standards of competence, or technical ability… But not only so, professional competence has to be joined with professional integrity.[6]

Nevertheless, the issue of self-regulation versus external restraint has continued to occupy medical and health care administrators over at least 30 years since Cochrane first embraced the concept of measuring both the effectiveness and the efficiency of care.[7] However, in reality, assessing the quality of care has turned out to be extraordinarily

1 *The Times*, 5 October 1943
2 Hoffenberg (1987)
3 Donaldson (2001)
4 Checkland, Marshall and Harrison (2004)
5 Hoffenberg (1987) p.83
6 Emmet (1970)
7 Cochrane (1971)

difficult.[8,9,10] Poloniecki dryly reminds us that 'half of all doctors are below average'[11] while Drife[12] has pointed out that deviations from average indicators tend to be regarded as substandard care as judged by efficiency standards, but could equally reflect the opposite. Assessment of care is too often reactive, retroactive and driven by outcomes, generally adverse, disproportionate to process.

Many attempts have been made to redress this balance by prospective assessment, whether this be called audit, quality assurance or peer review, but with limited penetration,[13,14,15] although this is improving. In Canada, where medicine is regulated at the level of the provinces, as opposed to nationally, peer assessment programmes such as those in Ontario[16] were largely voluntary, but Alberta[17] and now Nova Scotia[18] have recently adopted mandatory schemes.

Professional self-regulation has been haunted by George Bernard Shaw's cynical perspective in *The Doctor's Dilemma* (1906),[19,20] reinforced by well-publicised cases of deviant behaviour, most recently that of Shipman.[21] Indeed the Shipman case has continued to dominate thinking about professional regulation.[22,23] This leads to a concept of care based on a dichotomous view of competence as opposed to a more reality-based spectrum of quality, and ignores the important contribution of the environment to performance. This so-called 'bad apples'[24,25] premise to maintaining standards is exemplified by politicians like Waxman, who refer to 'a new willingness to… weed out incompetents'.[26]

Where patterns of care are examined, surprisingly high rates of variation have been described in procedures, outcomes and adverse events. Yet insistence on adversarial schemes[27] has led to litigation directed at peer reviewers and credentialing and disciplinary bodies in the United States, a move likely to defeat the purpose of measuring what we do[28,29,30] and necessitating legislation of immunity.[31]

---

8 Goldman (1992)
9 Epstein and Hundert (2002)
10 Naylor (2002)
11 Poloniecki (1998)
12 Drife (1987)
13 McLachlan (1976)
14 Duncan (1980)
15 Berwick (2005)
16 See the College of Physicians and Surgeons of Ontario website, Info-Physicians, Peer Assessment: http://www.cpso.on.ca/Info_physicians/peer2.htm (accessed 10 September 2006).
17 See the College of Physicians and Surgeons of Alberta website, Physician Achievement Review: http://www.par-program.org/ (accessed 10 September 2006).
18 See the College of Physicians and Surgeons of Nova Scotia website, Nova Scotia Physician Achievement Review: http://www.nspar.ca/ (accessed 10 September 2006).
19 Shaw (1946)
20 Donaldson (2003)
21 Smith J (2004)
22 Dewar and Finlayson (2001)
23 Elwyn (2006)
24 Berwick (1989)
25 National Steering Committee on Patient Safety (2002) Executive Summary, viii, Recommendation 5, p.14ff.
26 Waxman (1987)
27 Van't Hoff (1985)
28 Iglehart (1987)

Other sources of resistance come from organised medicine, such as the British Medical Association which at one point strenuously defended professional autonomy, stating that 'any supervision of the competence of an individual doctor… must be by the profession' and that the best guarantee of competence was 'the individual doctor's conscientious assessment of the standards of his treatment against the standard of his colleagues'.[32]

Fortunately, more constructive thinking has started to prevail, in which audit is seen 'as an educational exercise that may identify means of improving the treatment of patients'[33] and a realisation that accountability is not the equivalent of dogmatism. It has never been completely clear what aspects of care should be, and are actually, assessed. Some aspects of care are more readily assessed than others,[34,35] and what constitutes an adequate standard of care is frequently debatable,[36,37] particularly if we accept that one of the most critical aspects of care is mindfulness[38] – the awareness and reflection upon one's own limitations and how to deal with them. We must also keep in mind that technically, *self*-regulation is largely a myth in that the mechanisms for regulation are largely and increasingly invoked by the state.

Self-regulation and quality of care

Recently, and understandably, there has been a great deal of public interest in, and concern[39,40] about, a series of closely related issues: regulation of health professions, medical errors[41] and patient safety, and continuing quality improvement. Regulation and evaluation should meet a dual role – protecting and reassuring the public as to the maintenance of standards, and reassuring and supporting the profession as to the quality of care delivered.

An aspect of this that has been relatively overlooked, and not yet integrated well into the overall picture, has been the way in which health care systems handle problems, all too often by dealing with the aftermath and not the cause.[42]

> It is always easier to find a scapegoat than to change the culture of a working environment. But we must find the resources and muster the personal resolve to look at what we do in a systematic way, prospectively as well as retrospectively, expecting errors and developing non-blaming mechanisms for preventing them.[43]

---

29 Waxman (1987)

30 Curran (1987)

31 For example, US Supreme Court decision: Patrick v. Burget 108 S. Ct. 1,658 (1988) 486 U.S. 94 http://caselaw.lp.findlaw.com/scripts/getcase.pl?court=US&vol=486&invol=94 (accessed 8 October 2006).

32 British Medical Association, evidence to Royal Commission on the National Health Service 1977, cited in Hoffenberg (1987) p.92

33 Lister (1986)

34 Stern (1988)

35 Epstein and Hundert (2002)

36 Hoffenberg (1987) p.95

37 Double (2004)

38 Epstein (1999)

39 Johnston et al (2004)

40 Waite (2005)

41 Baker et al (2004)

42 Department of Health (1999) p.39

43 *CMAJ* editorial (2001)

One of the more profound influences on how we perceive quality of care, how things can go wrong and how we manage them, has been the emergence of an awareness of patient safety as a key issue. Many countries have tackled this in a formal way recently but the themes that emerge are common to all. In Canada,[44] as in the United Kingdom, Australia and the US, recommendations for the establishment of formal patient safety agencies have been accepted and implemented.

The Canadian National Steering Committee on Patient Safety report, *Building a Safer System,* refers to the need to 'Develop and implement responsive patient-focused programs for the receipt, review and management of concerns within health-care organizations',[45] and the need to '...develop a greater focus on improvement through education and remediation, vs blame and punishment, in legal, regulatory and human resource processes'.[46] Amongst the questions that were addressed was 'How can the manner in which the regulation and monitoring of health-care professionals and their institutions, and the legal systems, improve safety?'

One of the recommendations was the rejection of the term 'medical error', being associated with a 'culture of blame',[47] while the overarching conceptual model[48] saw the legal and regulatory processes as one ingredient of an integrated system, which included measurement, evaluation, education and communication. The emphasis was on tackling a legal and regulatory environment that has historically perpetuated fear of blame and litigation[49] rather than being based on continuous monitoring and correction.

There was recognition of the need for an open culture and for resolution as opposed to an adversarial system based on punishment and isolation. The current system does not encourage discussion of issues, due to a perceived burden of 'perfection'. Regulatory bodies are seen to be involved in a search for, and a need to cull 'bad apples'[50] rather than stressing education and remediation. The preferred system is based on continuous improvement and learning and is referred to as a culture of learning and safety[51] in contradistinction to a culture of blame.

Mechanisms for dealing with concerns

Regulatory bodies are still seen as having the responsibility for evaluation, addressing competence and performance and the correction of 'incompetence'.[52] Although restrictions on practice and withdrawal from practice are visualised as possible remedies, the preferred approach is stated to be identification and remedy of underlying problems.

Building a Safer System recognised the potential for devastating consequences to the individual resulting from hearsay or premature conclusions based on inadequate information and urged effective peer review. However in terms of 'non-punitive' reporting, the emphasis would appear to be on the reporter rather than on the reported, which seems unbalanced.

---

44 See the Canadian Patient Safety Institute website: http://www.patientsafetyinstitute.ca/index.html (accessed 10 September 2006).

45 National Steering Committee on Patient Safety (2002)

46 Ibid. viii Recommendation 8

47 Ibid. 7

48 Ibid. 11

49 Ibid. 12

50 Canadian Health Services Research Foundation (2006)

51 National Steering Committee on Patient Safety (2002) 15

52 Ibid. 16

Little is known about the general circumstances under which performance issues have arisen and their outcomes. Rosenthal[53] studied disciplinary procedures in the UK and Sweden from a sociological perspective and found a confusing, inefficient and inconsistent patchwork of formal and informal mechanisms. Although major reforms have been implemented in the UK since Rosenthal's study, there is little data on what effect these have had. Inconsistencies are aggravated by the fact that problems and assessment are handled within two-tier systems that are often poorly integrated and even inconsistent, arising from different legislative initiatives, a lower tier at a hospital or health authority level, and an upper tier at a jurisdictional licensing and regulatory level.

Another difficulty has been that of translating the rhetoric for constructive change into frontline managerial actions, which is essentially a culture change. Thus one finds commitments to change at a regulatory level:

> The College approaches complaints about physicians as problems to be solved. A complaint may provide the opportunity for a physician to change behaviour, or to improve some aspect of practice. In some instances… assessment and retraining may be required. Our experience is that the best outcome happens when the physician is a willing participant in the complaint process.… We prefer to work with the physician to identify the problem and to work towards a solution. We believe that the chances of long-term success with this approach are much higher than if disciplinary action is taken – action that may, in fact, be counter-productive to creating a positive change in physician behaviour.[54]

> We are changing the way the College currently monitors the performance of physicians. Specifically, we are moving from a reactive complaints and discipline model, to one which seeks to better guide the profession and prevent practice problems. The College wants to help physicians before any bad habits become entrenched into daily practice.[55]

The issues are likely to differ depending on clinical context, for instance between primary care and specialist practice and between community practice and academic medicine.

Academic medicine and academic freedom

The issues for academic physicians are a special case. They answer to two masters, hospital and university in an environment where free speech and academic and clinical freedom have been valued rights. The Canadian Association of University Teachers (CAUT) has addressed this issue several times,[56,57] and has a number of recent and ongoing inquiries into specific instances, through its Academic Freedom campaign,[58] a 'Task Force on Academic Freedom for Faculty at University-Affiliated Health Care Institutions', independent committees of enquiry,[59,60] and publications.[61]

---

53 Rosenthal (1995)

54 See the College of Physicians and Surgeons of Alberta website, Complaint Process: http://www.cpsa.ab.ca/complaints/attachments/boundary_complaints.pdf (accessed 10 September 2006).

55 See the College of Physicians and Surgeons of Ontario website, Info-Public, Peer Assessment: http://www.cpso.on.ca/Info_Public/factpeer.htm

56 Canadian Association of University Teachers (2004)

57 Canadian Association of University Teachers (2002)

58 See the Canadian Association of University Teachers website, Issues & Campaigns, Academic Freedom: http://www.caut.ca/en/issues/academicfreedom/default.asp

59 Ibid.

60 Canadian Association of University Teachers (2006)

61 Turk, Kirpalani and Guyatt (2005)

CAUT has noted widespread vulnerability and abuse, and in particular the use of termination and control of revenue to enforce social and academic acquiescence. It has stated that clinical academic staff must have the same rights and privileges as non-clinical academic staff. In particular it noted the need for security in terms of employment and income, and the triple jeopardy faced by the intermingling of university, hospital and practice plan personnel. It also found that disciplinary bylaws usually lack access to natural justice and procedural fairness, in striking contrast to grievance arbitration.

In the UK, a joint committee of the education and health departments has made similar recommendations.[62] They sought more explicit definition of accountability and appraisal given 'the peculiar problems faced by clinical academics who appear to have two posts with separate employers and yet actually have a single professional job.[63] They emphasise the need for a clear, harmonious and consistent framework at all stages of employment from selection and appointment. They stressed the same application to accountability, appraisal, and to the workings of any disciplinary process, noting that 'a clinical academic post is a single job held by a whole person, not two jobs held by two different half persons in one body'.[64]

One of the concerns expressed from the respective priorities of teaching hospitals and universities was that 'there is a very real risk that the pressures of service delivery… and of the delivery of education and research on universities will result in them growing further apart'.[65] The authors noted that 'the lines are traditionally blurred and the priorities interwoven'. However they were very much aware that different facets of the employment responsibility were subject to different lines of accountability.

Appraisal and performance review are at the heart of the document.[66] While there was agreement on a single appraisal process it was felt this should be a joint university/hospital function. With regards to disciplinary procedures,[67] as with appraisal, the emphasis is on managing, helping and remedy, rather than formal discipline. Interestingly, they suggest abandonment of older concepts of personal and professional or personal misconduct, in favour of appraisal of health, conduct and capability. It was envisaged that both parties would be intimately involved in all aspects of the process. The recommendations included the following:[68]

> …that the university and NHS body must establish absolutely clear and documented arrangements for dealing with the management of poor performance and for disciplinary matters of all types… Universities and NHS bodies should jointly prepare a formal agreement on the procedures for the management of poor performance and for discipline to be followed for senior NHS and university staff members with academic and clinical duties. As a minimum, these procedures should ensure joint working in the process from the time implementation of it is first contemplated; specify which body is to take the lead in different types of case; ensure suitable cross membership of disciplinary bodies; and be expeditious.

62 Follett and Paulson-Ellis (2001)
63 Ibid. p.6
64 Ibid. p.8
65 Ibid. p.10
66 Ibid. p.15
67 Ibid. p.19
68 Ibid. p.20

As a result of this the Department of Health developed a separate framework for academic clinical staff,[69] which essentially recognised the rights of both parties (universities and hospitals) to be engaged in any proceedings against a member of the staff.

A framework for reform

Only the UK has made a serious attempt to completely overhaul the mechanisms for dealing with performance issues amongst clinical staff following a series of well-publicised events and inquiries,[70,71,72,73] the intervention of a House of Commons committee[74] and internal reports describing the inadequacies of the existing system.[75,76] Liam Donaldson, then a Regional Medical Officer, and who was shortly to be appointed Chief Medical Officer, described the experiences of his own region, which rarely used formal mechanisms, and pointed to proposals for General Medical Council reform designed to shift the emphasis from punishment to remedy.[77] Criticism was mounting from a number of sources including the Society of Clinical Psychiatrists which produced a series of reports from 1990, describing the existing system as 'shocking' and 'a blot'.[78] Their data showed that less than a third of cases involved allegations of professional incompetence and that only 10 per cent of allegations were found to be justified. They commented on the severe health problems, including death, that resulted from suspensions.[79]

Although continually evolving since 1999,[80,81,82,83,84,85,86] a new framework only came into full operation in 2005, and it is therefore probably too soon to fully assess its effects although clearly it requires careful monitoring and evaluation. Philosophically it represents a major frame shift from a system based on concerns about individual performance to recognition of chronic system failures.

---

69 Department of Health (2005) 'Guidance on clinical academics' p.53

70 Savage (1986)

71 Donaldson (2003)

72 Smith (1998)

73 Kennedy (2001)

74 Public Accounts Committee (1995)

75 Donaldson and Cavanagh (1992)

76 Donaldson (1994)

77 General Medical Council (1992)

78 See the Society of Clinical Psychiatrists (SCP) website, Suspended Doctors Group: http://www.scpnet.com/Suspend.htm (accessed 10 September 2006).

79 Tomlin (1998)

80 Department of Health (1999)

81 Scottish Office, Department of Health (1999)

82 See 'Assuring the Quality of Medical Practice', a summary of the responses to Department of Health (1999), on the DoH website: http://www.dh.gov.uk/Consultations/ResponsesToConsultations/ResponsesToConsultationsDocumentSummary/fs/en?CONTENT_ID=4103036&chk=TGBDUb (accessed 10 September 2006).

83 Department of Health (2001)

84 See 'Doctors and dentists: discipline and suspension', Department of Health 2003–5, on the DoH website: http://www.dh.gov.uk/PolicyAndGuidance/HumanResourcesAndTraining/ModernisingProfessionalRegulation/DoctorsAndDentistsDisciplinaryFramework/fs/en (accessed 10 September 2006).

85 Department of Health (2005)

86 Ibid. Introduction and key changes

> Nevertheless, sometimes the failure may not be wholly attributable to one individual but may be symptomatic of organisational malaise. In determining remedial action, organisational factors need to be taken into account.[87]

A new system would need to be 'supportive and preventive', be proactive rather than reactive, and create a culture of prevention, recognition, and correction as 'an alternative to disciplinary action'. In criticising previous systems the framework noted the need to avoid precipitous actions, to utilise assessment at a distance and to be beware of the potential for abuse. It cautioned against those who seek to create inaccurate scenarios and those who saw performance issues as 'punishable offences', since 'the opportunity for re-education or improvement is then often permanently lost.'

For the first time, evidence-based best practices were utilised incorporating human resources principles such as appraisal.[88,89]

> Appraisal is a positive process to give someone feedback on their performance, to chart their continuing progress and to identify development needs. It is a forward-looking process essential for the developmental and educational planning needs of an individual. Assessment is the process of measuring progress against defined criteria… It is not the primary aim of appraisal to scrutinise doctors to see if they are performing poorly but rather to help them consolidate and improve on good performance aiming towards excellence.[90]

Assessment

This has necessitated establishing mechanisms for such management, such as the National Clinical Assessment Service (NCAS),[91] now appropriately part of the National Patient Safety Agency. Furthermore, to protect physicians, a provision was included whereby a doctor would be able to seek the assistance of the Authority in situations where they were concerned that they were 'the target of unjustified allegations'. A strong motivation was to reduce the incidence and frequency of suspensions (which it proposed renaming 'exclusions'), and legal involvement, for which the health system had been severely criticised.

> [The] Authority will endeavour to provide the doctor with a supportive environment … The focus will be very much on problem-solving, and where a problem with the doctor's performance is found, …answering the question 'what practical steps need to be taken so that this doctor can return to practice without risk to patients?'[92]

Systematic performance assessment entails establishment of good principles of management and systems. All too often, innovations or failures occur in system silos, without the ability to learn across the entire system.[93]

---

87 Department of Health (1999) p.19

88 See 'Appraisal for Doctors' on the NHS Clinical Governance Support Team website: http://www.appraisalsupport.nhs.uk/ (accessed 10 September 2006).

89 NHS Clinical Governance Support Team (2005)

90 Ibid. 59

91 National Patient Safety Agency. National Clinical Assessment Service. http://www.ncas.nhs.uk

92 Department of Health (2001) p.21

93 Degeling et al (2004)

> Tackling the blame culture – recognising that most failures in standards of care are caused by systems' weaknesses not individuals per se.[94,95]

> [NCAS involvement is to] recognise the problem as being more to do with work systems than doctor performance, or see a wider problem needing the involvement of an outside body.[96]

In a learning culture neither clinical nor management decisions can be based on opinion alone, and again, the potential for abuse was a central theme.

> Unfounded and malicious allegations can cause lasting damage to a doctor's reputation and career prospects. Therefore all allegations, including those made by relatives of patients, or concerns raised by colleagues, must be properly investigated to verify the facts so that the allegations can be shown to be true or false.[97]

Cultures of excellence not only value their workforce but let them know they are valued.[98]

> The focus is on helping doctors and dentists to keep up to date and to practice safely, not to punish them for any problems with clinical performance.[99]

In its 2004 Annual Report,[100] the NCAS stated that only 6 per cent of referrals required assessments, in 30 per cent of exclusions there was no basis, and measures undertaken included providing support to overworked doctors, helping with interpersonal skills, improving management support of physicians, and improving recognised training deficiencies. In the most recent statistics available, based on 1,772 cases,[101] referrals appear to be increasing, being at the level of about 1:120 practitioners. The overall approach taken is one of getting people back to work, and resolving differences.[102]

To carry out its stated functions, it was necessary to develop a toolkit for preventing and assessing performance concerns.[103] This provided both the evidence for best practice interactions,[104] as well as tools for management in handling performance concerns or allegations. The emphasis is on assessment as a learning exercise and how sound human resources practices result in improved clinical outcomes. As indicated earlier, health professionals today largely work in teams and within systems; performance improvement thus becomes a collective responsibility and exercise.

Better understanding of the factors affecting performance, and perceptions of performance leads to better management. Within this framework it becomes apparent that often performance problems:

---

94 Note: It is important to realise that moving away from *blame* does not mean abandoning *accountability*, which is a separate issue.

95 Department of Health (2005) Introduction and explanatory note, p.5

96 Ibid. I: Action when a concern arises, p.10

97 Ibid. I: Action when a concern arises, p.8

98 Kanter (1984)

99 Department of Health (2003)

100 NCAA (2004)

101 NCAS (2006a)

102 NCAS (2006b)

103 NCAS (2006c)

104 Csikszentmihalyi (1997)

> …have their origins simply in a clash of values between manager and clinician.
>
> Differences in work style are normally expected by colleagues and tolerated. But sometimes a different style will attract criticism and come to be seen as a sign of poor performance. If the person first categorising performance as poor is influential, then others may take the same view.
>
> Bullying can easily arise when people are intolerant and there is weak leadership. There is a large literature on bullying amongst health professionals, though this probably reflects growing awareness rather than increased occurrence… personality typing (perfectionism, self-criticism) also throws light on how colleague relationships can derail into victimisation and allegations of bullying when dominant or preferred work styles clash.[105]

This can often be unconscious. For instance an individual's enthusiasm can often make people around such a person feel demoralised. Furthermore, even when performance issues are established, good stewardship of human resources is appreciative of both humanity and efficiency:

> People with skills are expensive to replace. It makes sense to try to rebuild a career rather than scrapping probably still useful experience, skills and knowledge. 'Rebuilding' accommodates many possibilities – rebuilding a career path, trust, a working relationship or a pattern of clinical practice. A suitable and effective performance solution might need all four.[106]

However, changing a culture can be very challenging[107] and the difficulties are usually severely underestimated. In the most recent iteration of the Department of Health's attempts at reform, released in July 2006, appears this sobering statement (emphasis added):

> …it was clear that there was something of a climate of fear and retribution, so that any lapse in performance or simple human error was seen as punishable by suspension, disciplinary action and referral to the General Medical Council. **This remains the case today**.[108]

Discipline

It is unfortunate that disciplinary committees are often confused with committees of enquiry. The latter are supposed to be impartial bodies, predominantly concerned with enquiry into the truth and making recommendations without a specific presumption of blame. In contrast, the former represent a concept originally derived from the military, and can be defined as punishment intended to correct or train, or to be a deterrent.

Although the NHS framework recognises that disciplinary measures should only be used as a last resort, even then it bases these on the code of practice of the Advisory, Conciliation and Arbitration Service (ACAS)[109,110] in stating, inter alia:

---

105 NCAS (2006c) 'Investigating', subsection 8. http://www.ncas.nhs.uk/toolkit/investigating?contentId=2957&type=principle

106 NCAS (2006c) 'Rebuilding'. http://www.ncas.nhs.uk/toolkit/rebuilding

107 Scott et al (2003)

108 Department of Health (2006)

109 http://www.acas.org.uk

110 ACAS (2003) 'Core Principles of Reasonable Behaviour', p.6

> Use procedures primarily to help and encourage employees to improve rather than just as a way of imposing a punishment… Make sure that disciplinary action is not taken until the facts of the case have been established and that the action is reasonable in the circumstances… Where there appears to be serious misconduct, or risk to property or other people, a period of suspension with pay should be considered while the case is being investigated. This allows tempers to cool and hasty action to be avoided… any period of suspension should be as short as possible… Do not use suspension as a sanction before the disciplinary meeting and decision and treat employees fairly and consistently… Seek an external review if a disciplinary case is not concluded within [six] months… Recognise that events can move on and that formal disciplinary action, while initially appearing appropriate, may cease to be right. An alternative way of bringing the case to resolution must then be actively sought and found.

Given that many concerns in the health care workplace arise from interpersonal relationships and differences of opinion in areas of professional work steeped in uncertainty, disciplinary procedures are extraordinarily unsuited for dealing with these issues, which frequently escalate in classical conflict dynamics. Much of the literature around conflict deals with the roles of leadership and organisational culture.[111]

Organisational ethics: a Canadian case study

Given also that health care workplaces are usually relatively devoid of mechanisms to prevent and deal with these issues, it is all too tempting to inappropriately resort to extant disciplinary mechanisms with disastrous consequences. In one well-known long-running dispute in a Canadian teaching hospital,[112] the Health Authority's own internal Organizational Ethics Committee[113] expressed alarm at the ease with which this could happen, leading to insoluble conflict and widespread deleterious effects on morale.

> Indeed recent physician disciplinary proceedings have contributed to a culture of mistrust, insecurity, and even antagonism for a number of physicians and persons in administration and management roles.

This ethical analysis finds resonance with many of the issues derived empirically from management and conflict theory, human resources, and occupational psychology. The report noted that the situation that had arisen was:

> A clear marker for how fractured and distrustful some of these relationships have become…
>
> It is important that examination of due process and good governance with respect to physician discipline extends beyond the disciplinary bylaws. This issue includes mechanisms and processes available… for addressing problems with individual physicians in terms of patient care, teaching, research, and/or leadership. It also includes mechanisms and processes available to physicians to express grievances or concerns.
>
> These mechanisms and processes should be available to all early on when a dispute or question related to practice is identified and should offer less formal, less adversarial means for resolving and addressing what is at issue.

---

111 Wenzel (1986)

112 See CAUT, Issues & Campaigns, Academic Freedom, Gabrielle Horne at http://www.caut.ca/en/issues/academicfreedom/gabriellehorne.asp (accessed 10 September 2006).

113 Capital Health Ethics Committee (2005)

They describe the:

> ...stress, anxiety, and discomfort experienced by all involved parties when the bylaw process is initiated... which processes... can take on a life of their own in practice.
>
> The disciplinary bylaws should only be invoked or utilised in situations where physicians are doing (or not doing) something that has a *direct* impact on patient safety. [emphasis added]

Given the lack of resources for resolving differences of opinion or practice, the report noted how easy it was for issues to:

> ...escalate and be inappropriately framed as patient safety-related for lack of other suitable alternative mechanisms... the perception, and fear, is that the demand for accountability is a way in which to, in some cases inappropriately control these individuals.
>
> 'Disruptive physicians' – this label may be utilised as a mechanism for shutting out physicians who raise questions and challenge how things are done.

Unfortunately, despite these concerns and the issues raised, the dispute has continued since 2002 into the fifth year, despite an independent peer review by the Medical Staff Association that found no grounds for the actions taken.[114]

Summary

Appropriate understanding of human performance, the root causes of conflict, and human resources expertise have come slowly to health care, where reaction to public concerns about patient safety have been perceived as difficult to balance against employee rights, and the need for a healthy and safe workplace. Unfortunately this is ultimately counter-productive, and runs contrary to safety theory, since low staff morale ultimately leads to impaired delivery of services.[115]

Ultimately, disciplinary procedures should form a very small part of a comprehensive patient safety and continuous quality improvement orientated health care system. Ideally a system based on an open culture and improvement should not require a disciplinary component. Better understanding of human performance within systems leads to approaches that clearly identify conduct, capability, competence and collegiality issues, rather than an omnibus approach to workplace issues. Disciplinary procedures tend to be self-defeating, inefficient and ineffective, and are frequently misused.[116,117] They are required only as short-term emergency measures, and as a last resort, and careful attention to alternative measures should always be considered, preferably with the involvement of external expertise, not vested in the procedures and issues at hand. Organisations that are conflict aware and have built in resources for constructively managing conflict, perform most effectively.[118]

In the words of the Scottish Health Department in its approach to these issues, 'prevention [is] better than cure'.[119]

---

114 Sullivan et al (2005)
115 Marshall and Robson (2005)
116 Dearlove (2004)
117 Connor and Pearson (1989)
118 Robson and Marshall (2003)
119 Scottish Executive (2001)

References

ACAS (2003) *ACAS Code of Practice 1: Disciplinary and Grievance Procedures 2003.* Norwich: TSO. http://www.acas.org.uk/media/pdf/l/p/CP01_1.pdf (accessed 10 September 2006).

Baker GR, Norton PG, Flintoft V, Blais R, Brown A, Cox J, Etchells E, Ghali WA, Hebert P, Majumdar SR, O'Beirne M, Palacios-Derflingher L, Reid RJ, Sheps S and Tamblyn R (2004) 'The Canadian Adverse Events Study: The incidence of adverse events among hospital patients in Canada', *CMAJ*, 25 May 2004, 170(11): 1,678–86.

Berwick DM (1989) 'Continuous improvement as an ideal in health care', *N Engl J Med*, 5 January 1989, 320(1):53–6.

Berwick D (2005) '"A deficiency of will and ambition": a conversation with Donald Berwick', interview by Robert Galvin, *Health Aff* (Millwood), January–June 2005, Suppl Web Exclusives: W5-1-W5-9.

Canadian Association of University Teachers (2002) 'Policy Statement on Academic Appointments Held Jointly in a University and a Related Institution'. http://www.caut.ca/en/policies/jointappointments.asp (accessed 10 September 2006).

Canadian Association of University Teachers (2004) 'Defending Medicine: Clinical faculty and academic freedom'. http://www.caut.ca/en/issues/academicfreedom/DefendingMedicine.pdf (accessed 10 September 2006).

Canadian Association of University Teachers (2006) 'September 2006 CAUT Inquiry at Ottawa U', *Bulletin Online*. http://www.caut.ca/en/bulletin/issues/2006_sep/default.asp (accessed 10 September 2006).

Canadian Health Services Research Foundation (2006) 'We can eliminate errors in health care by getting rid of the "bad apples"', *J Health Serv Res Policy*, January 2006, 11(1):63–4.

Capital Health Ethics Committee (2005) 'Organizational Ethics Consultation Report. Organizational Ethics Consultation 2004-02. *Due Process and Good Governance*', May 2005. http://myweb.dal.ca/mgoodyea/files/organizationalethicsconsultationreport.doc

Checkland K, Marshall M and Harrison S (2004) 'Re-thinking accountability: trust versus confidence in medical practice', *Qual Saf Health Care*, April 2004, 13(2):130–5.

CMAJ editorial (2001) 'Error and blame: The Winnipeg inquest', *CMAJ*, 27 November 2001, 165(11):1,461, 3.

Cochrane AL (1971) *Effectiveness and efficiency: random reflections on health services.* London: Nuffield Provincial Hospitals Trust.

Connor GW and Pearson RG (1989) 'Use and abuse of summary suspension in medical staff disputes', *QRC Advis*, January 1989, 5(3):1, 4–6.

Csikszentmihalyi M (1997) *Finding Flow: The Psychology of Engagement with Everyday Life.* New York: Perseus.

Curran WJ (1987) 'Medical peer review of physician competence and performance. Legal immunity and the antitrust laws', *NEJM*, 316: 597–8.

Dearlove OR (2004) 'Suspension of doctors: GMC may be ultimate sacrifice', *BMJ*, 20 March 2004, 328(7441):709.

Degeling PJ, Maxwell S, Iedema R and Hunter DJ (2004) 'Making clinical governance work', *BMJ*, 18 September 2004, 329(7467):679–81.

Department of Health (1999) *Supporting Doctors, Protecting Patients*. London: Department of Health.
http://www.dh.gov.uk/PublicationsAndStatistics/Publications/PublicationsPolicyAndGuidance/PublicationsPolicyAndGuidanceArticle/fs/en?CONTENT_ID=4005688&chk=RXR/Rx (accessed 10 September 2006).

Department of Health (2001) *Assuring the quality of medical practice: Implementing 'Supporting doctors protecting patients'*. http://www.dh.gov.uk/assetRoot/04/08/46/19/04084619.pdf (accessed 10 September 2006).

Department of Health (2003) 'New framework for discipline and suspension – Joint statement of agreed principles'. http://www.dh.gov.uk/assetRoot/04/06/99/57/04069957.PDF (accessed 6 October 2006).

Department of Health (2005) *Maintaining high professional standards in the modern NHS.* http://www.dh.gov.uk/assetRoot/04/10/33/44/04103344.pdf (accessed 10 September 2006).

Department of Health (2006) *Good doctors, safer patients: Proposals to strengthen the system to assure and improve the performance of doctors and to protect the safety of patients*. A report by the Chief Medical Officer. http://www.dh.gov.uk/PublicationsAndStatistics/Publications/PublicationsPolicyAndGuidance/PublicationsPolicyAndGuidanceArticle/fs/en?CONTENT_ID=4137232&chk=KW63va (accessed 10 September 2006).

Dewar S and Finlayson B (2001) 'Dealing with poor clinical performance', *BMJ*, 13 January 2001, 322(7278):66.

Donaldson LJ (1994) 'Doctors with problems in an NHS workforce', *BMJ*, 1994, 308: 1277–82.

Donaldson LJ (2001) 'Professional accountability in a changing world', *Postgrad Med J,* February 2001, 77(904):65–7.

Donaldson LJ (2003) 'Commentary: The Doctor's Dilemma: A response', *Int J Epidemiol*, December 2003, 32(6): 915–16.

Donaldson LJ and Cavanagh J (1992) 'Clinical complaints and their handling: a time for change?' *Qual Health Care,* March 1992, 1(1):21–5.

Double DB (2004) 'Suspension of doctors: medical suspensions may have ideological nature', *BMJ*, 20 March 2004, 328(7441):709–10.

Drife JO (1987) 'Consultant accountability', *Brit Med J* (Clin Res Ed), 28 March 1987, 294(6575):789–90.

Duncan A (1980) 'Quality assurance: what now and where next', *Brit Med J*, 280: 300–2.

Elwyn G (2006) 'Dame Janet's disappointments', *Brit Med J*, 13 May 2006, 332: 1,161.

Emmet D (1970) *Rules, roles and relations*. London: Macmillan and Co Ltd.

Epstein RM (1999) 'Mindful practice', *JAMA*, 1 September 1999, 282(9):833–9.

Epstein RM and Hundert EM (2002) 'Defining and assessing professional competence', *JAMA*, 9 January 2002, 287(2):226–35.

Follett B and Paulson-Ellis M (2001) 'A Review of Appraisal, Disciplinary and Reporting Arrangements for Senior NHS and University Staff with Academic and Clinical Duties: A report to the Secretary of State for Education and Skills, September 2001'. http://www.dfes.gov.uk/follettreview/ (accessed 10 September 2006).

General Medical Council (1992) *Proposals for new performance procedures: a consultation paper*. London: GMC.

Goldman RL (1992) 'The reliability of peer assessments of quality of care', *JAMA*, 267: 958–60.

Hoffenberg R (1987) *Clinical Freedom: The Rock Carling Fellowship Lecture 1986.* London: Nuffield Provincial Hospitals Trust.

Iglehart JK (1987) 'Congress moves to bolster peer review: The Health Care Quality Improvement Act of 1986', *NEJM*, 316: 960–4.

Johnston RV, Boiteau P, Charlebois K, Long S and U D (2004) 'Responding to tragic error: Lessons from Foothills Medical Centre', *CMAJ*, 25 May 2004, 170(11):1,659–60.

Kanter R (1984) *The change masters*. London: Allen and Unwin.

Kennedy I (2001) *Learning from Bristol: the Report of the Public Inquiry into Children's Heart Surgery at the Bristol Royal Infirmary 1984–1995.* Cm 5207. London: The Stationery Office. http://www.dh.gov.uk/PublicationsAndStatistics/Publications/PublicationsPolicyAndGuidance/PublicationsPolicyAndGuidanceArticle/fs/en?CONTENT_ID=4009387&chk=LnDPof (accessed 10 September 2006).

Lister J (1986) 'The Politics of Medicine in Britain and the United States', *NEJM*, 315: 168–74.

Marshall P and Robson R (2005) 'Preventing and managing conflict: vital pieces in the patient safety puzzle', *Healthc Q*, 2005, 8 Spec No:39–44.

McLachlan G (ed) (1976) *A question of quality? Roads to assurance in medical care.* Oxford: Oxford University Press.

National Steering Committee on Patient Safety (2002) *Building a Safer System*. Ottawa: National Steering Committee on Patient Safety.
http://rcpsc.medical.org/publications/building_a_safer_system_e.pdf (accessed 10 September 2006).

Naylor CD (2002) 'Public profiling of clinical performance', *JAMA*, 287(10): 1,323–5.

NCAA (2004) *NCAA Annual Report and Summary Financial Statements 2003–4.*
http://www.ncas.nhs.uk/site/media/documents/1241_English_Annual_Report2003-04.pdf (accessed 10 September 2006).

NCAS (2006a) *NCAS Analysis of the First Four Years' Referral Data*.
http://www.ncas.nhs.uk/site/media/documents/1424_NCAS_First_Four_Years.pdf (accessed 10 September 2006).

NCAS (2006b) *BACK ON TRACK: Restoring doctors and dentists to safe professional practice. Framework Document.* October 2006.
http://www.ncas.npsa.nhs.uk/site/media/documents/1506_Framework.pdf (accessed 6 October 2006).

NCAS (2006c) 'NCAS Toolkit'. http://www.ncas.nhs.uk/toolkit/ (accessed 10 September 2006).

NHS Clinical Governance Support Team (2005) *Assuring the Quality of Medical Appraisal*.
http://www.appraisalsupport.nhs.uk/files2/Assuring_the_Quality_of_Medical_Appraisal.pdf (accessed 10 September 2006).

Poloniecki J (1998) 'Half of all doctors are below average', *BMJ*, 6 June 1998, 316(7146):1,734–6.

Public Accounts Committee (1995) 'Suspension of Dr O'Connell' The 40th report of the Committee of Public Accounts, session 1994–5. HC 322.

Robson P and Marshall P (2003) 'Using dispute resolution to resolve health care conflicts: An essential tool in hospital risk management', *Risk Management in Canadian Health Care*, January 2003, 4(7): 73–81.

Rosenthal MM (1995) *The incompetent doctor: behind closed doors*. Buckingham: Open University Press.

Savage W (1986) *A Savage Enquiry: Who Controls Childbirth?* London: Virago.

Scott T, Mannion R, Davies HT and Marshall MN (2003) 'Implementing culture change in health care: theory and practice', *Int J Qual Health Care,* April 2003, 15(2):111–18.

Scottish Executive (2001) 'Prevention Better Than Cure – Ensuring Safer Patients and Better Doctors'. Human Resources Directorate, Health Department.
http://www.show.scot.nhs.uk/sehd/mels/HDL2001_60.htm (accessed 10 September 2006).

Scottish Office, Department of Health (1999) 'Suspensions – a new perspective: Report of the short-life working group on suspension of medical and dental staff'. Circular PCS(DD)1999/7, 6 April 1999.

Shaw GB (1946) *The Doctor's Dilemma*. New York: Penguin.

Smith J (2004) *Safeguarding patients: lessons from the past — proposals for the future.* Command Paper Cm 6,394, 9 December 2004. London (UK): The Shipman Inquiry. http://www.the-shipman-inquiry.org.uk/fifthreport.asp (accessed 10 September 2006).

Smith R (1998) 'All changed, changed utterly. British medicine will be transformed by the Bristol case', *BMJ*, 27 June 1998, 316(7149):1,917–8.

Stern DT (1988) 'Practicing what we preach? An analysis of the curriculum of values in medical education', *Am J Med*, June 1988, 104: 569–75.

Sullivan JA, Yabsley R, Gray J and Janigan D (2005) *Report of the Peer Review Committee,* 12 December 2005. http://myweb.dal.ca/mgoodyea/files/reportofthepeerreviewcommittee.pdf (accessed 14 September 2006).

Tomlin PJ (1998) 'Society of Clinical Psychiatrists supports doctors who have been suspended', *BMJ*, 1998, 317: 811–12.

Turk J, Kirpalani H and Guyatt GH (2005) 'Has the corporatization of Canadian healthcare affected academic freedom?' *Royal College Outlook*, 2005 1(4): 14–16.

Van't Hoff W (1985) 'Audit reviewed: Medical audit in North America', *J Roy Coll Phys*, 19: 53–5.

Waite M (2005) 'To tell the truth: The ethical and legal implications of disclosure of medical error', *Health Law Journal*, 13:1–33.

Waxman HA (1987) 'Medical malpractice and quality of care', *NEJM*, 316: 943–4.

Wenzel FJ (1986) 'Conflict: an imperative for success', *J Med Pract Manage*, April 1986, 1(4):252–9.

Appendix

For more detailed discussion of some of the above issues, see:

Working Papers

Goodyear M (2005) 'Assessing the Quality and Appropriateness of Care'. http://myweb.dal.ca/mgoodyea/files/Assessingthequalityandappropriatenessofcarev2.doc

Goodyear M (2006) 'The Management of Concerns within Health Care Systems in the Context of Total Quality Management'. http://myweb.dal.ca/mgoodyea/files/concernsinhealthcare.doc

Goodyear M (2006) 'Effective Team Functioning in Health Care: A keystone of patient safety'. http://myweb.dal.ca/mgoodyea/files/teamfunction.doc

Goodyear M (2006) 'Conflict Management in Health Care Teams: A new paradigm – Safer care: Saving costs'. http://myweb.dal.ca/mgoodyea/files/conflict.doc

Publications

Goodyear M (2005) 'Physician, regulate thyself!' *CMAJ*, 30 August 2005, 173(5):465. http://www.cmaj.ca/cgi/content/full/173/5/465-a

A Personal Account of Suspension in the Twenty-first Century

Anonymous Surgeon

I am a consultant surgeon and had been in post for nearly ten years when I was summarily suspended from duty. Here are the facts: very serious allegations of both professional and behavioural misconduct were made against me by three of my immediate colleagues, all consultant surgeons. Independent assessment of the allegations was obstructed for nine months on the advice of the medical director. However, once due process was applied, it was judged that none of the concerns raised was justified and no re-training was necessary before I could resume full practice. In all, the work exclusion lasted 14 months. I then returned to full duties, working alongside my accusers, after a six-week 'running-in' period off site.

Well, that was easy. As a surgeon, I'm used to distilling hard facts and summarising and weighting the relative importance of issues, often from a morass of superfluous detail and emotional overlay. Writing the rest of this will be rather more difficult though. Some may see what follows as self-indulgent. I believe that by cutting the detail and emotion from actions such as these, we lose insight into the reason why so many doctors who go through an exclusion never return to work. It also accounts for why the majority of doctors without experience of suspension are unable to understand quite how devastating it is. I have never before written about what it was actually like. I have certainly done more confidential reports than I care to count on the events of the last few years – time lines of events for legal purposes, responses to allegations, defence of my actions to the GMC after subsequent malicious referral. I don't have to write this one and I'm not writing this for managers or lawyers or any professional bodies. I suppose I am writing this for myself. I am not going to be able to maintain detachment and I know I will have to revisit some of my darkest times. I have put off writing this for months, wrestling with the prospect. However, tonight is a good time, and it feels right that I do this now. It's time to move on. Don't misunderstand me, I will never forget, but it is now time to gather all the remaining baggage from this incident – the bits that I can't jettison, and try to move forward and regain some of my former strength: a catharsis, if you like.

It is now two and a half years since the assault. I look back on that period sometimes with bitterness, usually with anger, often with sorrow and occasionally with pride. I have been back at work for 15 months, working alongside my accusers, and while many acts have already been played in this drama in which I've been given the starring role, sadly, I believe that the finale has yet to come. That said, it seems I will have at least some control over plot direction for many of the final scenes, a very hard won right that won't necessarily turn this tragedy into a comedy. It has been a saga of wickedness, outright lies, power plays, discrimination, professional jealousy, wasted NHS resources, managerial incompetence, and at the root of it all, one doctor's lifestyle issues, flawed personality and ill health. I am angry at the cost of what amounts to criminal behaviour by medical colleagues, coupled with a lack of clinical governance and managerial accountability that should not be possible in a publicly funded health care organisation.

I am still in no position to divulge details of this sordid tale. Perhaps one day I will be (if nothing else, accurate and detailed diary keeping has given me a sense of purpose while riding the roller-coaster of a lengthy work-exclusion and the events that follow). However, what I can do now is to give some insight into how and why a doctor might so easily pass through the looking glass into a bizarre world of counter-intuition where principles are traded for political expediency. Where you might be surprised at who your friends turn out to be, and see allegiances switch seamlessly with a magician's sleight of hand. Where complete strangers can save your professional life (and in so doing, make you examine beliefs you've held since childhood). Where you obsess about other's motives and question your own sanity under the sheer weight of malice, lies and harassment. Where you are incredulous at the double standards and blatant discrimination. Where very senior managers have such confidence in your professional downfall that it obviates the need for accountability. Where you adapt or die, but must keep your core principles for survival to be worthwhile. Where you find the true meaning of support – if you don't know what it is, you've never really needed it. Where key people within the profession contribute to your recovery in ways that you will never be able to repay. Where you consider all the people who kept you going through the long, darkest time, helping you strategize, making you focus, stopping you drifting, making you strong enough to come through both the catastrophe itself and its difficult aftermath.

As I write, the clock strikes midnight on New Year's Eve. (A bit sad, you might think, but I'm comfortable with it.) My partner and nine-year-old son have already gone upstairs, my frail mother-in-law sleeps next door, but they know that I am starting to return to them after a significant absence. As a new year begins, I still sense the shadow of injustice nearby, but I draw strength knowing what I have come through. Coming as I do from an ethnic minority, working class background, achieving my childhood ambition to become a surgeon was a very remote possibility when it formed at the age of five. So while I do not take risks recklessly, I know I can play a long game in life and win because I've done it before.

The devastation that an incident of malicious accusation causes cannot be overestimated – to the health and welfare of the individual, their family, and the patients whose care is at the very least disrupted, and at worst irreparably damaged. It is particularly distressing when that accusation comes from within the profession. For this reason (as well as the more obvious need for public safety), it is crucial that local systems of clinical governance are in safe hands. I say to those whom I hope will never personally experience such a crisis, that the full range of human behaviour is within us all, doctors included. I understand that similar acts of corrupt governance occur from time to time among doctors in other regions, but it doesn't seem to have a name and it isn't spoken of openly. Perhaps I was naïve or just ignorant, but I'd not been aware of this kind of phenomenon before it happened to me. To me, there appear to be parallels between actions like these and the way the crime of rape has been viewed down the years. Clinical governance crimes like these between doctors are about power, not the protection of patients. It is not something that we are comfortable discussing, and it taints all it touches. There are long-term repercussions for the victim of such an attack and a common mind-set among casual observers is that the victim was asking for it.

I think I know what every one of you is thinking. Some will feel 'there but for the grace of God go I'. One or two will nod knowingly, able to predict what happens next with surprising accuracy, having seen it all before (either from the pitch or the stands). Many, however, will believe one or more of the following: 'no smoke without fire', 'we don't know all the facts', 'if negligence is disproved, this is about a breakdown in relationships, which is always 50–50', 'surely there has to be an inherent problem with a doctor who is suspended – even if there's nothing wrong with their clinical performance'. A few will think 'couldn't happen in my shop', and many will be ambivalent – 'don't tell me any more'. And I can understand all of these views, even if nice people wouldn't admit to many of them. And that is because they were probably my own, right up until 3pm on Wednesday 16 July 2003.

I was in the middle of a clinic – single-handed. Many grateful patients returning for follow-up, challenging new referrals still to come. My trusty clinical nurse specialist by my side, keeping the clinic's wheels greased, keeping reasonably to time and under control – then a knock on the door. Instead of the next patient, my clinical director – an affable lad, in post for two or three years. My houseman from long ago, when I had been his registrar. Now a consultant urologist, made clinical director of an infamously dysfunctional department of surgery by a desperate hospital management only a few months earlier. An inexperienced consultant, an inexperienced manager, a deliverer of messages. Slightly embarrassed, unsure of the protocol – so sorry to interrupt, could he have a word? Neither foe nor friend, just a man with a message. And what a message! Just three of us in the room: don't see any more patients, don't touch any more case records, the medical director is on his way to the hospital to suspend you.

A potent mix of emotion washes over me, leaving a physical aftermath: horror, shock, grief, panic, shame, terror, isolation and desperation. Nausea, deep, deep pain somewhere inside and uncontrollable tremor. As I'm led away in an almost dream-like state with clinic nurses and waiting patients looking on, I'm thinking 'contact' – who do I need to tell; who do I need? My colleague reassures me that she will deal with the remainder of the clinic patients. A momentary wry thought – after the battles I'd had single-handedly getting this nurse's extended role recognised and ratified for counselling, out-patient cancer follow-up, theatre assistance and flexible sigmoidoscopy. Months of protocol writing and exhaustive training were followed by departmental opposition then procrastination. And here was my clinical director apparently happy to let her see 'new' outpatient surgical referrals on her own without any specific training or assessment (presumably, the thought of a riot in the clinic waiting room swings it). I know she'll cope brilliantly and the irony evokes a harsh laugh. But what I hear sounds tainted by bitterness, the humour transient. And anyway, there is no-one I feel like sharing the joke with. So it dies, as many things I took for granted did that day.

I phone a surgical colleague who does well, calmly dispensing sensible and practical advice from 20 miles away. A nagging feeling – I think I can hear disbelief and uncertainly creeping into the conversation. It worries me, but then on momentary reflection I think it would worry me more if it wasn't there. And no wonder, because no other surgeon has been stopped working in these circumstances before in the region. I phone another colleague within the hospital. Soothing and reassuring, she'll join me soon.

I make my way to the venue where the really scary stuff starts. It's just a short walk from my clinic and miles away from the administrative offices and I pass an open doorway which leads into a small meeting room. No light is on, but sitting casually on the desk, almost by chance, is the general manager. It seems that I'm a little early for my own funeral. It is as though he has just been made aware of a flying visit by royalty (or a gathering lynch mob), and I am to be hastily briefed for an audience with the VIPs (or persuaded to acquiesce gracefully). Except he doesn't know how to prepare me because he's never been party to anything quite like this before. There is a heady atmosphere of apprehension and wariness and possibly something else... could it be shame or guilt, perhaps? I enter the room alone and I look this man in the eye and I still cannot believe this is happening. I have always made the greatest effort, gone the extra mile, been meticulous in my work – how can this be happening to me? I can feel hysteria coming on because I have told this man of impending serious jeopardy before and have been deflected, wrong-footed, fobbed off, put down and blind-sided albeit quite politely, such that I realise that until this moment I had presumed a greater insight and wisdom on his part, while in reality, he just wanted to bury bad news. Anger bites as I realise the heavy price I am about to pay for his determination to ignore the blindingly obvious and my explicit warning of it over the years. But perhaps all this is unfair on him… after all, his role within the organisation is probably that of messenger and here I am, lining up my sights. Not in a proactive, sanctimonious or hectoring way have I told him of serious problems with a colleague, but only when I've been obliged to: perhaps two or three occasions in five years. Like when a patient alleged that he was unfit to practise while on-call, which I handled precisely in accordance with GMC recommendations and defence society advice.

Except, on reflection, that isn't quite true. After all, I didn't follow *all* the advice of my defence society. The medico-legal adviser I had consulted two years previously about a colleague's fitness to practise, recommended at the time that I record the events, log them with the defence society, write an appropriate letter to hospital management, and maintain confidentiality – all of which I did. However, he went on to advise me that I should move to another post as quickly as I could, since he believed that I was in serious professional jeopardy. 'Not possible' had been my blithe response. I had only moved post three years previously and another move at this stage was not going to be feasible for both professional and social reasons. So I stayed put.

At the time, I also discussed my concerns of the colleague's fitness to practise with a senior colleague, having read the GMC's advice in such matters. When my senior colleague threatened to make me the 'Wendy Savage' of my own hospital if I didn't bury the concerns of my patient, I ensured that the threat was documented in independent contemporaneous notes, but didn't otherwise react. When a few weeks later I was unjustly attacked over my clinical performance, I robustly defended my position to the associate medical director and general manager, disproved the allegations and indicated that the unprovoked aggression and spurious accusations might have resulted from illness and life-style issues on my colleague's part, only when asked. The medico-legal adviser from a few years before happens to be my case-manager at the time that I am suspended more than two years later. In the months that follow, I am to ask him repeatedly how I can possibly have been so dismissive of the classical contributory factors of a disaster in the making.

As these thoughts tumble through my mind, I look at this general manager and I am in danger of losing control completely. But I work hard, choosing to forgo venting all the blinding anger at what his management team's approach has brought me, in order to prepare for the bigger challenge to come.

And then it seems the special party has arrived and is now ready for me. As I move into the adjoining room, a voice screams inside my head – is it possible that I have unwittingly done something (or omitted to do something) so terrible as to attract summary suspension? My inner sense of what constitutes a good doctor tells me that while none of us is infallible, my clinical approach borders on the obsessive: if I am found to have a problem, God help the rest of the department.

I still don't quite believe this is happening. I am reeling, but focus consciously on the words being uttered by the medical director who is sitting shoulder to shoulder with the human resources director behind a small table. I hear 'serious allegations', 'unable to give details', 'special leave, not suspension, although that could change once we have investigated further'.

Ever the helpful soul (I have chastised myself roundly over the years for this, but eventually concluded that without this inherent quality, I would probably not have succeeded, career-wise – automatic soothing and appeasement responses built in, adopts 'assistant' role unbidden, will tend to apologise when challenged, even if inappropriate). I offer to cancel the family holiday. I mentally note that I will already have to carry forward (or lose) two weeks of annual leave even if I leave for Spain in two days time as planned, but what the heck? 'There must be some mistake' I hear myself say 'surely I can help sort this out?' But I am told 'no' and I feel myself sliding toward the edge. This has been no administrative mistake or minor political manoeuvre. Terror grips me and I hear an involuntary cry. I get up from my chair wondering how they can investigate and decide on my future without any input from me whatsoever.

My next memory is more than an hour later in my office. I have no recollection at all of how I got there or what I did. I think I must have contacted the defence society, but to whom I spoke or what was said, I have no memory. Which isn't like me. Even under extreme pressure in a clinical setting, my recall is usually very good – blood results, clinical details, which GP, drugs and allergies – it is usually all there. I then flip into 'practical' mode and neatly dispatch the tasks I had planned to do prior to going on leave, and I can see myself in action and approve of the control in a detached sort of a way – I'm OK after all. I contact a GP about a patient due to receive 'bad news', trying to explain that I will no longer be able to deal with this in person now, trying to keep it together. Getting to a certain point, then losing it, yet determined to finish, to get the message across with a voice cracking with stress, breaking with distress.

As time goes on, it becomes obvious that I am still unfit to make the journey home. I feel incapable of facing my family (and myself, I suppose). But finally, at one in the morning, I think I might be safe to drive.

And so ends the first day of what is to become an ordeal that at times I think I cannot survive. I went on leave a couple of days later, and reached some of the lowest times then. I was still completely ignorant of the allegations, but learned from a colleague that a national newspaper seemed to have the inside track. Looking down from the third floor balcony of my Spanish holiday apartment onto the concrete below, I recognised that either I no longer had sound judgement (since I couldn't think of any clinical incidents or 'skeletons in cupboards' that might have triggered the action taken), or I had been stitched up so convincingly that it withstood what I assumed to have been rigorous internal scrutiny of the allegations prior to an exclusion being enforced. Either way, I was finished. My whole life spent growing a career in surgery, was now worthless.

To my shame, it wasn't the thought of my family that stopped me: it was the possibility that I might survive the attempt. And then the urge passed and has never revisited. Part of my coming to terms with this assault was to consider what might be worse than what I was going through. What if something happened to my partner or my son? Yes, that would definitely be worse, much worse. And whenever things looked bleak thereafter, I would take comfort knowing that as bad as things were, there are actually worse tragedies.

I strongly believe that our own life events improve the understanding we have of patients' problems and I now know some of the reflex psychological reactions to extreme and overwhelming adversity from personal experience. For example, I know what it is to cower in a corner in abject terror, like a dog being physically abused, when my personal space is invaded by a hostile medical manager. I know how it feels to steel myself into discussing the state I'm in with my GP, only to be turned away at the desk by his receptionist. I know what it is to lose every bit of self-respect and dignity, and then find something to justify going on. And yet I was fortunate. What if I hadn't had the overwhelming support of the consultant body in my hospital (apart from the obvious)? What if I hadn't been a doctor used to keeping good clinical notes? What if I hadn't the family I have, standing by me throughout? What if I hadn't benefited from the kindness and integrity of strangers? What if colleagues and acquaintances who owed me nothing, had decided to walk on by? I look back at how this might have turned out, and I know in my heart how lucky I've been.

1 2 3 4 **5** 6

Academic Freedom

Academic Freedom

Wendy Savage

Although academic freedom is generally thought of as one of the fundamental values of university life, it is rarely discussed or analysed in medical literature; this is unfortunate. As I said in my account of my suspension,[1] 'Academic freedom, the right to express opinions, is essential if we are to train doctors who can think'. The pursuit of knowledge in an objective way and its dissemination to the wider public are critically important, and they need to be defended in the sometimes hostile environment of today's universities.

There are four aspects of freedom in an academic environment: freedom to research, freedom to publish, freedom to teach and freedom to speak.[2] The increased 'managerialism' of our universities, and their emphasis on financial rather than intellectual considerations,[3] mean that all four are under threat. Some argue that tenure is important for the preservation of academic freedom[4] and many believe that the increasing use of short-term contracts for academic staff should be resisted.

Two cases from the University of Toronto have become widely known in this century. Both raise important issues. Dr Olivieri,[5] a respected haematologist, was conducting a trial under the auspices of the Canadian Medical Research Council and a drug company. She felt morally bound to inform her patients and the scientific community that the drug she was testing for the treatment of thalassaemia might be neither effective nor safe. She had earlier signed a confidentiality clause, and legal threats were issued by the drug company who wanted her not to inform her patients and questioned her analysis of the data. Only after protests made by international authorities did the University and the hospital adequately support her academic freedom and her responsibilities as a doctor.

Dr Healy, an academic psychiatrist from Swansea[6] had accepted the offer of a post at Toronto. The offer was withdrawn after he gave a lecture which raised the possibility that the selective serotonin re-uptake inhibitor (SSRI) group of antidepressants might cause suicide in some patients. The manufacturer of Prozac was a significant contributor to the University. The University authorities denied that their decision to withdraw the appointment had been affected by their relationship with the drug company, but many observers were extremely sceptical about their denials. Both cases demonstrate how dangerous to academic freedom working with the pharmaceutical industry can be.

Professor Arthur Schafer, a philosopher, has argued cogently[7] for a new system to liberate North American universities from their dependence on corporate funding which, he argues, compromises the integrity of researchers and creates a conflict of interest for universities.

---

1 Savage (1986) p.180

2 Keel Brooks (2004)

3 McLeod (2006)

4 Wright and Slovis (1997)

5 Olivieri (2003)

6 Healy (2003)

7 Schafer (2004)

Packham draws attention to the probable effect of the General Agreement on Trade in Services (GATS) in the UK.[8] 'The loss of higher aspirations, such as education of critically minded citizens in a democratic and civilized society would impoverish the university's research culture which demands honesty and openness to public scrutiny.... Publicly funded fundamental research would fade, leaving university research totally dependent for funds on the goodwill of industry and commerce. Present problems, such as the suppression of unwelcome results, and the use of questionable results to manipulate public opinion, would considerably increase.'

In the mid-1980s a group was formed to fight against attempts by the Department of Health and Social Security (DHSS) to control publication of results from research they funded. They founded the Association of DHSS-funded researchers (subsequently DH-funded) and managed to maintain their right to publish without interference from government.[9]

The relationship between professors and senior lecturers in medical schools is complicated because, while professors have more authority with regard to academic and administrative matters, senior lecturers are themselves consultants, and as such they are assumed to have the right to treat their patients as they see fit. It is perhaps surprising that I could find no references to this potentially difficult relationship in medical literature. At the enquiry into my suspension, Professor Grudzinskas stated '...if one holds an academic position then the clinical autonomy may have to be modified', although he did appear to retreat from this position under cross-examination by John Hendy.[10] The then dean added an appendix to his submissions to the Munro panel which is reproduced below. It confirmed my view that a professor did not have a right to interfere with my management of cases merely because he would have done things differently.

> This case has raised the issue of the relationship between a Professor and a Senior Lecturer in a clinical unit. It is accepted in the University that on matters of organized teaching and administration of a department a Professor has a right to demand co-operation. It is accepted that a Senior Lecturer may well disagree with a Professor on academic issues and that this may be beneficial provided the disagreement does not lead to personal animosity and that ludicrously extreme views are not put forward. However, there is little guidance as to whether or not a Professor has authority over the clinical practice of a Senior Lecturer who holds an Honorary Consultant Contract in his or her own right; it is usually accepted in the Health Service that all consultants are equal and independent and have the right to investigate and treat patients as they see best. On the other hand, Professors and Readers have in their contracts that their appointments are conditional upon the Health District in which the teaching hospital is situated granting them clinical facilities; Senior Lecturers have no such clause in their contract and can only use the clinical facilities allocated by the Health District to the Professor.
>
> But Mrs Savage had an Honorary Consultant Contract and access to the beds and other clinical facilities of the Academic Unit of Obstetrics and Gynaecology for six years before Professor Grudzinskas arrived.

---

8 Packham (2003)

9 DHSS-funded researchers. Personal communication with Alison Macfarlane and Gerard Draper, August 2006.

10 Savage (1986) pp.120–1

> Most people take the view that she is a consultant in her own right and clinically independent of the Professor although subject to him as regards the organization of her teaching, her participation in it, and in the running of the Academic Department of Obstetrics and Gynaecology.

The Research Assessment Exercise has been heavily criticised,[11] and the movement towards critical mass, with large departments joining together to work on particular areas of research such as molecular biology and drug therapies, suggests that the days of the maverick individual thinker may be numbered. I think this will be detrimental to some aspects of research, and that it will diminish the standing of our universities in the long term.

Women are under-represented at the top of medical academia. Just two of the 32 medical schools in the UK have a woman as dean and seven of them have no women professors at all.[12] Only recently, after pressure from the then president of the Medical Women's Federation and her successors, has this issue been addressed by the Council of Heads of Medical Schools (CHMS).[13] The Athena project, which has been surveying women in science and technology in an attempt to improve their career progression, is surveying medical academics at the time of writing.[14]

In this section, Anne Maclean writes about the 'great battle of Swansea'. Her discussion of the fundamental values of academic life and of the dangers of turning our universities into corporations, based as it is on her own struggle for professional survival, is as relevant today as when it was written in 1998.

References

British Medical Association (BMA) Health Policy and Economic Research Unit (at the request of the Medical Academic Staff Committee) (2004) *Women in Academic Medicine: Challenges and Issues*. London: BMA.

Council of Heads of Medical Schools (CHMS) (2006) *Clinical Academic Staffing levels in the Medical and Dental Schools: Data Update*. London: CHMS. http://www.chms.ac.uk

Healy D (2003) 'In the grip of the python: conflicts at the university–industry interface', *Science & Engineering Ethics*, 9:59–71.

Keel Brooks A (2004) 'Protecting America's secrets while maintaining academic freedom', *Academic Medicine*, 79:333–42.

McLeod D (2006) 'Research funding changes undercut science and maths', *The Guardian*, 15 June 2006. http://www.guardianunlimited.co.uk

Olivieri NF (2003) 'Patients' health or company profits? The commercialisation of academic research', *Science & Engineering Ethics*, 9:29–41.

Packham DE (2003) 'G.A.T.S and universities: implications for research', *Science and Engineering Ethics*, 9:85–100.

Savage W (1986) *A Savage Enquiry: Who Controls Childbirth?* London: Virago.

---

11 Williams (1998)

12 BMA (2004)

13 CHMS (2006)

14 http://www.Athenaproject.org.uk

Schafer A (2004) 'Biomedical conflicts of interest: a defence of the sequestration thesis-learning from the cases of Nancy Olivieri and David Healy', *Journal of Medical Ethics*, 30:8–24.

Williams G (1998) 'Misleading, unscientific and unjust: the United Kingdom Research Assessment Exercise', *BMJ*, 316:1,079–82.

Wright SW and Slovis CM (1997) 'Tenure track in emergency medicine', *Annals of Emergency Medicine*, 30:622–5.

Academic Freedom and Blowing the Whistle

Anne Maclean

The character and ethos of the present system of higher education in the United Kingdom is deeply inimical to the existence of academic freedom. For that very reason it is more than ever necessary that such freedom should be acknowledged, defended and exercised. In the first part of this chapter I shall maintain that the protection afforded by the principle of academic freedom extends to academic 'whistle-blowers'; and in the second part I shall use aspects of a recent *cause célèbre* – the 'great battle' at the University of Wales Swansea – to illustrate and support my claim.

The higher education system, as it now stands, is the product of the Thatcherite assault on universities and other educational institutions which began in 1980 and culminated in the Education Reform Act of 1988. The Act itself, it must be said, incorporates the principle of academic freedom. In clause 202(2) (a) of Part IV, the newly established University Commissioners are instructed to have regard to the need:

> ...to ensure that academic staff have freedom within the law to question and test received wisdom, and to put forward new ideas and controversial or unpopular opinions, without placing themselves in jeopardy of losing their jobs and privileges they may have at their institutions.

The Committee of Vice Chancellors and Principals doubtless regarded the inclusion of this clause as a victory for universities; as a safeguard of academic freedom, however, its effectiveness is greatly reduced by the fact that the Act also provides for the dismissal of academics 'by reason of redundancy' (and not, as hitherto, only for 'good cause'). The redundancy provision, bad enough in itself, must be viewed in the context of the larger purposes served by the Education Reform Act as a whole; which must be considered as an instrument for transforming – not to say destroying – the traditional university system.

As traditionally conceived, a university is a community of individuals engaged in the advancement of learning, knowledge and understanding and in the transmission of these things to the next generation. It is, quite simply, an academic institution. Thus the work of university teachers, researchers and scholars is properly governed by academic purposes and objectives and informed by academic values and priorities. It belongs to the nature of a university, so understood, that it should be relatively independent and self governing; and that it should be administered so as to serve and promote the academic activities and interests of its members.

It is to such a conception of a university that there belongs, as a necessary feature, the notion of *academic freedom*. This has been defined recently as 'the right of teachers in universities and other sectors of education to teach and research as their subject and conscience demands'; and declared to be 'an integral aspect of open societies'.[1]

1 O'Hear (1995) pp.3–4

John Griffith, Emeritus Professor of Public Law at the University of London and former Chancellor of the University of Manchester, discusses the importance of academic freedom in a pamphlet published in opposition to the education policies of the Thatcher government. He points out that, although the arguments for academic freedom are broadly the same as those for free speech, discussion and enquiry in society at large, '...the general case for "free speech" and free access to its results...has a special application to teaching and research':

> Whatever else they may be designed to do, academic institutions of all kinds and at all levels must be critical. They must be committed to re-examining accepted knowledge, assumptions and practices. It is their job... to nurse scepticism and to apply it to established beliefs and the present order of things and to do so systematically.[2]

Academic freedom is essential, Griffith argues, if universities and other academic institutions are to perform their sceptical and critical duties.

Thus one of the central functions of universities, as traditionally understood – the function of criticism – requires the existence of academic freedom as a condition of its performance. However, as previously stated, the Education Reform Act of 1988 was the culmination of an assault on universities as traditionally understood. It was the final and crucial stage of a process whereby the Thatcher government sought to transform universities as defined above into very different institutions – ones more in keeping with that government's totalitarian ambitions and comprehensive market ideology.

In short: the point of the Thatcher government's reform of education was to change universities from academic institutions pursuing academic objectives into corporations serving purposes ultimately external to those of academic activity as such – managed in the way that business corporations are managed and funded so as to necessitate their mutual competition and, at the same time, facilitate their control and direction by the State.[3]

In the Thatcherite view, academics are made for universities and not universities for academics. The Jarratt report of 1985 maintains that a university is 'first and foremost' a corporate enterprise 'to which subsidiary units and individual academics are responsible and accountable'.[4] A corporate enterprise must have a corporate purpose; and the White Paper of 1987 indicates clearly the Thatcherite conception of the primary purpose of universities and other institutions of higher education. It is the *extra*-academic purpose of meeting 'the demand for highly qualified manpower' and thus serving 'the economic requirements of the country'.[5]

The function of a university is not, it would seem, to *educate* its students – that is, impart knowledge to them, acquaint them with the finest achievements of human intellect and culture, expand and enrich their imagination and their understanding. Rather, it is to *train* them in the skills required by industry, business and commerce, in accordance with

---

2 Griffith (1987)

3 The last of these points cannot be enlarged upon here. For discussion of it, see the pamphlet by John Griffith (1987) mentioned above, and also his *Universities and the State: The Next Steps* (1989). The first part of the present paper is greatly indebted to Professor Griffith's work.

4 Jarratt (1985) 3.41

5 The command paper *Higher Education: Meeting the Challenge* (Her Majesty's Stationery Office, 1987) adds that '[T]he Government and its central funding agencies will do all they can to encourage and reward approaches by higher education institutions which bring them closer to the world of business.'

the government's perception of the needs of the economy. Of course this perception will change from time to time; here is one reason, at least, for the introduction of the redundancy clause and the increasingly prevalent and iniquitous practice of employing university teachers and researchers on short-term contracts.

For the last twenty years then, universities and other institutions of higher education have been in the process of becoming – primarily – training schools for business, industry and commerce. Evidently, such organisations are most unlikely to discharge the critical and sceptical functions described by John Griffith. It is difficult to envisage them 're-examining accepted knowledge, assumptions and practices', except within the narrow limits defined by their role as servants of the economy; and they will surely be discouraged from applying 'scepticism' to 'established beliefs and the present order of things'. They are there to *service* the present order of things, by supplying it with a workforce that is skilled, efficient, well trained – and intellectually compliant. It will be neither necessary nor desirable for the members of this workforce to be taught how to think for themselves; they might ask awkward questions about the way things are.

It will be clear, I think, that academic freedom is hardly a prerequisite of the proper functioning of 'academic' institutions as conceived above. Quite the reverse: it constitutes a serious danger to it.

Academic freedom, to repeat, involves the freedom to advance 'new ideas and controversial and unpopular opinions'; to 're-examine accepted knowledge, assumptions and practices'; and to criticise 'established beliefs and the present order of things'. The scope of this freedom thus extends well beyond the content of academic subjects; the unpopular opinions academics have a right – indeed, a duty – to express may concern the present state of society and social institutions – *including, of course, universities themselves.*

There are certainly plenty of such opinions to be expressed. In my experience, the vast majority of lecturers, scholars and researchers are angry and disgusted by the fate that has befallen institutions of higher education. Every day they face the demoralising consequences of the Thatcherite 'reforms'; for example, too few lecturers trying to teach and examine too many students, many of whom are poorly qualified and have little interest in the subjects they are supposed to be studying; a massive overload of pointless and time-wasting bureaucratic procedures, frequently involving facile and confused attempts to quantify the inherently qualitative; a steady decline in real academic standards; a contempt for traditional academic subjects and a subordination of academic concerns to economic and financial ones. It is essential that, instead of submitting to this state of affairs in silence, academics publicise and condemn it.

It must be emphasised that this is not just a matter of making general statements, important though they are; it is also a matter of citing the instances which support them. It will be necessary, on occasion, to draw attention to particular states of affairs within particular institutions. Thus a lecturer may be compelled, in certain circumstances, to question the academic integrity of a course or degree programme, or to criticise the standards of teaching and examining involved in it.[6] For obvious reasons, the institution concerned is likely to be the lecturer's own employer.

6 I repeat: in certain circumstances. These include, as was the case in Swansea, the failure or obstruction of attempts to remedy matters through appropriate internal procedures.

The principle of academic freedom, I am arguing, sanctions the putting forward by academics of 'controversial and unpopular opinions' about what is happening, not only in society at large or universities in general, but in the very institutions in which they work. In other words, it sanctions in an academic context what is popularly known as 'whistle-blowing'.

It will be obvious, I think, that this particular exercise of academic freedom stands to bring individual academics into serious conflict with the institutions which employ them. Universities, as mutually competing corporations, will take the attitude to whistle-blowers that we expect of such corporations – namely that of denying their claims and penalising their 'disloyalty'. As everyone knows, if an employee of a manufacturing company publishes the defects of a particular product that employee is almost certain to be dismissed – after all, the company will lose business to its competitors and profits will suffer. One might have expected quite different attitudes to prevail in an academic context. But universities do not merely serve the commercial world in the way already indicated – more and more they belong to that world, offering rival products (modules) to the relevant consumers (would-be students), dependent for state funding upon the cost of making the products (developing and teaching the modules) and the number of consumers they attract (student places filled). An academic whistle-blower, therefore, is likely to receive from her institution much the same treatment as the company employee just referred to.

We can now appreciate the full significance of the idea that universities are to be run as if they were business corporations. Business corporations are *managed*; the system of management is a hierarchical one; and at the top of the hierarchy is a chief executive – the managing director – who has ultimate authority over the activities of all of the corporation's staff. This system of line management has now been imposed upon universities, with vice chancellors as chief executives and other university officers and heads of department occupying the subordinate managerial positions.

Thus any academic contemplating whistle-blowing must be prepared for the worst as far as her own position is concerned. Furthermore, new statutes and contracts of employment in higher education increasingly contain clauses destructive of or detrimental to academic freedom, especially when exercised in the manner under discussion: clauses creating an offence of 'bringing [an institution] into disrepute', for instance, or imposing a duty upon employees not to speak to the media. And finally, the use of short-term contracts, whose renewal depends upon the approval of the institution and/or head of department concerned, militates against the willingness of academics to speak their minds, even in private.

It would seem then, that in the eyes of their employers, academics should be – at least outwardly – as intellectually compliant as the workforce it is now their business to train. This must not be accepted. Lecturers, scholars and researchers must continue to discharge their duty of criticism; they must strenuously defend the principle of academic freedom; and they must unite in support of any of their number penalised for saying what she thinks.[7]

---

7 One good consequence of the Swansea affair was the creation of CAFAS, the Council for Academic Freedom and Academic Standards. This organisation exists to defend academic freedom, campaign against the decline in academic standards, investigate allegations of malpractice and support victimised individuals. Further information and an application form for membership may be obtained from: http://www.cafas.org.uk; email: shakti81@aol.com; telephone: 01932 840928.

II

In May 1993 a report by Sir Michael Davies, acting on behalf of the Visitor of the University of Wales (the Queen), effectively brought an end to what Sir Michael himself described in the report's subtitle as 'the "Great Battle" in Swansea'.[8] The battle had begun over three years earlier, when a group of lecturers, including the present author, complained to the University of Wales about the conduct of the board of examiners for the taught degree of MA in Philosophy and Health Care at the University College of Swansea (later renamed the University of Wales Swansea).[9] The complainants alleged that the standards of teaching and examining for this degree were seriously inadequate; and in particular, that the examining board had awarded the MA to a dissertation known by at least some of its members to be largely copied from the published writings of others.

The struggle which followed the lodging of this complaint involved the suspension by the College of two of the complainants, the enforced resignation of another – myself – and four pre-Davies enquiries. One of these, that of the Calvert Committee, was discredited and overturned by the Davies report; two others, the reports of Morgan and Swinnerton Dyer, found the complaint to have had – in the words of Sir Michael Davies – 'substantial justification';[10] and the Davies report itself ordered that the complainants be reinstated. The Centre for Philosophy and Health Care was required to revise the taught MA programme and reform its academic practices.

The length of the dispute and the complexity of its history forbid any detailed recounting of it here; for that, readers are referred to the Davies report itself. In what follows I shall concentrate on those aspects of the Swansea story which relate to the claims made in this chapter; it is a story which illustrates both the vital importance of academic freedom and the serious threat to it which present circumstances pose.

The issue of academic freedom came to the surface very quickly when the failure of the University of Wales to conduct its promised enquiry into the complaint against the examining board precipitated the affair into the public arena via an interview with the complainants in the *Guardian* newspaper. Ironically, it was Swansea's then Principal, Professor Brian Clarkson, who emphasised the protection afforded to the whistle-blowers by the principle of academic freedom. When asked publicly whether disciplinary action would be taken against them, he replied: 'We have such a thing as academic freedom and that is meant to allow all people to raise questions of genuine academic concern'.[11]

Notwithstanding this, Professor Clarkson himself suspended me from my teaching duties for refusing to retract opinions attributed to me in the *Guardian*; and shortly thereafter he recommended to the College Council that I be dismissed for 'good cause'. At this point, faced with two separate disciplinary proceedings, the 'good cause' and the Calvert Committee (see below), and with the University of Wales having failed to honour

---

8 Davies (1994)

9 The unit responsible for the taught MA programme, the Centre for the Study of Philosophy and Health Care – then attached to the Department of Philosophy – was, in fact and spirit, a child of the Thatcher years. It purported to give 'relevance' to the ultimate academic subject, philosophy, and it attracted both large numbers of students and funding from external sources. The authors of *Academic Standards under Pressure* (Cohen and Williamson, 1991) called it 'a paradigm of the priorities that are now supposed to govern universities'.

10 Davies (1994) p.115

11 BBC Radio Wales, 7 October 1990, quoted in Davies (1994) p.114

its promise of investigating my original complaints, I was persuaded to resign. Two of the other complainants, Michael Cohen and Colwyn Williamson, were suspended pending an enquiry into retaliatory grievances made against all three of us by the chairman of the examining board we had complained about, Professor DZ Phillips. This enquiry, chaired by Professor Harry Calvert, eventually recommended that 'good cause' proceedings be brought against Mr Williamson and that Mr Cohen be reprimanded and warned that similar proceedings would be brought against him should he continue to behave as he had done.

The Davies report endorsed the description of these events by the Association of University Teachers as Professor Phillips being allowed to 'get his retaliation in first'.[12] My aim in rehearsing them here is to illustrate and support my point about the treatment academic whistle-blowers must expect to receive now that a commercial ethos has been substituted for an academic one. Swansea's Principal, as we saw above, spoke of academic freedom; but his actions expressed the mentality of the 'chief executive', as did the following remark attributed to him by the *Times Higher Education Supplement* of 14 June 1991:

> If this had happened in a company, and I had been managing director, those people would have been up the road the moment they kicked up the fuss they did. They would have taken us to an industrial tribunal, but they would have been off the payroll.

When the memorandum recommending 'good cause' proceedings against me was placed before the Council of the College, it contained the following passage:

> In the Principal's view, the issue is nothing to do with academic freedom, but with Mrs Maclean's breach of duty of co-operation, fidelity and utmost good faith towards the College...

This illustrates a remark made by Anthony O'Hear, whose definition of academic freedom was quoted earlier in this paper; namely, that 'one should never underestimate the ingenuity of academics themselves in justifying denials of academic freedom to their colleagues'.[13] A further instance is provided by a letter sent by my then colleagues in the Centre for the Study of Philosophy and Health Care to all members of the University College of Swansea, immediately after the Principal had announced his intention of bringing proceedings against me. The letter sought to persuade its readers that, contrary to what they might suppose, my dismissal would not constitute an offence against academic freedom. They were urged not to regard freedom as an 'absolute' and not to confuse it with 'licence'. Above all, they were informed, academic freedom is not a licence to 'denigrate colleagues' by accusing them of 'lowering academic standards'.

The protection afforded whistle-blowers by the principle of academic freedom, then, is vulnerable to sophistry and self-delusion on the part of academics themselves – their ability, when their personal interests are involved, to invent reasons for saying that no such principle is at stake.

Nevertheless, the turning point in the Swansea dispute came through a further exercise of academic freedom – the publication by Michael Cohen and Colwyn Williamson, after quitting the Calvert proceedings in disgust, of a pamphlet entitled 'Academic Standards under Pressure: the Case of Swansea'.

---

12 *Times Higher Education Supplement* of 14 June 1991 quoted in Davies (1994) p.86

13 O'Hear (1995) pp.3–4

This pamphlet, which detailed the original complaints against the examining board of the Centre for Philosophy and Health Care and recounted the story of the dispute up to that time, generated an enormous amount of sympathy for the complainants' cause within the academic community; for example, on 22 March 1991 a letter in support of it signed by fourteen Professors of Philosophy appeared in the *Guardian* newspaper. The combination of pressure and embarrassment compelled the University of Wales to conduct the independent enquiry which it had promised almost a year earlier. It was the findings of this enquiry – by Sir Peter Swinnerton-Dyer – which prevented the implementation of the Calvert Committee's recommendations and caused the whole matter to be referred to the University's Visitor, represented by Sir Michael Davies.

I come finally to the Davies report itself. Sir Michael's recommendations have already been mentioned; what needs to be stated here is that 'academic freedom' was one of the grounds he cited for those recommendations (the others being 'natural justice' and the fact that the complainants had 'some substantial basis' for their criticisms). Quoting clause 202(2) of the Education Reform Act – see earlier in this chapter – Sir Michael says that in his opinion 'the Visitor should be guided by these principles [of justice and academic freedom]'. He goes on to remark:

> Of course, they do not mean that academic staff have unrestricted licence – obviously not.
>
> They have to obey the law, Criminal and Civil, and there are other circumstances which may place them 'in jeopardy of losing their jobs'. The Establishment says that the critics at Swansea have indeed overstepped that line. *However, in drawing that line, in my opinion the fact that it is a line to be drawn in an adult academic world and not in a commercial jungle is of profound importance.*[14]

To this should be added Sir Michael's comment on the remark attributed to Swansea's Principal by the *Times Higher Education Supplement* (quoted earlier):

> The point is that neither the University of Wales nor the University College of Swansea is a 'company' in the profit making or any other sense. They are academic institutions. I believe that this has not always been remembered in Swansea.[15]

I have argued that academic freedom is not only an essential feature of academic institutions; its exercise in, among other things, blowing the whistle, is vital if we are to succeed in retaining the distinction upon which Sir Michael insists. And succeed we must.

---

14 Davies (1994) p.114; italics added

15 Ibid.

References

Cohen M and Williamson C (1991) *Academic Standards under Pressure*. Council for Academic Freedom and Democracy.

Davies M (1994) *The Davies Report: The 'Great Battle' in Swansea*. Thoemmes Press.

Griffith J (1987) *The Attack on Higher Education*. Council for Academic Freedom and Democracy.

Griffith J (1989) *Universities and the State: The Next Steps*. Council for Academic Freedom and Democracy.

Her Majesty's Stationery Office (1987) *Higher Education – Meeting the Challenge* (White Paper). London: HMSO.

Jarratt A (Chairman) (1985) *Report of the Steering Committee for Efficiency Studies in Universities*. London: CVCP.

O'Hear A (1995) 'Academic Freedom', in Honderich (ed.) *The Oxford Companion to Philosophy*. Oxford: OUP.

6

What Women Want

What Women Want

Wendy Savage

From my own experience of caring for pregnant women I believe that the majority of women want a normal birth cared for by people they know and trust. They need peace and quiet in order to concentrate on the instinctive nature of giving birth. If one looks at animal behaviour, cats and dogs tend to go into a quiet dark place to give birth, and cows and sheep may stop labouring if moved. We are mammals, and it seems likely that we instinctively want to behave in the same way. It therefore seems plausible that the underlying reason for the increase in intervention in hospital practice is that we have set up a system which is antipathetic to the needs of women, for peace, quietness and privacy.

The modern British labour ward, where women hear the sounds of other women giving birth and of telephones and bleeps going off, and where the lighting is usually harsh fluorescent strips, could almost be designed to interfere with the natural process of labour. Add to these the frequent interruptions by midwives coming to 'get the keys' to the drug cupboard (often without knocking on the door), changes of midwifery staff, the doctor's round when five or six people enter the woman's room and discuss her 'case', and it is hardly surprising that in some hospitals almost half the women require labour to be strengthened by a synthetic version of oxytocin, the natural hormone which makes the uterus contract.

Continuity of carer

Ideally women would like to be looked after during labour by one or two people whom they have got to know during the antenatal period.[1] In the past this was achieved by having a domiciliary midwife, sometimes supported by her general practitioner. The close personal relationship built up was probably the reason why, in the 1958 perinatal mortality survey, although the numbers were small, the district midwives achieved better outcomes than the hospital group; this was despite having a higher proportion of poorer patients and doing fewer blood tests.[2] The addition of a midwife to the general practitioner improved his results, but the lesson drawn by obstetricians was not that midwives had good results but that GPs had less good results than expected. They therefore encouraged women to have their babies in hospital under the care of obstetricians, a policy also supported by Cranbrook in the government report on maternity services.[3]

One of the difficulties in researching this area is that the choices available to women are limited now that the vast majority of births take place in hospital, so women who have a standard hospital birth may not know what they are missing. Although most women are satisfied with their birth, in the 1994 survey 98 per cent of those who had a home birth were happy with their decision compared with 90 per cent of those having a hospital

1 House of Commons Health Select Committee (1992) paragraph 49, XV, Vol.1

2 Butler and Bonham (1960) Table 19, pp.68–9

3 Ministry of Health (1959)

birth. Ninety-five per cent enjoyed their home birth compared with 76 per cent in hospital.[4] In a recent Canadian study, significantly more women who delivered at home were satisfied with the experience compared with those giving birth in hospital.[5]

The work of Green et al[6] showed that women who felt in control were more likely to be satisfied with their birth experience than those who felt they had not made decisions and had lost control.

Ina May Gaskin's *Spiritual Midwifery*[7] has sold 750,000 copies, and the midwives whom she led at the Farm in Tennessee showed amazingly good results. I suggested to Ina May that she get a public health physician to compare their outcomes from 1971–89 with one of the national surveys of birth in the US, and this study was published in 1992. When matched for variables such as age, parity and social class, the women delivered at home or in the homelike surroundings at the Farm had a perinatal mortality rate (the number of stillbirths and deaths in the first week of life per 1,000 births) of 10, while that for the comparison group was 13.3, although this was not statistically significant.[8] The caesarean section rate (CSR) was significantly lower (1.5 per cent v 16.5 per cent). Continuity of carer, attention to diet, a holistic approach and flexibility allowed each woman to be treated as an individual and for her psychological needs to be met. Ina May, a self-taught lay midwife, lectures all over the US in medical and midwifery schools and has made videos of births including vaginal breech births.[9]

The Vision 1976

Thirty years ago, the Association of Radical Midwives (ARM) was formed, following a letter to *The Sunday Times* from three pupil midwives who had come from the USA, Canada and Australia to train in what they had thought was the home of midwifery. They were shocked by what they found. This was just after the induction rate had risen to its peak in 1974 of 40 per cent in England and 45 per cent in Wales. Oliver Gillie and his team at *The Sunday Times* ran a campaign against this unnecessarily high rate of intervention, which had shocked the public, and the rate began to fall. The 1974 NHS reorganisation (the first) had brought the domiciliary (now called community) midwives, previously employed by local authorities, under the same management as the hospital midwives and, as the home birth rate fell, their work changed so that they lost the holistic care of women and became postnatal 'nurses'. In hospitals they were in danger of becoming 'obstetric handmaidens', and in many places morale was low.

The ARM published their *The Vision* in 1976. The third edition of the *The Vision*,[10] published in 1986 (the year after the WHO published its consensus statement 'Birth is not an Illness'),[11] set out a ten-year plan to achieve their goals:

- The woman was to be the centre of care
- The relationship between mother and midwife was fundamental to good care

4 Chamberlain, Wraight and Crowley (1997) Table 7.6, p.136 and Table 9.2, p.168
5 Janssen, Carty and Reime (2006)
6 Green, Coupland and Kitzinger (1988)
7 Gaskin (1977)
8 Durand (1992)
9 Gaskin (2003) and http://www.inamay.com
10 Association of Radical Midwives (1986)
11 World Health Organisation (1985)

- The midwife was unique in her way of working 'with women'
- There needed to be a publicity campaign to put the midwife back in her rightful place in the community and change the perception of the public
- There should be continuity of care for all women
- Midwives' skills should be fully utilised
- There should be provision of community-based care and choice for all women
- Maternity services should be accountable to women
- Care should cause no harm to mother or baby.

They envisaged that in ten years' time, 60 per cent of midwives would be working in the community in groups of two to five, based in a variety of settings: community or health centres, shops, houses, hospitals etc. The midwife would be recognised as the portal of entry for pregnant women into care and midwives would care for the majority of healthy pregnant women who fell within 'normal limits'.

So what happened to this vision? My own suspension in 1985 on false charges of incompetence caused an outcry amongst local GPs and women, who saw that the underlying struggle was about a women's right to have her baby 'where, when and how' she wanted as one of the local GPs, Mary Edmondson, put it.

The publicity and the subsequent enquiry raised the awareness of the public about what was happening to maternity services, and the late Audrey Wise was able to persuade the Health Select Committee to look at the way they were organised. The Winterton report[12] in 1992 followed by Julia Cumberlege's Expert Committee report in 1993, *Changing Childbirth*,[13] appeared to make the ARM's vision government policy.

The Winterton and Cumberlege reports

The 1991–2 Health Committee of the House of Commons, chaired by Nicholas Winterton, for the first time took evidence from women and also visited Holland to see how their services were organised. Luke Zander, who has written the foreword to this book and was one of my staunch supporters, was an advisor to this committee. They were disturbed by the conflict that often existed between the different professionals, and emphasised that the woman should be at the centre of care. They did not accept the view that hospital was the safest place to give birth. Their report[14] identified what I have summarised as the 'Five Cs': women should have *choice* and *control* over where and how they give birth, there should be *continuity of care* and *carer*, and *co-operation* and *communication* between professionals should be improved.

In response to the Select Committee's report, the government established an Expert Maternity Group, chaired by Baroness Cumberlege. The group took evidence from a number of organisations, visited maternity units and commissioned a Mori survey of women who had recently given birth. The only option explained fully to the majority of them was hospital birth in a consultant unit. Seventy-two per cent would have liked the option of a different kind of care, of whom 44 per cent wanted a midwife-led 'domino' delivery (short stay in hospital for six hours after birth, with the midwife accompanying

12 House of Commons Health Select Committee (1992)

13 Maternity Services Committee, Department of Health (1993)

14 House of Commons Health Select Committee (1992)

them home and often assessing at home initially). Twenty-two per cent (that is 16 per cent of the whole sample of women) said they would like the option of discussing home birth – 20 years after the rate had fallen to 1 per cent and after 30 years of obstetric propaganda about how dangerous it was.[15]

In 1993, the group published *Changing Childbirth*. Midwives were to be put at the centre of care, and indicators of success in achieving the desired goals were spelt out. It was envisaged that within five years:

1. All women should be entitled to carry their own notes
2. Every woman should know one midwife who ensures continuity of her maternity care – the named midwife
3. At least 30 per cent of women should have the midwife as the lead professional
4. Every woman should know the lead professional who has a key role in the planning and provision of her care
5. At least 75 per cent of women should know the person who cares for them during their delivery
6. Midwives should have direct access to some beds in all maternity units
7. At least 30 per cent of women delivered in a maternity unit should be admitted under the management of the midwife
8. The total number of antenatal visits for women with uncomplicated pregnancy should have been reviewed in light of the available evidence and RCOG guidelines
9. All frontline ambulances should have a paramedic able to support the midwife who needs to transfer a woman to hospital in an emergency
10. All women should have access to information about the services available in their locality.

It appeared that a radical reorganisation of childbirth was about to happen. Sadly, it has not. The big failure in 1993 was that the implementation of these proposals was to be 'cost neutral'. This meant that no money was available locally. A Changing Childbirth Implementation Team at the Department of Health sent out newsletters, and furious activity erupted throughout the country as midwives and managers tried to follow the suggestions. Divisions within the Royal College of Midwives (RCM) meant there was no coherent strategy. The influence of powerful professional interests, the institutionalisation of midwives, the turmoil in the NHS (which has been repeatedly reorganised since 1989), coupled with a new government which had different priorities, have meant that, despite many good pilot projects, care has improved for very few women. In some places, such as Tower Hamlets, the minority of women who had an excellent domiciliary service lost it as team midwifery was introduced, because midwives inexperienced in home birth lacked confidence. Home births, which had fallen to 1 per cent, rose to a peak of 2.2 per cent in 1999 then fell slightly to 2.1 per cent in 2000–2. In 2004 the rate rose to 2.3 per cent and in Wales to 3.3 per cent.[16]

Midwifery shortages result in poor care and receive much negative publicity, yet we have 92,000 trained midwives in this country, only 32,745 of whom intend to practise

15 Maternity Services Committee, Department of Health (1993) p.70

16 Office of National Statistics (2006) FMI Series 2002–4

in 2005. This is 2,000 fewer than in 1992, and the proportion of part-timers increased from 40.5 per cent in 1994 to 54.3 per cent in 2005, which further reduced midwifery hours.[17] When one looks at the number of midwives employed in the NHS there should be enough: 24,784 were employed in 2005 in England and Wales, or 18,928 FTE (the equivalent number of full-time midwives, by hours worked). Assuming that the proportion of part-timers is similar throughout the country, the table below shows that in England there are on average 32.4 births a year per midwife. In Scotland there are 21.5, Northern Ireland 22.9 and Wales 26.8. The range in England is from 27.6 in the North West to 38 in the Eastern region and 36.7 in the East Midlands.

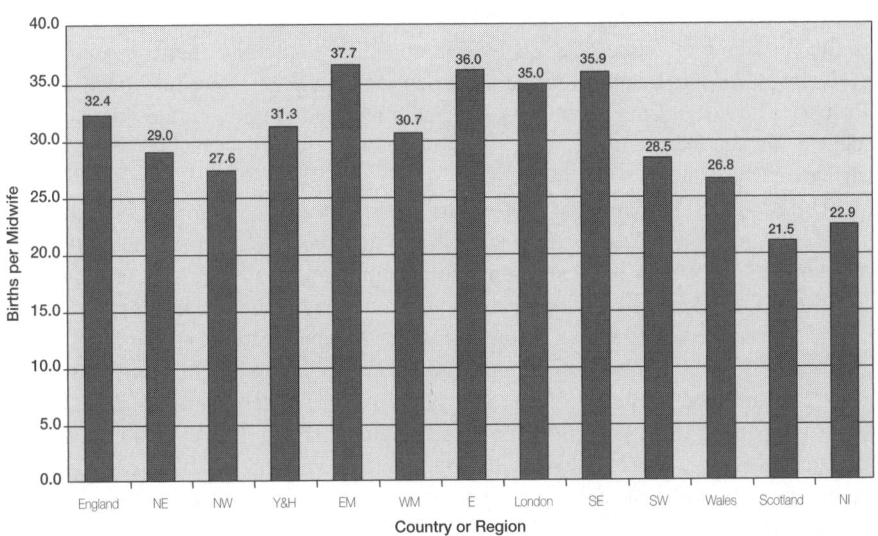

Data sourced from Maternity Services Committee, Department of Health (1993) and House of Commons Health Select Committee (1992)

Even allowing for managerial time there are fewer than 40 births per midwife. This is less than one a week allowing for holidays and study leave, which would not be an excessive workload if midwives were able to organise their time properly.[18]

The solution – primary and secondary care midwives

The key person in providing maternity care for healthy women is the midwife. The current situation, with midwifery shortages, poor deployment and midwives leaving the profession because of frustration, will never change whilst all midwives are managed from the hospital. The labour ward will always take priority over the community.

My solution to these problems and my vision for the twenty-first century is for midwives to recognise that medicine is becoming more specialised and to organise themselves, as has the medical profession, into primary and secondary care midwives.[19] There would be a national contract for those who do not want to work independently and

17 Nursing and Midwifery Council (2006)

18 The Information Centre (2006); Office of National Statistics (2005); NISRA (2005); General Register Office for Scotland (2006)

19 Savage (2003)

community midwives would deliver many women in hospital, at least initially, and would have rights of access to hospital beds.

Primary care midwives would work in the community, either independently or with contracts from PCTs, in small groups of two to five as envisioned by the ARM, and as has been shown to work by the South East London Midwifery group led by Nicky Leap, even when transferred to NHS management.[20] The Independent Midwives Association (IMA) have proposed to government a community midwifery model, 'one mother, one midwife', which would fit in with this idea.[21] Secondary care midwives would work in hospital, and some could specialise.

A campaign to change things in this way needs to be mounted by user organisations representing women, midwives and the RCM. The first National Service Framework (NSF) was set up to improve and standardise treatment for cancer. Maternity was added to the children and young people's NSF in 2005. The maternity standard sounds like *Changing Childbirth* and might be a vehicle for change.[22] There may need to be a Primary Midwifery Care Agency established for a limited time, to draw up contracts and look for suitable premises. Some ring-fenced money will be needed to get this radical change off the ground.

The All-Party Parliamentary Group for Maternity meets regularly, but has been ineffective in changing policy, despite the briefings it receives from the Maternity Care Working Party, which has user and multidisciplinary professional representation. Ministers of Health come and go, speak in platitudes and nothing changes.

With what seems to me to be the disastrous mismanagement of the NHS in the summer of 2006, small well-loved maternity units which provide the care that women want, like and need, are being closed throughout the country, despite the strenuous efforts of women and staff to keep them open.[23] In August 2006, 14 out of 43 units were threatened with closure.[24] Elizabeth Manero has written an excellent guide to campaigning against closures with a summary of the legal background and NHS organisation.[25]

Fifty years after the National Childbirth Trust and AIMS (Association for the Improvement of Maternity Services) were formed, the maternity services, whilst achieving safe outcomes for the baby, prevent the majority of women from experiencing birth in the fulfilling way that is their right. Sheila Kitzinger, Janet Balaskas, Caroline Flint, Mary Cronk and the Independent Midwives Association in this country have shown that it is possible.[26]

In this section, Beverley Beech from AIMS writes from her experience of dealing with distressed women for almost 30 years, and Professor Jane Sandall looks at the question of what women want from a more academic viewpoint.

I have dealt with the question of who decides about services in the introduction to the first section of this book, as it is bound up with the question of power.

---

20 Sandall, Davis and Warwick (2001)

21 Independent Midwives Association (2006a)

22 Department of Health (2006)

23 Robotham and Hunt (2006)

24 National Childbirth Trust (2006)

25 Ibid.

26 Kitzinger (2005); Kitzinger (2006); Balaskas (2004); Flint (1995); Cronk (1998); Independent Midwives Association (2006b)

References

Association of Radical Midwives (1986) *The Vision*, 3rd edition.

Balaskas J (2004) *New Natural Pregnancy: Practical Wellbeing from Conception to Birth.* Stroud, Gloucestershire: Gaia books.

Butler NR and Bonham DG (1960) *Perinatal Mortality*. Edinburgh & London: E & S Livingstone.

Chamberlain G, Wraight A and Crowley P (1997) *Home Birth; The report of the 1994 confidential enquiry by the National Birthday Trust Fund*. Carnforth (UK) and New York (USA): Parthenon Press.

Cronk M (1998) 'Keep your hands off that Breech', *Aims Journal*, Vol.10, No.3. http://www.aims/journal/vol10no3/handOffbreech/htm

Department of Health (2006) *National Service Framework for Children, Young People and Maternity Services*. London: DoH.

Durand AM (1992) 'The safety of home birth: The Farm Study', *Journal of the American Public Health Association*, 82:450–2.

Flint C (1995) *Midwifery Teams and Case Loads*. Oxford: Butterworth – Heinemann (now part of Elsevier).

Gaskin IM (1977) *Spiritual Midwifery*. Tennessee, USA: The Book Publishing Company.

Gaskin IM (2003) *Ina May's guide to childbirth*. London: Random House.

General Register Office for Scotland (2006) Scottish Births 2005. http://www.scotland.gov.uk/Topics/Statistics/Browse/Population-Migration/TrendBirths

Green J, Coupland VA and Kitzinger JV (1988) *Great Expectations: A prospective study of women's expectations and experiences of childbirth*. Cambridge: Child Care and Development Group.

House of Commons Health Select Committee (1992) *Second Report on the Maternity Services* (The Winterton report). London: Her Majesty's Stationery Office.

Independent Midwives Association (2006a) Community Midwifery Model. http://www.independentmidwives.org.uk/article155.html

Independent Midwives Association (2006b) Statistics. http://www.independentmidvives.org.uk/article155.html

The Information Centre (2006) Hospital and Community Staff (HCHS) England 1995–2005, Tables 1.2a and 2.2a for employed midwives. http://www.ic.nhs.uk/pubs/nhsstaff/nonmeddetailtab/file

Janssen PA, Carty EA and Reime B (2006) 'Satisfaction with planned place of birth among midwifery clients in British Columbia', *J Midwifery Womens Health.*

Kitzinger S (2005) *The Politics of Birth*. London: Elsevier.

Kitzinger S (2006) *Birth Crisis*. London: Routledge.

Maternity Services Committee, Department of Health (1993) *Changing Childbirth*, (The Cumberlege report). Report of the expert maternity group chaired by J. Cumberlege. London: HMSO.

Ministry of Health (MoH) (1959) *Report of the Maternity Services Committee* (The Cranbrook report). London: HMSO.

National Childbirth Trust (2006) *Local campaigns for midwife-led birth centres*. http://www.nct.org.uk/about/campaigns/birth#local

Northern Ireland Statistics and Research Agency (NISRA) (2005) http://www.nisra.gov.uk/demography/default.asp?cmsid=20_22&cms=demography_Vital+Statistics&release=

Nursing and Midwifery Council (2006) *Statistical analysis of register 2005.* http://www.nmc-uk.org.uk

Office of National Statistics (2005) Births, selected background data, England and Wales. http://www.statistics.gov.uk/statbase/Product.asp?vlnk=14408

Office of National Statistics (2006) *Birth Statistics: Birth and patterns of family building*. Series FM1. London: HMSO.

Robotham M and Hunt S (2006) 'Birth centre closures: Avoiding long term costs for short term savings?' *British Journal of Midwifery*, 34:376–7.

Sandall JM, Davis J and Warwick K (2001) *Evaluation of the Albany Midwifery Practice, Kings College Hospital London.* Obtainable from Prof Sandall, Women's Health Research Group, Health and Social Care Research Division, King's College, Waterloo Bridge Wing, 150 Stamford Street, London, SE1 9NH.

Savage W (2003) Editorial, *Brit Jour Midwifery*, Vol.11, p.646.

World Health Organisation (1985) 'Appropriate Technologies for Birth', *Lancet*, 2:436–37.

What Services do Women Want and Who Decides on the Kind of Care that is Offered to Them?

Beverley Beech

The majority of women no longer see birth as a normal, physiological process during which a small minority of women and babies encounter problems and complications which need medical attention. Instead, it is viewed as a disaster about to happen, and anyone who emerges unscathed and physically and emotionally intact is considered lucky. This perception of the dangers involved persuades most women that the only safe place to give birth is in a hospital, surrounded by doctors, nurses and all the paraphernalia of modern medicine. They are totally unaware of how highly political childbirth has become.

Because the majority of women no longer birth at home, surrounded by their family and friends, most women never see a normal birth. Instead, they rely on what they are told in hospital-based antenatal classes, television, films, books, newspapers and magazines.

The huge range of damaging effects resulting from inappropriate medicalised deliveries remains unaddressed and concealed from the majority of women, and the unjustified levels of caesarean operations are excused by claims that women are 'choosing' them.

By centralising and medicalising birth, health professionals have ensured that women are kept largely in ignorance of the potential for normal birth, midwives are largely compliant with the medical model, and those campaigning for change have little influence on the decision- and policy-making committees.

Historical pressures

For hundreds of years, and in all cultures, men were not permitted to attend births. Over the centuries, male practitioners inveigled their way into the birthing room and gradually gained control. They did so by applying and controlling access to so-called science and technology and by undermining women's confidence in their own bodies.

The gradual domination and control of childbirth and maternity care by male practitioners has been well researched and documented by Jean Donnison.[1] It became fashionable to have a male physician in attendance at home but the poor or destitute in the big cities, whose home conditions were usually utterly appalling, had to rely on charitable lying-in hospitals where the risk of death from puerperal fever was considerable. During the nineteenth century a Doncaster surgeon, Robert Storrs, commented: '...the extent to which these institutions increase the danger of childbirth is now well known'.[2]

By 1865, Queen Charlotte's Hospital, which was acknowledged to have 'a great

1 Donnison (1988)

2 Storrs (1843)

reputation as a school of obstetric practice', had a maternal mortality rate of 40.0 per thousand compared with rates of 3.5 per thousand in the outdoor midwifery department of St George's Hospital and 6.0 per thousand in the lying-in wards of 39 metropolitan workhouses.[3]

In the 1950s, just over a third of women gave birth at home and by 1968 this had decreased to less than one-fifth. In 1970 the Peel report, without any evidence to support its claim of safety, concluded: 'We think that sufficient facilities should be provided to allow for 100 per cent hospital delivery. The greater safety of hospital confinement for mother and child justifies this objective'.[4] No-one asked women whether they wished to leave the comfort and safety of their own homes. Ironically, one of the early campaigns of the Association for Improvements in the Maternity Services (AIMS), founded in 1960, was for more maternity beds, so that, at a time of bed shortages, those women who needed, or wanted, to give birth in hospital would be able to do so.

The Peel report's recommendation, however, was soon interpreted as a directive to force all women to give birth in hospital. Any woman who chose to give birth at home faced increasing hostility and professional antagonism. The received opinion was that birth outside hospital was dangerous.

The hospitalisation of childbirth has led to a huge increase in intervention and a failure to recognise the effects that medicalisation has on the process of giving birth. As the World Health Organisation has said:

> By medicalising birth, i.e. separating a woman from her own environment and surrounding her with strange people using strange machines to do strange things to her in an effort to assist her (and some of this may occasionally be necessary), the woman's state of mind and body is so altered that her ways of carrying through this intimate act must also be altered and the state of the baby born must equally be altered. The result is that it is no longer possible to know what births would have been like before these manipulations. Most health care providers no longer know what 'non-medicalised' birth is.
>
> This is an overwhelmingly important issue. Almost all women in most developed countries give birth in hospital, leaving the providers of the birth services with no genuine yardstick against which to measure their care... The entire modern obstetric and neonatological literature is essentially based on observations of medicalised birth.[5]

Individual women

Medical professionals have been highly successful in undermining women's confidence in their ability to give birth by stressing the risks and claiming that without their involvement untold damage or disaster would occur. When untold damage and disaster do occur the women are often persuaded that there was nothing more that could have been done, or that the disaster was unavoidable, particularly as they had given birth in hospital. Yet, when the evidence is carefully examined, as Julia Allison demonstrated in her research of district midwifery practice in the post-war period up until the 1970s, community midwives had far better outcomes than any of the local hospitals, despite attending at home many very high-risk women who had been refused a hospital bed.[6]

---

3 Donnison (1988)
4 Peel (1970)
5 WHO (1985)
6 Allison (1996)

Today, a young woman rarely has any contact with pregnancy and birth until she herself becomes pregnant. Her information is not gained by being with pregnant and birthing women who have had good experiences, but via magazines, films, TV and newspapers where birth is all too often presented as a painful, dangerous and life-threatening experience from which mother and baby are saved only by the timely intervention of heroic medical men. The constant diet of traumatic births (graphically portrayed in such films as *Gone with the Wind* and *Dracula*) together with the medical profession's constantly reiterated view that 'no birth is safe except in retrospect' results in cohorts of young women who are fearful of childbirth.

Those images are then compounded by negative anecdotal stories from friends, relatives and colleagues who were delivered in high-technology units, unaware of the high levels of avoidable and unnecessary interference that take place there. And woe betide any woman who starts asking questions. A mother who enquired about the statistics for the maternity units in her area of South Wales received the response, 'Who are you to be asking?' from the two midwives she separately approached for help.

Even when women are well informed and know their rights, most of them will be very reluctant to make choices that might antagonise their attendants and are unwilling to unburden themselves with a midwife they have barely met.

> If you tried to invent a system designed to undermine women's confidence in themselves and their bodies you'd come up with the one we have now. I never ever lay awake at night wondering whether I'd got too much protein in my urine, but I did spend many lonely hours worrying about whether I'd be able to cope with motherhood, whether I'd like the baby, would it wreck my marriage, would my mother-in-law be able to keep her nose out, would I lose my financial independence etc etc etc, and I don't remember ever feeling I could discuss any of this with any of the midwives I met at the antenatal clinic. How could I? To discuss any of this would be to confide in someone, and you don't confide in someone you've only just met.[7]

Undermining midwives

With the majority of women having been forced into hospital for birth, the midwives too were required to practise in hospital. Over the years their midwifery skills were undermined, devalued, and diminished to such an extent that today some student midwives reach their final year of training without ever having seen a normal birth.

In 1976 a group of student midwives, distressed about the shortcomings in their training and practice decided to create the Association of Radical Midwives to try and reclaim their skills, resume their role as 'with women' and strengthen the partnership between mothers and midwives.

The struggle to be 'with women' and respect the natural flow of birth is a difficult one, and bullying within the profession is rife.[8] Those midwives who rock the boat and do not comply with hospital protocols find themselves continuously having to justify their practice, yet rarely do the obstetric nurses who intervene without good cause have to justify their interventions.

NHS midwives are in the unenviable position of attempting to work from a woman-centred perspective (a perspective systematically denied to them), empower women from

7 Hayes (1998)
8 Hadikin and O'Driscoll (2000)

a disempowered position, respect when they are frequently disrespected, nurture without being nurtured themselves, offer choice when they have few choices, and provide 'unbiased' information (as though this existed) that they cannot act upon because of local policies which constrain them. The NHS midwife has become the 'piggy-in-the-middle', caught between policies, employers, colleagues and women.[9]

Although the majority of midwives will claim that they are the woman's advocate, few of them are. Many of those NHS midwives who fail to comply with the medicalised values imposed in the majority of maternity units are persecuted and bullied. Those midwives who really do advocate for women often find themselves before disciplinary hearings.

As a result of understaffing, stress, bullying and the refusal to allow them to practise midwifery, midwives are leaving the profession in droves and some of them are now practising as independent midwives because, as one midwife when asked why she was leaving a profession that she loved said: 'because I am no longer prepared to abuse women in the hospital system'. But working outside the NHS comes at a price: almost every single independent midwife has at some time been reported to the Nursing and Midwifery Council, and the majority of those who have been through the disciplinary procedures and found innocent of the charges have left the profession deeply traumatised by the experience.

Consumer involvement

Women's dissatisfaction with the services on offer in the 1960s and 70s encouraged women to organise. While many individual women struggled to ensure some control of their pregnancy, labour, and birth, others, often those who had already experienced birth, gathered together to campaign collectively to improve maternity care for all. The two foremost childbirth organisations in the UK, the Association for Improvements in the Maternity Services and the National Childbirth Trust were both established around 1960. While, in the early days, the National Childbirth Trust primarily focused on preparing women for childbirth, AIMS concentrated on persuading the NHS to change its practices.

During the 1970s, when induction of labour became commonplace, Jean Robinson challenged the necessity for intervening in so many labours,[10] and when the consumers asked for the research evidence to support the high levels of episiotomy in most hospitals (over 90 per cent for first time mothers) the midwives were enabled to carry out research which showed that episiotomy did not prevent tears, and should not be carried out routinely.[11]

In 1972 a Newcastle mother, Margaret Whyte, decided that she would campaign against the current practice of forcing all women into hospitals. She started the Society to Support Home Confinement, wrote a four-page leaflet telling women what their rights were and suggested a standard letter that a woman could send to the hospital stating her intention to give birth at home. AIMS joined with the Society to campaign for home births on the grounds that a woman has the right to choose a home birth, in spite of medical opinion that any woman wanting to do so must be out of her mind.

It was not until 1980, when Marjorie Tew, a respected statistician, published her

9 Edwards (2005)
10 Robinson (1974)
11 Sleep (1984)

study comparing mortality statistics by place of birth, that childbirth groups changed tactics and campaigned for home birth on the grounds of safety. She found that in every single risk group it was safer to be born at home.[12]

In 1992, a House of Commons Select Committee investigated maternity care. For the first time ever, lay people were invited to present evidence and, as a result, the Committee's investigations revealed how inappropriate centralised obstetric care was for the majority of women.

> ...this Committee must draw the conclusion that the policy of encouraging all women to give birth in hospitals cannot be justified on grounds of safety.

The report went on to say that:

> ...there is a widespread demand among women for greater choice in the type of maternity care they receive, and that the present structure of maternity services frustrates, rather than facilitates, those who wish to exercise that choice.[13]

Fourteen years later, little has changed. The Government responded by focusing on 'choice' and 'women-centred care' which has become the mantra for maternity care in the new millennium. Choice and women-centred care are illusions, as any woman who tries to exercise choice outside the menu prepared by health professionals will soon discover. As Ruth Sharples Weston observed:

> We do not have women-centred care we have consultant-centred care... with consultant-centred care a doctor who you may never see or meet dictates the choices you can make for birth. The consultant is the top of the hierarchy, the centre of the wheel. The service we receive revolves around their interests, wants, needs and foibles. The needs and wants of the birth woman are subjugated to him/her.[14]

Those women who want to birth at home still face an uphill battle. While the rhetoric of 'choice' suggests that home birth is available, the reality is that women are coerced and manipulated and misled. While in the past women could be sure of a midwife attending them at home, today practically every trust in the UK has an unwritten policy of telling women who book a home birth that 'should we be short of staff when you go into labour you will have to come into hospital'. It is only the women who insist that they are staying put who achieve a home birth and the trusts then claim that 'few women want to birth at home'.

In 1994 the UK Central Council for Nursing, Midwifery and Health Visiting, issued advice to midwives because of the problems women were having arranging a water birth. 'Water birth should... be viewed as an alternative method of care and management in labour and as one which must, therefore, fall within the duty of care and normal sphere of the practice of a midwife.' Twelve years later women are still being told that there is no guarantee that a water birth will be available, and that if the midwife who is qualified is not available they will have to get out of the water.

When anaesthetists wanted midwives to take over the topping up of epidurals the midwives adopted the proposals overnight, but AIMS has never had a case of a woman refused an epidural because the midwife was not trained to top it up.

12 Tew (1980)

13 Health Committee (1992)

14 Sharples Weston (2005)

As Nadine Edwards has shown in her book *Birthing Autonomy*, women are manipulated, bullied, coerced and guided into making choices that their carers want rather than deciding upon what they want for themselves.[15]

Effecting change

Over time, childbirth groups have progressed from being viewed as an irritating source of uppity women, to the present day, when no official body can produce anything without having 'consulted' the users.

Alongside the rhetoric of 'choice' came the need to demonstrate that women were 'consulted' and no organisation worth its salt produces anything without going through a consultation process. While, in many instances, it is a paper exercise and there is little or no intention of listening to what it is said, it does offer the users an opportunity to influence decisions and some changes have resulted. The National Institute for Clinical Excellence (NICE) actively includes and recruits lay involvement in drafting its clinical guidelines and actually provides some financial assistance to enable groups to take part. However, the deluge of 'consultation' has resulted in user groups becoming overwhelmed and, because the majority of consultations do not fund user involvement, the quality of the responses they receive is often inadequate. Expecting users to respond, often within a very short time frame, on top of dealing with the day-to-day work of their groups, is another form of abuse.

Even though women have succeeded in taking one step forward in the battle to improve maternity care from a woman's perspective, women's voices are still not heard in the corridors of power. Despite nominal representation on local trust boards, maternity services liaison committees, Royal Colleges and the Department of Health, women are a minority influence. They may well be able to affect the provision of new curtains for the labour ward, but where it matters most – the power base, where crucial decisions are taken about the provision of care – women have barely a toehold. Just as lawyers quickly learned to use a female barrister to defend a rapist, so health professionals soon learned to appoint a token woman to speak 'for women'. However, if she really speaks for women and makes a fuss, or is too critical, she soon finds herself out of a job. Such pressures can inhibit plain speaking, but in spite of this lay members have spoken out. Jean Robinson, a lay representative on the General Medical Council, published a book, *A Patient Voice at the GMC*,[16] which drew attention to the activities of this body and the difficulties a lay member had in effecting change.

Challenging a dominant ideology takes time, patience, and multiple strategies. Women initially asked nicely, in the belief that if the effects of unnecessary medical intervention were explained to the professionals they would understand and alter their practice. The women were dismissed on the grounds that the professionals knew better.

The profession's claim that their practice was based on research resulted in the users asking to see the research evidence. What they found came as a terrific shock – very little maternity practice was based on good research evidence. The users changed tactics, they started to read and challenge the research and advise individual women who were not happy with what they were told to ask for the evidence and say: 'Thank you for your advice, I would like to see the research paper upon which it is based and after I have read

15 Edwards (2005)
16 Robinson (1988)

it I will decide whether or not to act on what you have recommended'.

Midwives, skilled at doing good by stealth, would 'accidentally' drop the scissors when required to do a routine episiotomy, or not call the obstetrician because 'suddenly the baby emerged'. Women would avoid going to a hospital appointment thereby avoiding a browbeating session with the doctor, or call the midwife to a home birth at the last minute so that she would arrive too late to intervene.

Women, faced with a hospital birth and meeting a midwife they had never seen before, wrote their own 'birth plans' but that initiative backfired when hospitals devised birth plans for themselves. Later research revealed that those women who went into hospital with a birth plan ended up with more interventions than those who did not put their intentions on paper.[17] It has been speculated that the increased interventions may have been provoked because the attendants resented being told what to do by the women.

Finally, there is confrontation. When all else has failed the time comes to stand up and challenge the status quo. Despite the Government's desire to see community-based care; despite research showing far better outcomes for women and babies when women have individualised, community-based midwifery care; despite the rhetoric that care should be women-centred; despite the government's assurance that small maternity units would not be closed down; despite huge local opposition; the system persists in being doctor-centred and pursues the medical profession's aim of establishing more large, centralised obstetric units.

It took less than a decade to force the vast majority of women into hospital for birth and 40 years to change the perception that home birth is dangerous. Unless we challenge the current plans for centralised obstetric care it may well take another 40 years to get the majority of women out of large centralised hospitals. Women and midwives are a potentially powerful group – if only they will get together and realise the potential they have.

References

Allison J (1992) *Delivered at Home*. Chapman and Hall.

Donnison J (1988) *Midwives and Medical Men – A history of the struggle for the control of childbirth*. Historical Publications.

Edwards NP (2005) *Birthing Autonomy*. Routledge.

Hadikin R and O'Driscoll M (2000) *The Bullying Culture*. Books for Midwives Press.

Health Committee (1992) *Second Report, 1991–2 Session, 'The Organisation of Maternity Services'* Vol.1. London: HMSO.

Hayes K (1998) Personal Communication of February 1998.

Jones MH, Barik S, Mangune HH et al (1998) 'Do birth plans adversely affect the outcome of labour?' *British Journal of Midwifery*, Vol.6, No.1, pp.38–41.

Peel, Sir J (1970) *Standing Maternity and Midwifery Advisory Committee, Domiciliary Midwifery and Maternity Bed Needs*. HMSO.

Robinson J (1974) 'A time to be born', *The Times*, 12 August.

17 Jones et al (1998)

Robinson J (1988) *A Patient Voice at the GMC – A lay member's view of the General Medical Council*. London: Health Rights.

Sharples Weston, R (2005) 'Liberating Childbirth', *AIMS Journal*, Vol.17, No.3, pp.6–9.

Sleep J (1984) 'Episiotomy in normal delivery', *Nursing*, 2, p.614.

Storrs R (1843) General Register Office.

Tew M (1980) 'Is home a safer place?' *Health and Social Service Journal*, 89: 702–5.

World Health Organisation (1985) *Summary report on the Joint Interregional Conference on Appropriate Technology for Birth*. (ICP.NCH 102/m02s) Regional Office for Europe, World Health Organisation.

Who Decides What Women Get in Childbirth?

Jane Sandall

About 601,000 births took place in England in 2004–5; the majority of them took place in the NHS with 0.5 per cent in the private sector. Maternity care remains one of the few areas of health care that still embodies the original collective vision of the NHS. It is an equaliser, where women of all social classes and from all ethnic and cultural backgrounds have the possibility of receiving the same service. In the UK, a range of policies have driven changes in the organisation and delivery of maternity care, and thus the choices available to women. *The Winterton Report* and the government's response, *Changing Childbirth*, used the views and experiences of women in their recommendations.[1] Both reports concluded that there should be less focus on mortality rates as the major outcome measure and recommended a move towards a 'woman-centred' approach that offered women choice in place, type of service and 'continuity of care'. *Changing Childbirth* ignored the wider range of social and environmental effects on health highlighted in *The Winterton Report* in favour of a strategy that treated maternity care as a vehicle for the expression of consumer values (Streetly, 1994). Viewed through this lens, policymakers used the argument of women's interests to pursue particular management aims. Not surprisingly, the implementation of the *Changing Childbirth* policy has been patchy, and pilot schemes were not mainstreamed.

More recently, Parliamentary Reports on maternity care have expressed concerns yet again regarding lack of real choice in place of birth, rising caesarean section rates, inequalities in care, and about the maternity staff shortages as well as the huge variation in services across the country.[2] These concerns have informed the *National Service Framework for Children, Young People and Maternity Services*.[3] The key vision in this ten-year programme espouses the following principles and philosophy:

- That services are viewed from the perspective of a woman's journey through the system
- That for the majority of women, pregnancy and childbirth are straightforward processes and events, facilitated by health professionals, during which medical interventions should only be recommended if they are of demonstrable benefit to mother and/or child
- That the provision of information about choices and service provision in pregnancy and childbirth are paramount
- That services should be community-based, woman-centred, and ensure a non-interventionist service for women at low risk, focusing on normal childbirth
- That services for childbirth should be provided as close to home as possible within a

1 House of Commons (1992); Department of Health (1993)

2 House of Commons Health Committee (2003a, 2003b and 2003c)

3 Department of Health (2004a)

clinical network that provides an appropriate level of care for women and babies with complications.

What do women want?

> In a civilised country, the fourth richest in the world, is it not reasonable to expect that every mother giving birth should be accompanied by a midwife, a knowledgeable and skilled professional, to accompany her through what can be a traumatic and frightening experience?
>
> Baroness Cumberlege
>
> *House of Lords Debate on Maternity Care, January 2003*

Women's birth experiences can influence how they feel about themselves, their relationship with their baby and their future parenting. Research that has asked women what they would like has been criticised as promoting the status quo because, in general, service users tend to value the kind of care they have experienced over innovations of which they have no experience.[4] Bearing this caution in mind, general desires that arise from this research are: [5]

- To have trust and confidence in staff providing intrapartum care
- To have one-to-one care from a named midwife throughout labour and birth whom they have got to know and trust throughout pregnancy
- To receive personalised care and be treated with kindness, support and respect
- A pleasant and safe birth environment
- To receive adequate information and explanations about choices for childbirth, including pain relief and hospital practices
- To be listened to and have real choices in place and type of birth
- To have access to medical help if complications arise.

It has been argued that only the more vocal women make the above demands. However, women who are disadvantaged and socially excluded require similar services but are less likely to be listened to, or to get them.[6] So what is the current situation in 2006? Who decides what type of service women get and how is the decision made? These questions will be considered through looking at a number of critical issues.

Choice – where?

Around 2 per cent of births took place at home and 5 per cent on midwife/GP wards. There is a very small increase in the numbers of women who are birthing out of hospital (home birth, midwife led units, GP units) with wide geographical variations in the availability of community midwife led units and home birth ranging from 0–45 per cent.[7] Community-based, midwife-led birth centres provide locally accessible and low-tech care. In the DoH-funded evaluation of the Edgware Birth Centre over 90 per cent of

4 Teijlingen et al (2003)

5 Garcia et al (1998); Gready et al (1995); Green et al (1998); Lavender (2003)

6 Singh and Newburn (2001); McCourt and Pearce (2000)

7 Office for National Statistics (2006)

women cited as prime attractions (of the birth centre) 1) the relaxed and homely atmosphere, 2) the freedom to do what felt right for them during labour and delivery and 3) having their own room from the time of arrival until the time of leaving. Interventions in labour were significantly reduced in women using the birth centre when compared to a similar group of women at 'low risk' who planned to have their babies at local maternity hospitals.[8] Overall, a Cochrane Review found that there appeared to be some benefits from home-like settings for childbirth, although increased support from caregivers is a more important factor than pretty wallpaper.[9] In addition, if midwife-led units aim to replicate home, why not make the provision of birth at home a reality where women really do have control over their space and health professionals are truly guests.

What kind of birth?

A strategy for 'normal' birth based on current evidence aims to promote a culture of the expectation of normality in childbirth among society and professionals as a means of effecting improved outcomes for mother and child.[10] In 2004–5, an estimated 48 per cent of women gave birth without intervention. (Defined by ONS as without induction, without the use of instruments, not by caesarean section and without general, spinal or epidural anaesthetic before or during delivery.) This compares with 56 per cent in 1991–2. It is unknown how many women nationally gave birth without a wider range of interventions, but local studies indicate that it could be as low as 25 per cent using the following criteria in addition to the ones above (ARM, acceleration, episiotomy).[11] There are unexplained variations in childbirth interventions and caesarean section rates,[12] along with variations in the use of effective interventions, despite the introduction of evidence-based clinical guidelines and strong evidence from the Cochrane Library.[13] Such variations carry social, psychological and economic costs.[14] In addition, more needs to be known about the short- and long-term impact of mode of delivery on the baby.[15]

The proportion of women having a caesarean increased from a level of under 3 per cent in the 1950s to 12 per cent by 1990, reaching 23 per cent by 2005. There is some evidence that the birth environment and organisational culture are important factors in contributing to a woman-friendly space, and in improving 'normality' in childbirth.[16] There is evidence in other fields that staffing levels and skill mix have a beneficial impact on outcomes.[17] It is unknown whether the same pattern occurs with midwife staffing numbers, but lack of such important evidence has implications for how maternity services are staffed and by whom.

There is some evidence that guideline-driven care is effective in changing the process and outcome of care provided by professions allied to medicine. However, caution is needed in generalising findings to other professions and settings.[18] The National Institute

8 Saunders et al (2000)
9 Hodnett (2003)
10 National Childbirth Trust (2003a)
11 Downe, McCormick and Beech (2001)
12 RCOG Clinical Effectiveness Support Unit (2001)
13 Wilson et al (2002)
14 Tracy and Tracy (2003)
15 Bewley and Cockburn (2002)
16 Ontario Women's Health Council (2002)
17 Rafferty et al (2006)
18 Thomas et al (2003)

for Clinical Excellence guidelines have been developed for antenatal care for healthy pregnant women, caesarean section, induction of labour and electronic fetal monitoring, with new guidelines being developed on intrapartum care, postnatal care and postnatal depression. However, the social and political shaping of the construction of these powerful multi-professional guidelines has gone unexamined. The majority of current guidelines focus on the scope of midwifery practice, and the implementation of guidelines and the impact on practice and women's experiences of care have been largely unevaluated. In particular, guidelines that advocate the non-use of a technology such as routine electronic fetal monitoring for women at 'low risk' seem to be heavily contested in practice.

Managing pain

Support from the midwife may include helping the woman to make informed choices about her pain relief, helping her choose among pharmacological and non-pharmacological methods. A woman's reactions to labour pain may be influenced by the circumstances of her labour, including the environment and the support she receives. Preparation for childbirth during pregnancy has been shown to reduce the need for pain relief in labour.[19] The use of coping skills in labour is associated with definite benefits in terms of women's experience of pain and emotional distress. Many women in labour value the use of mobility and water, and alternative methods. Coping skills are easily disrupted by changing environment and after procedures such as monitoring or examinations.[20] In 2004–5, about 20 per cent of women had an epidural before or during delivery, 2 per cent had a general anaesthetic and 12 per cent a spinal anaesthetic. Epidural analgesia is very effective in reducing pain during labour, although there appear to be some potentially adverse effects. Further research is needed to investigate beneficial and adverse effects and to evaluate the different techniques used in epidural analgesia.[21]

Improving safety

Whilst childbirth has become increasingly safe for most women, there is still no such thing as zero risk for childbearing women as the Health Commission enquiry at a London Hospital has shown.[22] A small number of women die due to failure to detect the severity of illness and effect optimal treatment, failure to seek advice from appropriately experienced staff, failure of experienced staff to attend, and poor communication and teamwork. However, just over 50 per cent of direct maternal deaths are due to having some form of substandard care in which a different treatment may have affected outcome.[23] Maternal deaths should not be regarded as the only indicator of substandard care as valuable lessons can also be learnt from the numerically much larger numbers of near misses and serious morbidity,[24] and the level of chronic morbidity that incapacitates women still remains unrecognised.[25]

There are some clear indications for delivery in hospital units with appropriate levels of expertise. However, the evidence that formal risk scoring is helpful in predicting poor

---

19 Hodnett (2002); Simkin (1995)

20 Spiby et al (1999)

21 Howell (2003)

22 Healthcare Commission (2006)

23 CESDI (1997)

24 Waterstone et al (2003)

25 Bick and MacArthur (1995); MacArthur, Lewis and Knox (1991); Thompson et al (2002)

outcome is less clear cut, and labelling may result in unwarranted interventions.[26] A wide range of criteria are currently used to determine who may be considered low risk and plan to give birth either in a midwife-led unit or at home.[27]

Recent public inquiries, the acceptance by medical and professional institutions of the need for more robust and publicly demonstrated forms of professional regulation, an apparent declining trust in public services and professionals, and the proliferation of new health care regulatory bodies, indicate that these issues have become highly charged topics of public concern. The Bristol enquiry and the Ayling and Neale enquiry reports[28] indicate that major work is needed on the problem of cultures within the health service that prohibit professionals from reporting concerns to one another across professional boundaries. The National Patient Safety Agency has taken forward the issues raised in *An Organisation with a Memory*[29] and *Building a Safer NHS for Patients*[30] stressing a systems-led approach to changing those aspects of NHS culture that contribute to organisational disincentives to learning from errors. However, in practice, a blame culture and scapegoating continue in a field where litigation risk is high.

Continuity of care

Support by midwives in labour can be provided either by a midwife whom the woman has not met, or as part of a model which provides continuity of care throughout pregnancy, birth and the postnatal period. Continuity of care can be defined in a range of ways.[31] There is evidence that continuity of care in complex organisations may be associated with increased patient safety.[32] Women tend to express a preference for what they have experienced,[33] and women who had a known carer in labour were considerably more likely to say this was important to them than women who had not.[34] There is strong evidence that women who receive care from a team of midwives do not develop a relationship of trust or value care in the same way, and that such care has less impact on childbirth outcomes.[35,36] There is a small amount of evidence that caseload models of care are more sustainable for the midwifery workforce than team midwifery due to a greater degree of control over work organisation and job satisfaction.[37] A review of costs of caseload care found that costs depend on location of care, caseload size and staffing costs. Such models of caseload midwifery care, which have been set up to serve disadvantaged women,[38] and involve midwife community-based case loading,[39] are being evaluated through the Sure Start programme.[40] Outcomes from caseload models

26 Anderson and Blott (2003)
27 Campbell (1999)
28 Department of Health (2004b and 2004c)
29 Department of Health (2000)
30 http://www.publications.doh.gov.uk/buildsafenhs/
31 Freeman (2000)
32 Cook, Render and Woods (2000)
33 Hundley et al (2002)
34 Garcia et al (1998); Allen, Bourke Dowling and Williams (1997); Gready, Newburn and Dodds (1995)
35 Green, Renfrew and Curtis (2000)
36 Kaufman (2000)
37 Sandall J (1998 and 1999)
38 Hutchings and Henty (2002); Sandall, Davies and Warwick (2001)
39 Davies and Evans (1991); Sandall, Davies and Warwick (2001); Marks, Siddle and Warwick (2003)
40 Hutchings and Henty (2002)

include a higher rate of home births, reduction in the use of epidural anaesthesia and pharmacological analgesia, lower oxytocin augmentation, lower rate of caesarean section, lower rates of episiotomies, lower rate of inductions, higher rates of breastfeeding and more positive responses to the experience of pregnancy and birth.[41] There is some evidence that women at low risk who choose their place of birth once labour has commenced have good birth outcomes, and that labour assessment programmes, which aim to delay hospital admission until active labour, may benefit women with term pregnancies.[42] Such a model of care reduces the number of women coming into hospital too soon. This is best achieved within a caseload midwifery model that conducts early labour assessment at home.

Woman-centred care

Women have complained of depersonalised and 'production line' care. In one national study, two-thirds of women were left without professional support at some time during labour, and 25 per cent said this worried them.[43] Women in labour have need for companionship, empathy and help as well as skilled professional care and frequently the midwife is the person who will provide this. There is now cumulative evidence from a systematic review of randomised trials that one-to-one continuous support for a woman in labour can both reduce intervention rates and improve maternal and neonatal outcomes.[44] Support may be provided by a range of professional and lay people. A policy of continuous support during labour improves outcomes of labour but may increase short-term marginal health care costs. Costs are likely to be considerably more where additional external staff are employed solely to provide support. The results are sensitive to the costs of interventions in labour.[45] Thus, the role of maternity assistants and of doulas (whom women pay themselves), will be a contentious one for midwives.

Working in partnership with women

In addition, a smaller percentage of women reported 'having a say' in childbirth interventions compared to other aspects of maternity care. Partnerships are achieved through empowering women and their families and by full involvement in choices about their care. Women report a lack of real choice and information about provision of services for out-of-hospital birth, at home and in midwife-led birth centres.[46] There is evidence of ad hoc service reconfigurations that have had more negative than positive effects from the perspective of women and their families.[47] There is little evidence how reconfiguration affects accessibility for geographically isolated or disadvantaged groups.[48] It is important that women and their families are able to access and transfer within the system, and that they should know to whom, and where they would be referred if a problem arose. In order to keep care locally accessible and provide high-quality care,

---

41 The North Staffordshire Changing Childbirth Research Team (2000); Page et al (1999); Homer, Davis, Brodie et al (2001); Benjamin, Walsh and Toub (2001); Sandall, Davies and Warwick (2001)

42 Lauzon and Hodnett (2003)

43 Audit Commission (1997)

44 Hodnett et al (2003)

45 Henderson, Mugford and Hodnett (Unpublished)

46 Lavender and Chapple (2003)

47 National Childbirth Trust (2003b)

48 Gulliford et al (2001)

clinical networks offer the potential for women to move in a systematic pathway through the system, which may be configured in a range of service models such as a hub-and-spoke model of a specialist tertiary centre surrounded by midwife-led units or community-based group practices and secondary care.[49]

There is increasing evidence that user involvement in the commissioning and evaluation of services improves quality. Interventions to promote patient-centred care within clinical consultations may significantly increase the patient-centredness of care. However, there is limited and mixed evidence on the effects of such interventions on patient health care behaviours or health status; or on whether these interventions might be applicable to providers other than physicians.

Care of women with medical complications should be provided by multidisciplinary teams. However, there is little evidence as to which organisation and patterns of care produce the best outcomes in women with a high-risk pregnancy.[50] Good evidence is now needed about the optimum patterns of care for women in this group. A maternity clinical network may mirror the developing neonatal services-managed clinical networks.[51]

Conclusion

In the light of current changes what are the key issues facing maternity services today? Changes in workforce deployment such as the Changing Workforce Programme, revisions to medical training, the European Working Time Directive, maternity staffing standards and neonatal service reconfigurations are all altering professional practice boundaries.[52] This has resulted in the introduction of maternity support workers, of senior medical staff taking on direct care, extending the roles of nurses and midwives to include activities usually undertaken by junior doctors, and the promotion of midwifery-led care.[53]

Midwives will be expected to work in more autonomous ways, taking on new areas of responsibilities which will require new knowledge and new areas of expertise and development of clinical skills. The scope of midwifery practice of UK midwives is already broad compared to many other countries. There were 30,000 practising midwives and 2,000 consultant obstetricians in the UK in 2003. In 2004–5, about 36 per cent of births were attended by hospital doctors and 64 per cent by midwives. The overall balance between the professions has changed steadily since 1989–90 when 24 per cent of births were attended by doctors and 76 per cent by midwives. This shift reflects the changing pattern of delivery method. Virtually all spontaneous births are conducted by midwives, while doctors conduct caesareans and virtually all instrumental deliveries.[54]

Midwives will be expected to be exercising independent clinical judgement, both in initial history taking and diagnosis, referral and intervention in pregnancy and childbirth. They will be expected to develop new knowledge such as expertise in pre-conception care, early pregnancy care, maternal and newborn screening, perinatal mental illness, and new clinical skills such as emergency obstetric and newborn life support skills,

49 Hibbard et al (1993)

50 Anderson and Blott (2003)

51 Scottish Executive (2003)

52 RCOG, RCM (1999)

53 Modernization Agency, Working Time Directive, Future Healthcare Network, NHS Confederation (2004)

54 Office for National Statistics (2006)

examination of the newborn, and new management skills such as managing a birth centre, managing a caseload, managing a group practice, running groups, working with voluntary groups and service uses, effective health promotion techniques, peer review and practice audit techniques, leading and managing a team and ability to understand and critique evidence. Midwives will need to develop their leadership skills for working within a multi-agency context at both a strategic and operational level.

Under current consideration are the employment of nurses in HDU areas and postnatal wards, the future role and responsibilities of maternity assistants in hospital and the community. Looking abroad, UK midwifery could either move down an American route, where midwives supervise the work of labour room nurses and provide a wider service overall in terms of women's health needs, or to a model such as that in New Zealand, where many midwives work in community-based practices, and women choose their lead maternity carer who gets paid directly by the state. The problem with this, and the Dutch system, is that when women develop complications, care is handed on to tertiary care providers. It can be argued that women are the losers here in a system where midwifery jurisdiction is so tightly bounded. The NSF has provided a philosophy and underlying principles of care and provides the opportunity for midwives to develop their practice in partnership with women. The major issue is whether enough midwives wish to, and are equipped to rise to the challenge.

References

Allen I, Bourke Dowling S and Williams S (1997) *A Leading Role for Midwives – Evaluation of Midwifery Group Practice Development Projects.* London: Policy Studies Institute.

Anderson E and Blott M (2003) 'What is "best practice" in terms of the organisation and delivery of services for women with medical and/or obstetric complications', Commissioned unpublished review. Oxford: NPEU.

Audit Commission (1997) *First class delivery: Improving maternity services in England and Wales*. London: Audit Commission.

Benjamin Y, Walsh D and Toub N (2001) 'A comparison of partnership caseload midwifery care with conventional team midwifery care: labour and birth outcomes', *Midwifery*, 17:234–40.

Bewley S and Cockburn J (2002) 'II. The unfacts of "request" caesarean section', *BJOG*, 109(6):597–605.

Bick D and MacArthur C (1995) 'The extent, severity and effect on health problems after childbirth', *British Journal of Midwifery*, 3:31.

Campbell R (1999) 'Review and assessment of selection criteria used when booking pregnant women at different places of birth', BJOG, 106:550–6.

CESDI (1997) *4th Annual report, Intrapartum related deaths*. London: CESDI.

Cook RI, Render M and Woods DD (2000) 'Gaps in the continuity of care and progress on patient safety', *BMJ*, 320:791–4.

Davies J and Evans F (1991) 'The Newcastle Community Midwifery Care Project and evaluation', *Midwives, Research and Childbirth*, Vol.II. London: Chapman and Hall.

Department of Health (1993) *Changing Childbirth, Part 1: Report of the Expert Maternity Group*. London: HMSO.

Department of Health (2000) *An organisation with a memory, Report of an expert group on learning from adverse events in the NHS chaired by the Chief Medical Officer*. London: DoH.

Department of Health (2004a) *National Service Framework for Children, Young People and Maternity Services*. London: DoH.

Department of Health (2004b) *Committee of inquiry, independent investigation into how the NHS handled allegations about the conduct of Clifford Ayling, submitted to the Secretary of State for Health on 15 July*, Cm 6298. Norwich: TSO.

Department of Health (2004c) *Committee of inquiry to investigate how the NHS handled allegations about the performance and conduct of Richard Neale, Submitted to the Secretary of State for Health on Thursday 19 August 2004 by Her Honour Judge Matthews QC*, Cm 6315. Norwich: TSO.

Downe S, McCormick C and Beech BL (2001) 'Labour interventions associated with normal birth', *British Journal of Midwifery*, 9, 10:602–606.

Freeman G, Shepperd S, Robinson I, Ehrich K and Richards S (2000) *Continuity of Care. Report of a Scoping Exercise for the National Coordinating Centre for NHS Service, Delivery and Organisation R&D*. London: NCCSDO.

Garcia J, Redshaw M, Fitzsimons B and Keene J (1998) *First Class Delivery, A National Survey of Women's Views of Maternity Care*. London: Audit Commission, NPEU.

Gready M, Newburn M and Dodds R (1995) *Choices – Childbirth options*. London: National Childbirth Trust.

Green JM, Coupland V and Kritzinger JV (1998) *Great expectations, A prospective Study of Women's Expectations and Experiences of Childbirth*. Cheshire: Books for Midwives Press.

Green J, Renfrew M and Curtis P (2000) 'Continuity of care: what matters to women, review of the evidence', *Midwifery*, 16:186–96.

Gulliford M, Morgan M, Hughes D et al (2001) *Access to Health Care, Report of a Scoping Exercise for the NCCSDO*. London: King's College.

Healthcare Commission (2006) *Investigation into 10 maternal deaths at, or following delivery at, Northwick Park Hospital, North West London Hospitals Trust, between April 2002 and April 2005*. London: HCC.

Henderson J, Mugford M and Hodnett E (Unpublished) 'Cost Consequences of Continuous Support During Labour: Economic Implications of The Results of a Systematic Review of Trials'. Oxford: NPEU.

Hibbard BM, Dawson A, Boyce J et al (1993) 'A paramedic based emergency domiciliary obstetric service: the South Glamorgan experience', *British Journal Obs & Gynae*, 100(7): 618–22.

Hodnett ED (2002) 'Pain and women's satisfaction with the experience of childbirth: a systematic review', *Am J Obstet Gynecol*, May 2002, 186 (5 Suppl Nature):S160–72.

Hodnett ED (2003) 'Home-like versus conventional institutional settings for birth' (Cochrane Review). In: *The Cochrane Library*, Issue 2, 2003. Oxford: Update Software.

Hodnett ED, Gates S, Hofmeyr GJ and Sakala C (2003) 'Continuous support for women during childbirth' (Cochrane Review). In: The Cochrane Library, Issue 3, 2003. Oxford: Update Software.

Homer CSE, Davis GK, Brodie PM et al (2001) 'Collaboration in maternity care: a randomised trial comparing community-based continuity of care with standard hospital care', *BJOG*, 108,1:16–22.

House of Commons Health Committee (2003a) *Provision of Maternity Services, Fourth Report of Session 2002–3*, Vol.1. London: The Stationery Office.

House of Commons Health Committee (2003b) *Inequalities in access to Maternity Services, Eighth Report of Session 2002–03,* Vol.1. London: The Stationery Office.

House of Commons Health Committee (2003c) *Choice in Maternity Services, Ninth Report of Session 2002–03,* Vol.1. London: The Stationery Office.

Howell CJ (2003) 'Epidural versus non-epidural analgesia for pain relief in labour' (Cochrane Review). In: *The Cochrane Library*, Issue 2, 2003. Oxford: Update Software.

Hundley V, Penney G, Fitzmaurice A, van Teijlingen E and Graham W (2002) 'A comparison of data obtained from service providers and service users to assess the quality of maternity care', *Midwifery*, 18 (2):126–35.

Hutchings J and Henty D (2002) 'Caseload midwifery practice in partnership with sure start: changing the culture of birth', *MIDIRS Midwifery Digest*, 12, supplement 1, S38–S40.

Kaufman K (2000) 'Have we yet learned about the effects of continuity of midwifery care?' *Birth*, 27,3:174–6.

Lauzon L and Hodnett E (2003) 'Labour assessment programs to delay admission to labour wards' (Cochrane Review). In: *The Cochrane Library*, Issue 2, 2003. Oxford: Update Software.

Lavender T (2003) 'Report to the Department of Health Children's Taskforce from the Maternity and Neonatal Workforce Group – January 2003'. http://www.advisorybodies.doh.gov.uk/maternitywg/report-jan03.pdf#search=%22tina%20lavender%22 (accessed 6 September 2006).

Lavender T and Chapple J (2003) *Evaluation of Different Models of Maternity Care. The views of Women and Midwives*. London: DH.

MacArthur C, Lewis M and Knox E (1991) *Health after Childbirth*. London: HMSO.

McCourt C and Pearce A (2000) 'Does continuity of carer matter to women from ethnic minority groups?' *Midwifery*, 16: 145–54.

Marks MN, Siddle K and Warwick C (2003) 'Can we prevent postnatal depression? A randomised controlled trial to assess the impact of continuity of midwifery care on rates of postnatal depression in high risk women', *Journal of Maternal-Fetal and Neonatal Medicine*, 12, 1–9.

Modernization Agency, Working Time Directive, Future Healthcare Network, NHS Confederation (2004) 'Survey of models of maternity care. Towards sustainable WTD compliant staffing and clinical network solutions'.

National Childbirth Trust (2003a) *The NCT Birth Policy*, 12 Principles. London: NCT.

National Childbirth Trust (2003b) *Reconfiguring Maternity Services, Views of User Representatives*. London: NCT.

The North Staffordshire Changing Childbirth Research Team (2000) 'A randomised study of midwifery caseload and traditional "shared care"', Midwifery, 16:295–302.

Office for National Statistics (2006) *NHS Maternity Statistics, England: 2004–05.* London: Government Statistical Service.

Ontario Women's Health Council (2002) *Attaining and maintaining best practices in the use of Caesarean sections, An analysis of four Ontario hospitals*, Report of the Caesarean section working group of the Women's Health Council. http://www.womenshealthcouncil.on.ca

Page L, McCourt C, Beake S, Vail A and Hewison J (1999) 'Clinical Interventions and outcomes of One-to-One midwifery practice', *Journal of Public Health Medicine*, 21:243–8.

Rafferty A, Clarke SP et al (2006) 'Outcomes of variation in hospital nurse staffing in English hospitals: Cross-sectional analysis of survey data and discharge records', *Int Jnl Nursing Studies*.

RCOG Clinical Effectiveness Support Unit (2001) *The National Caesarean Section Audit Report*. London: RCOG.

RCOG, RCM (1999) *Towards safer childbirth. Minimum standards for the organisation of labour wards, Report of a Joint Working Party*. London: RCOG.

Sandall J (1998) 'Occupational burnout in midwives: new ways of working and the relationship between organisational factors and psychological health and well being', *Risk, Decision and Policy*, 3(3): 213–32.

Sandall J (1999) 'Team midwifery and burnout in midwives in the UK: practical lessons from a national study', Original article, *MIDIRS Midwifery Digest*, 9, 2:147–51.

Sandall J, Davies J and Warwick C (2001) *Evaluation of the Albany Midwifery Practice Final Report*, Nightingale School of Nursing and Midwifery, King's College London.

Saunders D, Boulton M, Chapple J, Ratcliffe J and Levitan J (2000) *Evaluation of the Edgware Birth Centre*. London: North Thames Perinatal Public Health Service.

Scottish Executive (2003) *Implementing a Framework for Maternity services in Scotland*. Edinburgh: Stationery Office.

Simkin P (1995) 'Reducing pain and enhancing progress in labour: a guide to non-pharmacologic methods for maternity caregivers', *Birth*, 22,161–71.

Singh D and Newburn M (2001) *Access to maternity information and support, the experience and needs of women before and after giving birth*. London: NCT.

Spiby H, Henderson B, Slade P et al (1999) 'Strategies for coping with labour: does antenatal education translate into practice?' *J. Advanced Nursing,* 29:388–94.

Teijlingen ER, Hundley V, Rennie A, Graham W and Fitzmaurice A (2003) 'Maternity satisfaction studies and their limitations: "What is, must be best"', *Birth*, 30, 2:75–82.

Thomas L, Cullum N, McColl E, Rousseau N, Soutter J and Steen N (2003) 'Guidelines in professions allied to medicine' (Cochrane Review). In: *The Cochrane Library*, Issue 2, 2003. Oxford: Update Software.

Thompson J, Roberts C, Currie M and Ellwood D (2002) 'Prevalence and persistence of health problems after childbirth: associations with parity and method of birth', *Birth*, 29:83–94.

Tracy SK and Tracy MB (2003) 'Costing the cascade: estimating the cost of increased obstetric intervention in childbirth using population data', *BJOG*, 110:717–24.

Waterstone M, Wolfe C, Hooper R and Bewley S (2003) 'Postnatal morbidity after childbirth and severe obstetric morbidity', *BJOG*, 110(2):128–33.

Wilson B, Thornton J, Hewison J, Lilford R, Watt I, Braunholtz D and Robinson M (2002) 'The Leeds University Maternity Audit Project', *International Journal for Quality in Health Care*, 14:175–81.

Summary and Policy Implications

Wendy Savage

As Luke Zander wrote in his preface, although there have been some positive initiatives in maternity care over the past 20 years the issues raised by my case remain unresolved. The chapters in this book show that problems remain in all areas.

'Birth and power' and 'what women want'

These two issues are intertwined: women cannot have the kind of birth they want and are capable of achieving unless they have some control over the way that services are provided. What women want is to be supported by one or two people they know and trust to give birth in an environment in which they feel they are in control and are safe. They hope to have a live healthy baby and come through the experience in the best condition possible for embarking on motherhood. Women still do not control childbirth and the services that have evolved over the last sixty years are unsuitable and unsustainable. The caesarean section rate continues to increase year on year without any sign of it falling and home birth is still not seen as a reasonable alternative by many professionals or managers. The ostensible reason for treating birth as a potential medical emergency, rather than as a profound personal experience rooted in the family, is that it is very dangerous. Yet 95.5 per cent of babies were born alive in 1946 and by 1970 this had risen to 97.6 per cent and birth trauma (when the baby was damaged by being forced down the birth canal) as a cause of perinatal death had virtually been eliminated. By 1980, over 99 per cent of babies of 28 weeks gestation and over survived the 'dangerous' experience of birth.

My solutions to the problem of inappropriate care are firstly to ring-fence the budget for maternity services. Surely the birth of healthy children is essential for the nation's welfare and their mothers need to be in the best possible condition to care for them. Without protection of the budget, other services such as cancer or heart disease, which are major causes of mortality, will be seen as more important. The recent reduction in the recruitment of midwives, despite the service already being understaffed, confirms the need for this to be done.

Secondly, midwives need more independence, in order to be able to provide the care that they want to give and women want to receive. The Dutch system, where still one-third of women have their babies at home, is a rare example in developed nations of strong independent midwifery with good outcomes for mother and child. I am not sure just what is needed to enable community care to regain its status and important role in the care of pregnant women. Perhaps adopting the 'one mother – one midwife' approach would be enough. Perhaps we should adopt my proposal that primary and secondary care midwives should work co-operatively, as GPs and hospital doctors do. I suggest that a pilot study of alternative methods of deploying midwives in different regions should be set up and successful models then extended to the whole NHS. The excellent results of the South East London Midwifery Group now working as the Albany practice at King's College Hospital show that high home birth rates, high breast feeding rates and lower CS rates can be achieved with midwives working in a way that gives personal continuity of care for women without being too stressful for the midwives themselves. The new National Service Framework for maternity care has good principles but the implementation needs to be overseen by an independent midwifery task force with enough power to ensure that things happen.

I think that midwives should regain their own regulatory body as they are very different from nurses, who outnumber them by 20 to 1 on the Nursing and Midwifery Board.

Lastly, we need to look at the way birth is treated in the national curriculum. Too often, frightening videos of women giving birth in a hospital setting are shown to teenagers, filmed purely from the medical viewpoint; and so the beauty and power of a woman giving birth with a supportive midwife at home is lost.

Accountability

Despite all the talk of openness and transparency our health bodies are not democratically elected, are increasingly subservient to Whitehall and with some notable exceptions are remote from the community they serve. Although the government talks about increasing local freedom to make decisions I believe that without elected members of trusts, who live locally, use the service and report back to the people who elected them, things will only get worse. As Onora O'Neill says, we need less rhetoric about openness and transparency and more honesty.

Her thoughts for improving accountability of public bodies are:

> Intelligent accountability, I suspect, requires more attention to good governance and fewer fantasies about total control. Good governance is possible only if institutions are allowed some margin for self-governance appropriate to their particular tasks, within a framework of financial and other reporting. Such reporting, I believe, is not improved by being wholly standardised and relentlessly detailed, and as much that needs to be accounted for is not easily measurable, it cannot be boiled down to a set of stock performance indicators. Those who are called to account should give an *account* of what they have done, and their successes and failures, to others who have sufficient time and experience to assess the evidence and report on it. Real accountability provides substantial and knowledgeable independent judgement of an institution's or professional's work.

As far as doctors are concerned I believe the pendulum has swung too far. Whilst 20 years ago doctors were rarely called to account, they now face too many systems of accountability in a climate where honest human error seems unrecognised. The current consultation about regulation of the medical profession ends on 10 November 2006. I have grave reservations about many of the proposals, which seem diametrically opposed to the sentiments expressed in this paragraph and which were also expressed by the Chief Medical Officer (CMO) himself in earlier publications.

Incompetence

Incompetence has been rare in the medical profession up until now. However, reduced hours of working coupled with changes in the teaching and training programme will either lead to narrowly competent specialists (as in the former Soviet Russia) or to an increase in the number of incompetent doctors. I believe that the leaders of the profession need to assert themselves and reclaim control of training and teaching. I disagree with the CMO's suggestion that undergraduate education should be overseen by a renamed Postgraduate Medical Education and Training Board. This has enough to do reorganising the postgraduate training without interfering with undergraduate education and imposing a sterile uniformity on medical schools. As professionals, we must not allow the government to gain control of the standards and content of education and the lay voice should be included as it is now by having independent governors.

Disciplinary procedures for doctors

The CMO clearly understands that most medical errors are due to systems' failures and that the way to improve the situation is by investigation to understand what went wrong and retraining – not by blaming and shaming. However, in the aftermath of the shortcomings exposed in Bristol and Alder Hey, managers appear to be far too ready to consider the use of immediate suspension – especially considering that the NCAS can find alternative measures to deal with the problem in 85 per cent of the cases. The changes in the disciplinary procedures, as highlighted by John Hendy's chapter, mean that doctors have lost the protection of an independent enquiry panel looking at whether the charges for which they are being disciplined are justified. The British Medical Association needs to renegotiate the framework with the Department of Health and the policy of individual trusts being responsible for disciplining doctors should be reconsidered.

In addition, to prevent the collusion between managers and doctors leading to inappropriate suspensions, consideration should be given to regulating managers. A regulatory body could set standards and discipline managers who breach them. The current practice does not inspire confidence in the medical profession or the public. Frequently, managers accused of inappropriate actions, for example illegal phone-tapping or falsifying their qualifications, lose their jobs in a blaze of publicity only to be quietly reinstated somewhere else when the furore has blown over.

Academic freedom

Academic freedom is in jeopardy as our universities yield to the siren call of the market and consumerism and the pressure from government to produce a compliant workforce. Vigilance to maintain academic standards is essential and joining CARAL might be one way of helping to uphold them. Baroness O'Neill's paragraph about accountability also applies to the way that the Research Assessment Exercise and the Teaching Quality Assessment do little to encourage academic freedom and innovative thought.

Conclusion

Twenty years have passed since my suspension was fiercely debated for months within the medical profession. The media covered the childbirth issues accurately throughout the prolonged period until I was reinstated. Yet the underlying issues are as alive today as they were then. Women need to take control of childbirth, academics need to make sure their voices are heard in universities and in the training of medical students and doctors need to challenge the way their hospital colleagues are disciplined if we are not to lose highly skilled doctors unnecessarily.

I would like to thank all those who contributed to this re-examination of the issues and all those at Middlesex University Press who produced the book. I have found writing this book difficult as it re-awakened many of the feelings of being trapped in a situation which I could not control, particularly when I returned to work in 1986. Any errors are my own.

Finally I would like to thank all those women in Tower Hamlets and the childbirth organisations, my patients and the GPs and midwives of Tower Hamlets. Within the medical school I received particular help and support from the late Professor David Ritchie, Professor Sheila Hillier, Professor David Wingate and Professor Irene Leigh and on my return to work Professor Mal Salkind and the Academic Department of General Practice.

Appendix

Wendy Savage's Submission to the Joint Working Party on Disciplining Doctors, 1987

16 May 1988

Dear Ms James,
I was invited to make comments on the HM(61)112 procedure currently being reviewed by the BMA in conjunction with the DHSS.

Firstly, there are the deficiencies of the procedure itself and secondly, the manner in which it is used in practice. Lastly I will make some suggestions for improving the system.

1.1 The procedure is out of line with modern employment law in that a prima facie case is built up secretly, before the accused doctor is aware that there are any complaints about his or her competence or conduct.

1.2 The responsibility for deciding whether or not a prima facie case exists lies in the hands of the Regional/District Chairperson who is advised by the respective General Manager and Medical Officer. In the case of the Region, the evidence collected by these people is usually indirect, relies heavily on unsworn testimony of the colleagues of the accused doctor and their altruism or lack of it is hard to ascertain. In the case of Teaching Districts the manipulation of people in essentially subordinate positions within the medical hierarchy, is well shown by my own case.

1.3 The way in which outside expertise is brought into the decision-making process is not spelt out and as in my case the unwritten rule that a close colleague should not be used to give impartial advice, may not be followed.

1.4 The access to notes in order to build up a case seems to break professional confidentiality for patients and trust between colleagues and the way these notes are used, in many cases without ensuring that the patient's name is removed before photocopying and sending to outside experts, lawyers etc seems quite wrong.

2.1 The way in which the defence organisations operate to protect their members from claims from patients does not make them well suited to deal with these employment problems. They must keep the doctors in 'watertight compartments' which can mean, as in my case, that the Regional Assessor was being advised by the MDU that there was no reason why he should not give an assessment of my cases whereas another person in the MDU knew that we met regularly at monthly meetings and that he had been closely involved with training both the Professor, who had collected the evidence against me, and one of the chief witnesses who testified about my alleged incompetence, the lecturer.

2.2 The defence organisations normally use their own firm of solicitors who have a very large case load and the leisurely time scale accepted in medico-legal cases can irretrievably damage the accused doctor's position, particularly if s/he has been suspended.

2.3 The defence organisations may assess the case on inadequate evidence and take a judgement that it is not in the interests of their members to fight a case in which the chance of success is not high. This is not good enough for a doctor faced with the loss of her or his profession. If the doctor goes to the BMA, the Industrial Relations Officers who do a good job may not have sufficient 'muscle' to protect the doctor and reference to Committees may delay crucial decisions. The BMA Legal Advisor cannot cope with the details of 40 cases a year in addition to his other work.

2.4 Suspension is often used inappropriately and because there are no guidelines as to how the suspended doctor should be treated, they are banned from the hospital precinct, not allowed to carry out duties such as teaching, research or administration that could still be usefully performed. The resulting isolation coupled with the instructions from lawyers not to discuss the situation with anyone leads to demoralisation of the accused doctor and allows gossip and rumour to thrive.

2.5 The standard of proof accepted by the Chairperson is often considerably less than would be accepted in a Court of Law.

2.6 The pressure on Regional Legal Advisors often leads to delay in instituting the case, with cancellations at the last minute which increase the doctor's demoralisation and frustration.

Alternatively the seriousness of the charges is not understood by the doctor who may not prepare the case or be represented adequately and then finds her or himself facing the permanent loss of her or his job.

I believe that the BMA has accepted this procedure despite its faults because, quite rightly, it feels that it should be difficult to dismiss a doctor because of the monopolistic position of the NHS as an employer, the rigidity of the career structure and the problem faced by a doctor who is dismissed by the NHS in finding alternative employment. In the private sector s/he may well face the same colleagues who have heard all about the case 'privately' and have accepted the 'verdict', and s/he is usually untrained for any other position and often too old to retrain. So dismissal by the NHS at age 50 means premature retirement of a skilled person whose training has been heavily underwritten by the State. However in my opinion it is wrong to sacrifice a few people for the job security of the many and it does not seem the way for us to behave having said that we will discipline ourselves as a profession.

3. Suggestions for improving the situation

I sincerely hope that the working party that is conducting this review has at least one and preferably two members from outside the charmed circle of the medico-legal world. Unless there are experts in employment law from different fields I believe the review will be fundamentally flawed. Medical employment must be seen in the context of the wider world.

3.1 The doctor should be told by the appropriate person as soon as a query is raised about her or his competence or conduct and her or his side of the story heard. If after this interview a problem has been agreed by both sides, a formal written warning should be given, and the steps necessary to deal with this discussed by both parties. If the problem continues, the doctor should be warned that evidence will now be formally collected and if patients are to be used, they should be told why and their consent should be sought before their case notes are used.

3.2 In the event of such a problem, the doctor should have access to legal advice through a new body to be set up under the control of the GMC or the BMA. The doctor would be entitled to select her or his own solicitor from a panel agreed by the defence organisations, who would continue to fund the doctor's defence.

3.3 The Regional/District Chairman in the event of a Tribunal or Enquiry being held should have to convene this within a stated period of time – three or at most six months – so that a decision about the doctor's future would be made within at most nine months or a year.

3.4 The Enquiry or Tribunal procedure should be in public and the witnesses should give evidence on oath. The rules of evidence should apply.

3.5 Suspension for any period other than a few days (ie to allow a dangerous situation to be assessed) should be referred to a panel of senior doctors maintained by the GMC/BMA who would decide having heard the evidence, whether or not the doctor's behaviour warrants such a measure. S/he should then be told clearly the reasons for this by the panel, the steps necessary to resolve the situation and how long this should be for. The suspended doctor should be usefully employed in the hospital if at all possible.

If the underlying reason for the problem is mental illness then the doctor must be told this and helped to obtain treatment.

3.6 Changing the consultant contract so that there are more short-term contracts of five to seven years could alleviate the underlying problem of conflict between colleagues which, as a deputy secretary of the BMA said, lay behind many accusations of misconduct or incompetence. Given a system as outlined above, this could work and even be welcomed by doctors, who like most of the population are less likely to stay in one place for 30 years now than when the NHS began 40 years ago.

3.7 Doctors who put forward a malicious case against one of their colleagues should be subject to summary dismissal by the RHA/DHA.

Wendy Savage

A Savage Enquiry

Who Controls Childbirth?

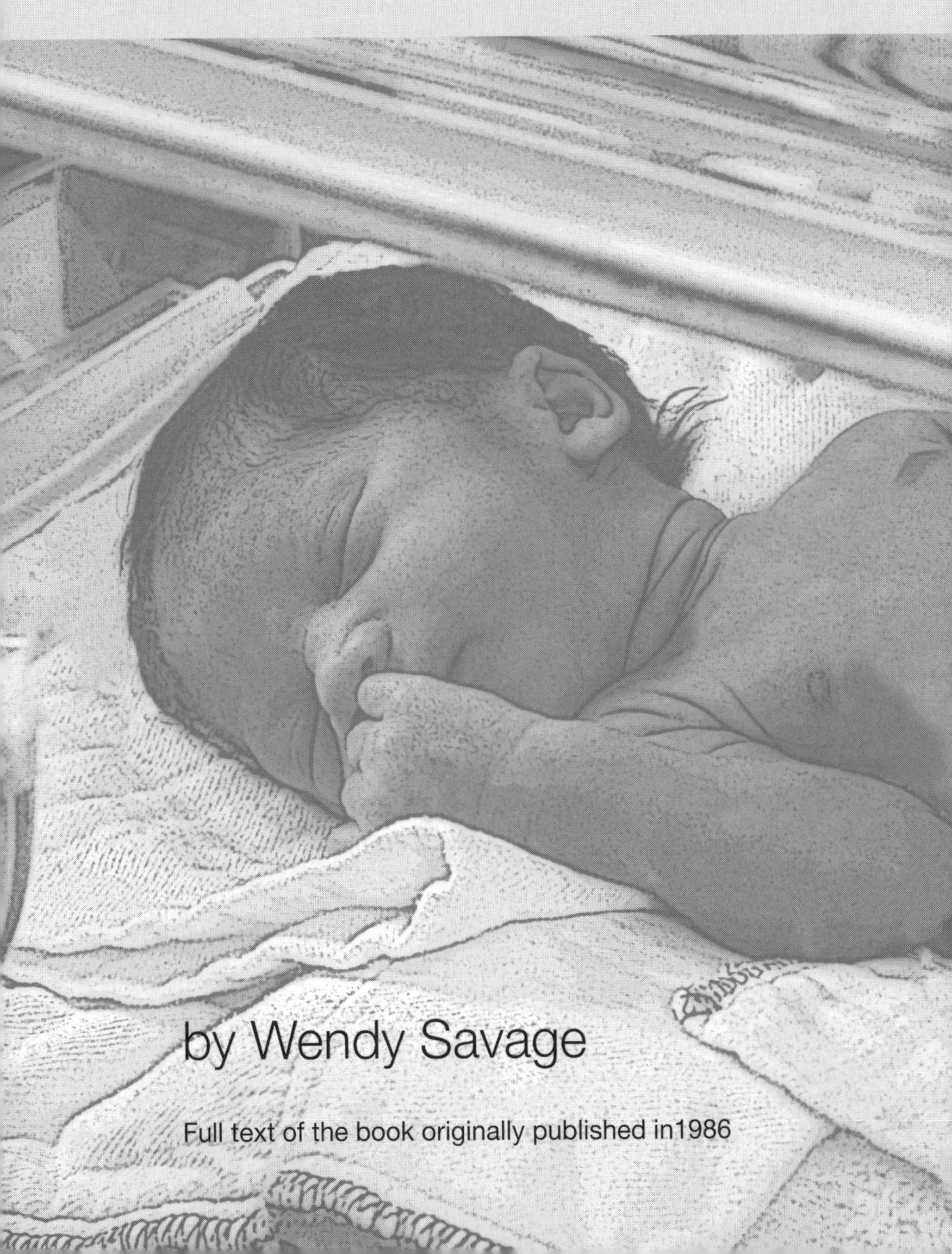

by Wendy Savage

Full text of the book originally published in1986

To all those who have known doubt, perplexity and fear
as I have known them,
To all who have made mistakes as I have,
To all those whose humility increases with their knowledge
of this most fascinating subject,

THIS BOOK IS DEDICATED

Ian Donald wrote this dedication when he was Regius Professor of Midwifery at the University of Glasgow for his book *Practical Obstetric Problems* (Lloyd Luke 1955). When I was working in Nigeria in 1964–7 his book was invaluable and I was delighted and honoured when he gave me permission to use his words for this book. I think myself fortunate when I worked in Nairobi from 1967–9 to have been trained by Glaswegians, as in general the Scottish contribution to obstetrics has been notable, and in particular Ian Donald's immense clinical knowledge has been complemented by his pioneering work with ultrasound.

AND IN ADDITION

This book is dedicated to the women of the world who face the uncertainty of childbirth with such optimism and courage.

Originally published by VIRAGO PRESS Ltd 1986

Contents

Acknowledgements 210
Dramatis Personae 212
Chronology 216
INTRODUCTION 217
CHAPTER 1 Suspension 219
CHAPTER 2 The Making of an Obstetrician 223
CHAPTER 3 Return to the London 231
CHAPTER 4 The Hidden Agenda 245
CHAPTER 5 The Muted Response of the Medical Establishment 259
CHAPTER 6 The Public Protests 267
CHAPTER 7 The Legal Battle 273
CHAPTER 8 The Five Cases 279
CHAPTER 9 The Run-up to the Enquiry 291
CHAPTER 10 The Enquiry Begins 295
CHAPTER 11 Expert Witnesses for the Prosecution 309
CHAPTER 12 I Defend My Practice 315
CHAPTER 13 Expert Witnesses for the Defence 325
CHAPTER 14 The Long Wait 337
CHAPTER 15 Birth and Power 343
APPENDIX I List of Charges 349
APPENDIX II General Conclusions of the Panel's Report 354

Acknowledgements

This book would not have been written without the assistance and friendship of Jane Leighton who, as a socialist and feminist, understood the medico-political issues so well; the support and enthusiasm of Debbie Owen, and the flexibility and encouragement of all the Virago staff. Brian Raymond has read numerous drafts rapidly and efficiently, and given me suggestions for more elegant phrases. Judi Dooling, Marianne Kilchenman and Barbara Smith have helped with some of the typing and Jane Hawksley redrafted chapter 2. I would like to thank them all for their help.

My thanks also to all those who have read parts of the manuscript and made suggestions comprehensively and fast despite their busy lives: Eva Alberman, Beverley Beech, Alex Campbell, Iain Chalmers, Peter Dunn, Myra Garrett, Sue Hadley, Marion Hall, Marky Hayton, John and Pauline Hendy, Edmund Hey, Peter Huntingford, Tony Jewell, James McGarry, John McGarry, Collette O'Neill, Heather Reid, David Ritchie, Christine Smith, Gordon Stirrat, Alec Turnbull, Sid Watkins, David Widgery. Some of their ideas and changes I have incorporated, but any inaccuracies are my responsibility and the sentiments are my own.

Brian Raymond encouraged me to start writing, and I would like to thank him and all those others who have made it possible to write this account of what was an important event in my life, but one which has far-reaching implications beyond myself.

I have had such strong and continuing support from too many people to name all of them individually, but I would like particularly to thank Luke Zander and Ron Taylor whose understanding of the principles of justice and own personal integrity have been an example to all doctors, and Sheila Hillier, Eva Alberman, Helen Bender, Alyson Hall, Irene Leigh, Colin Murray-Parkes, Frances Marks, Graeme Snodgrass, and Elizabeth Watson of the London Hospital and Medical College whose personal confidence in me has helped enormously. My thanks, too, to Mary Edmondson, Erica Jones, John Robson, Kambiz Boomla, Jane Taylor, Jo Shawcross, Liz Hodgetts, Alex Mills, Viv Taylor, Roseanna Pollen, Anna Livingstone, Tom Kalloway, Bernard Taylor and Michael Liebson and all the other Tower Hamlets GPs who, with the midwives, in particular Jane Grant and Debbie Hughes, have worked so hard for my reinstatement and expressed their trust in me long before I was cleared.

Sheila Kitzinger and Iain Chalmers as well as providing moral support helped me with references, and the librarians at the Royal College of Obstetricians and Gynaecologists and all the library staff at the London Hospital Medical College have been efficient and sympathetic.

Phillipa Micklethwaite as President of the National Childbirth Trust, Beverley Beech of AIMS, Ruth Evans of the Maternity Alliance and Ron Brewer, Secretary of the Tower Hamlets CHC, have all been very helpful. The Support Group have worked immensely hard, and Sue Hadley, Heather Reid and Myra Garrett deserve special thanks. The Appeal Fund Committee did enormously well to raise over £60,000 for my legal costs and deal with the press whilst many of them were coping with young families as well as demanding jobs. I am sad that Sam Smith, who worked so hard, died a week after the enquiry finished and so missed the end of the story. My thanks to them all, and also the hundreds of people who have written to me, sent me cards and flowers and books, and the thousands who donated money and signed the petition presented to the DHSS.

Katy Simmons, Bob Moore, Joseph Winceslaus, Felicity Challoner, Alison Spankie, Melanie Davies, John MacVicar, Michael Moore and Mary McNabb were amongst those who gave affidavits for the High Court case and I am grateful to them for doing this at such short notice.

I would also like to thank the expert witnesses who appeared on my behalf at the enquiry, and gave hours of their precious time. They and my lawyers did this freely, and took on the task of defending me with no guarantee of payment, because of the principles involved.

I am grateful to the journalists in all the different types of media who have followed the case with interest and informed people about the issues; the MPs who have supported me in the House of Commons and outside; the many organisations who have publicised the struggle in their newsletters, and the unions and constituency Labour Parties, CHCs and women's groups who have spread the news and often sent contributions.

Lastly, I would like to thank my children for their support and understanding, in particular Wendy who kept my press-cuttings up to date, and Jay who bore the brunt of the phone calls and my preoccupation with the fight, and also the man who, like them, never doubted my competence – and whose advice and loving help (which included the meals I had not time to cook) kept me going during the lonely struggle before my suspension in April 1985.

Wendy Savage
Islington, 1 August 1986

Dramatis Personae

TOWER HAMLETS HEALTH AUTHORITY

Chairman	*Francis Cumberlege*
District Administrator till December 1985	*Sotiris Argyrou*
District Medical Officer	*Jean Richards**
District General Manager from 3.2.86	*John Alway*

PANEL OF ENQUIRY

Chairman	*Mr Christopher Beaumont*
Professor of Obstetrics and Gynaecology in Dundee	*Peter Howie*
Consultant Obstetrician and Gynaecologist, Rugby	*Leonard Harvey*

LAWYERS

Regional Legal Adviser till 30.6.86	*Terry Dibley*
Counsel for Tower Hamlets Health Authority	*Ian Kennedy QC* *James Badenoch*
Barrister instructed by the Medical Protections Society representing all the London Hospital doctors who gave evidence at the enquiry	*Mr Conlin*
Solicitors for Wendy Savage	
Until 28.5.85	*James Watt* and *MAMS Leigh* of Hempsons
From June 1986 to present	*Brian Raymond* of Bindman and Partners
Counsel for Wendy Savage	*John Hendy*
Medico-legal expert retained by Hempsons	*Professor Geoffrey Chamberlain*, St Georges Hospital

LONDON HOSPITAL MEDICAL COLLEGE (LHMC)

Dean, January 1983 to 30.9.86	*Mike Floyer*, Professor of Medicine*
Professor of Surgery to 30.9.85 and Dean July 1981 to December 1982	*David Ritchie*
Chairman of the Academic Division of Surgery	*John Blandy*, Professor of Urology*
Chairman of the Academic Board 1.10.85 to 30.9.86	*Harry Allred*, Professor of Dentistry, and Dean of Dental Studies. DHA member
Chairman of the Final Medical Committee and Medical Council	
February 1982 to January 1985	*Sid Watkins*, Professor of Neurosurgery
February 1985 to present	*Sam Cohen*, Professor of Psychiatry

* denotes a graduate of the London Hospital Medical College

LONDON HOSPITAL

Department of Obstetrics and Gynaecology

Senior Consultant	*John Hartgill**
Chairman of the Division of Obstetrics and Gynaecology	*Trevor Beedham**
Consultant	*David Oram*
Senior Registrar	*Paul Armstrong*
Registrars	*Toby Fay, Hani Youssef, Gillian Robinson*

Department of Paediatrics

Senior Lecturer in Paediatrics	*Roger Harris*

JOINT APPOINTMENTS LHMC AND ST BARTHOLOMEW'S MEDICAL COLLEGE

Professor of Obstetrics and Gynaecology	*Jurgis Gediminis Grudzinskas (Gedis),* based at LHMC and London Hospital
Professor of Reproductive Physiology	*Tim Chard*, based at Bart's
Senior Lecturer in Obstetrics and Gynaecology	*Wendy Savage*, based at LHMC and London Hospital (Mile End)*
Lecturer in Obstetrics and Gynaecology	*Tony Nysenbaum*
Professor of Clinical Epidemiology	*Eva Alberman*, based at LHMC*

ST BARTHOLOMEW'S HOSPITAL

Senior Consultant in Obstetrics and Gynaecology until December 1985	*Gordon Bourne*, Regional Assessor in Obstetrics for North East Thames Region. Expert witness at the enquiry in February 1986

GENERAL PRACTITIONERS IN TOWER HAMLETS

Dr Sam Smith, retired. Founder of St Stephens Road practice. Treasurer of Appeal Fund*

Mary Edmondson, General Practitioner Obstetrician (GPO), Steele's Lane Health Centre. Secretary of Appeal Fund

Tony Jewell, GPO, South Poplar practice. TUC nominee on the DHA. Chair of Appeal Fund*

WENDY SAVAGE SUPPORT CAMPAIGN

Chair	*Beverley Beech* of the Association for Improvements in the Maternity Services AIMS) and Health Rights
Vice-Chair	*Ron Brewer*, Secretary of the Community Health Council (CHC)
Members of Executive Committee	*Sue Hadley* and *Heather Reid* of National Childbirth Trust (NCT), *Myra Garrett* of Tower Hamlets Health Campaign (THHC), *Kate Parkin, Lucy Micklethwaite*

* denotes a graduate of the London Hospital Medical College

Other Supporters — *Luke Zander*, Senior Lecturer in General Practice, St Thomas's, *Sheila Kitzinger*, anthropologist, author and natural childbirth teacher

EXPERT WITNESSES CALLED BY THE HEALTH AUTHORITY: 'THE PROSECUTION'

John Dennis: Professor of Obstetrics and Gynaecology, Southampton, Regional Assessor in Obstetrics for Wessex
Gordon Bourne: see above

EXPERT WITNESSES CALLED BY WENDY SAVAGE: 'THE DEFENCE'

Peter Dunn: Reader in Child Health, University of Bristol
Alexander Campbell: Professor of Paediatrics, University of Aberdeen
Iain Chalmers: Director of the National Perinatal Epidemiology Unit
Marion Hall: Consultant Obstetrician and Gynaecologist and Honorary Senior Lecturer, University of Aberdeen
Edmund Hey: Consultant Paediatrician, Newcastle
James McGarry: Consultant Obstetrician and Gynaecologist and Honorary Clinical Lecturer, University of Glasgow
John McGarry: Consultant Obstetrician and Gynaecologist, North Devon District Hospital, Barnstaple
Gordon Stirrat: Professor of Obstetrics and Gynaecology, University of Bristol
Ron Taylor: Professor of Obstetrics and Gynaecology, United Medical School of St Thomas's and Guys', London

* denotes a graduate of the London Hospital Medical College

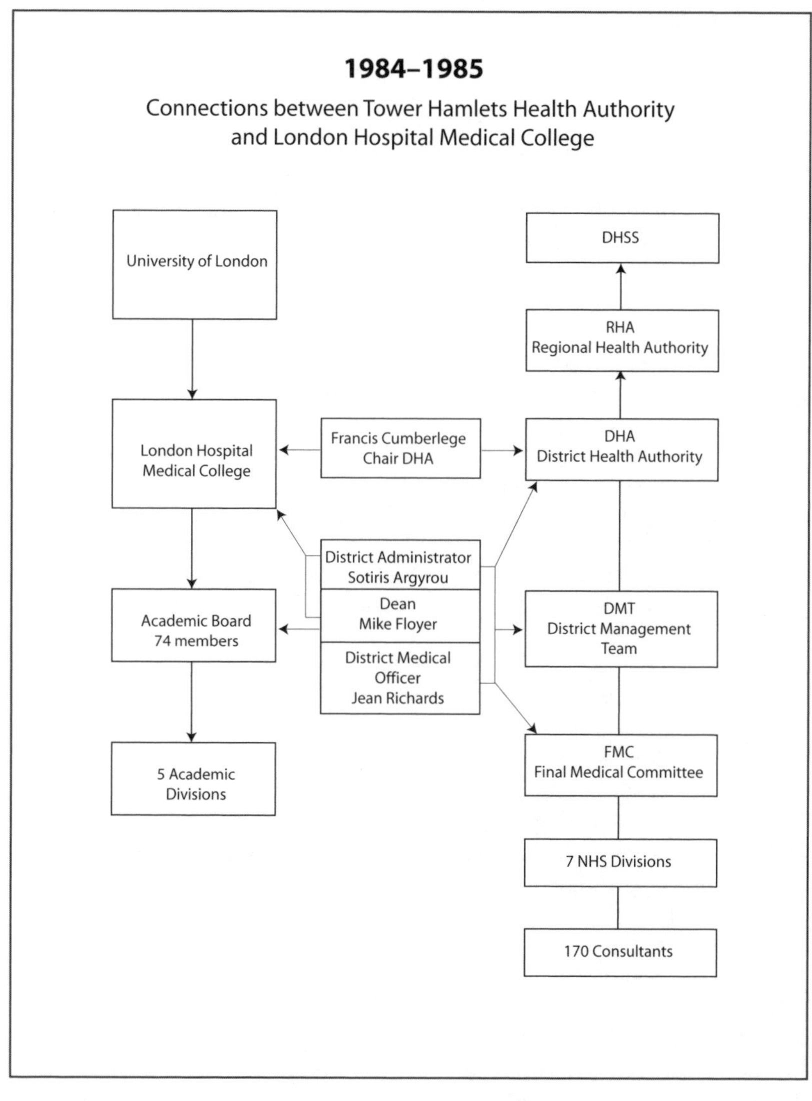
1984–1985
Connections between Tower Hamlets Health Authority and London Hospital Medical College
University of London
London Hospital Medical College
Academic Board 74 members
5 Academic Divisions
Francis Cumberlege Chair DHA
District Administrator Sotiris Argyrou
Dean Mike Floyer
District Medical Officer Jean Richards
DHSS
RHA Regional Health Authority
DHA District Health Authority
DMT District Management Team
FMC Final Medical Committee
7 NHS Divisions
170 Consultants

Chronology

August 1977	Wendy Savage appointed Senior Lecturer in Peter Huntingford's department
July 1981	Peter Huntingford leaves. Trevor Beedham appointed
Jan 1983	Gedis Grudzinskas and David Oram appointed
Jan 1984	District Health Authority decide to centralise obstetric and gynaecological services at Whitechapel
20.2.84 and **19.3.84**	Grudzinskas writes to Wendy Savage re employment
26.4.84	Baby U born
3.5.84	Baby U dies
21.5.84	Trevor Beedham's letter to Gedis Grudzinskas which served as a formal request to the District Administrator for an enquiry into the U case
21.8.84	Wendy Savage notified by District Administrator of Us' formal complaint through Community Health Council
24.9.84	Wendy Savage and Roger Harris see Us with secretary of Community Health Council
27.9.84	Jean Richards, District Medical Officer, mentions HM (61)112 and possibility of sending U case notes to Gordon Bourne
4.10.84 and **12.10.84**	Wendy Savage sees Dean of London Hospital Medical College, who tells her: 'One case not enough for a 112'
24.4.85	Suspended
13.6.85	March on District Health Authority in protest
28.6.85	Wendy Savage replies to criticisms of cases to Chairman of DHA
5.8.85	High Court application to be heard in vacation accepted
15.8.85	Decision taken to proceed to HM (61)112 enquiry, communicated to Wendy Savage's lawyers, Bindmans
2.9.85	High Court judge turns down hearing for a breach of contract
3.2.86	Enquiry begins
8.3.86	Enquiry ends
9.7.86	First part of report received by Brian Raymond and Wendy Savage
10.7.86	Second March organised by Support Group, press conference
21.7.86	Wendy Savage and Brian Raymond receive Part 2 of report
24.7.86	Tower Hamlets Health Authority vote unanimously to reinstate Wendy Savage, Cumberlege holds press conference
10.10.86	Wendy Savage returns to work as practising obstetrician and gynaecologist

Introduction

> ***She should have been a good and agreeable girl and made sure she got on with her colleagues. If she had played her cards right she would have found being a woman was to her advantage and her male colleagues might have been prepared to do her more favours.***
>
> Senior obstetrician quoted in *Sunday Times*, 9 March 1986

I was suspended from my post as Honorary Consultant in Obstetrics and Gynaecology to the Tower Hamlets Health Authority on 24 April 1985, on the grounds of alleged incompetence, after twenty-five years in medical practice. I realised then what millions of other people in this country already know – that the loss of your job is a shattering experience. I was lucky not to have to share their financial anxieties, as I was suspended on full pay as Senior Lecturer in Obstetrics and Gynaecology at the London Hospital Medical College; but the allegation of professional incompetence, and the abrupt ending of my active role of looking after patients and teaching students, was devastating.

The loss of my job was like a bereavement. Powerful, confusing, and shifting emotions swept over me – disbelief (can this really be happening?), sadness, guilt, self-doubt, anger.

Attempting to deal with these emotions in a totally unfamiliar situation – as a client of lawyers, a person responding to events over which she has no control – was a sharp contrast to my usual role of the autonomous doctor, making daily decisions close to life and death; an independent woman in command of her own world. The added and unsought responsibility of responding to media attention and finding that I had become a public figure, a spokesperson for the pregnant woman, has not been easy. It has only been possible because of the immense support I have had. That support has helped me to sustain my inner conviction that I must fight back and win this battle, not only for myself but for all women.

Over the years I have been practising, I have learnt that women need to be able to talk as equals with doctors, to be informed of the choices available to them and encouraged to make up their own minds about becoming pregnant, or continuing with a pregnancy. I have realised how important it is for a woman to feel in control of the birth process if she is going to emerge as a confident parent. I have become increasingly aware of the deficiencies in the care that we, as obstetricians, provide for pregnant women.

Pregnancy is not an illness. I belong to the school of thought which believes that every pregnancy is normal unless there are indications that something is wrong. Those at the opposite end of the obstetric spectrum believe that no pregnancy is normal, except in retrospect. This attitude, together with the labelling of women as high risk on the basis of statistical, rather than individual information, leads to a situation where too many women are forced to attend hospital clinics, rather than having the more personal care of the midwife or a general practitioner closer to home. I feel that as the risks in childbirth become smaller, statistical methods of predicting (on the basis of her age, number of children or income) which woman will lose her baby have limited use. In my view, if you look at each woman as an individual, and plan her care with her, you will get the best result.

I and many of my supporters saw my suspension as part of the continuing struggle about who controls childbirth, and it was on this ground that we chose to fight. It was only about the issues of choices in childbirth that I was prepared to speak publicly, but at a deeper level, I knew that this battle was about the way doctors relate to and work with each other, and about the fact that I am not a member of the 'establishment' and saw no reason to conform to the medical profession's unwritten, but well understood 'party line', especially if I thought this was not in the interests of patients.

These issues do not lend themselves to the shorthand, confrontational approach of the media, and at first I felt they were best resolved privately. Up to the time that the enquiry started in February 1986 I hoped, somewhat idealistically, that it would be possible to accomplish this. But the aggressive way that the Health Authority case was conducted, the initial response of my accusers in the face of the expert opinions of obstetricians and paediatricians who supported my disputed management, and the report of the panel which exonerated me, have convinced me that the medical politics which underlie my suspension need to be revealed.

This book has been written for a number of reasons. First, so that my supporters can fill in the gaps in the story which they followed in the newspapers, and to express my gratitude for their trust in me and what I was fighting for.

Second, although I know it will upset many members of the medical profession, who feel we should not wash our dirty linen in public, I hope that doctors who read this will understand that the actions of my colleagues at the London Hospital were not significantly different from those taking place every week in other hospitals and medical academic units in this country. I believe such behaviour arises from the way we, as a profession, have organised ourselves. We also need to look closely at what it is in the training of doctors and the institutions we have set up – the British Medical Association, the Royal Colleges, the General Medical Council – which made it so difficult for the leaders of our profession to act effectively against the injustice of my suspension, despite the immediate, strongly expressed support from local patients and GPs. We need to make positive changes in the regulations for disciplining doctors which will prevent a repetition of the damaging, prolonged, bitter and expensive battle which has taken place over the last fifteen months. I hope that my colleagues at the London Hospital will accept this as a constructive attempt to understand the issues and actions which lay behind my suspension.

Third, for myself, there is a need to work through, and make sense of, this extraordinary experience. Right at the start I made the decision that I was not going to conduct myself as a 'guilty' person because I knew that the charge was false. I was going to carry on going into work, doing teaching and research as far as possible and accept invitations to talk about obstetrics and gynaecology as if there was no threat to my professional livelihood or slur on my reputation hanging over me. I hope, by sharing this ordeal with others, that I will be able to put the horrific part of these fifteen months behind me, and take forward the good things: the trust, friendship and generosity of those who have supported me.

25 July 1986

Chapter 1

Suspension

'Now for the evidence,' said the King, 'and then the sentence.' 'No!' said the Queen, 'first the sentence, and then the evidence!' 'Nonsense!' cried Alice, so loudly that everybody jumped, 'the idea of having the sentence first!'

Lewis Carroll, *Alice's Adventures under Ground*

Tuesday, 23 April 1985

A telephone call interrupts my gynaecology clinic at Mile End Hospital. I am seeing the ninth of the fifteen women booked for this morning. She is about my age – fifty – with a common problem for women approaching the menopause. She thought her periods had stopped and then, a year later, she had some bleeding. Women know that this may be a sign of cancer and it is always difficult for the doctor both to allay their fears and yet do the necessary D and C (dilation and curettage – scraping of the inside of the womb to make sure there is no abnormal growth there). I am listening to the woman and am irritated to be interrupted at a delicate stage of the consultation by a nurse saying that Dr Richards is on the telephone and wants to make an appointment to see me. I ask her to tell Dr Richards the times when I will be available and resume the conversation.

We try to create as much privacy as possible at the Mile End clinic. If the woman agrees to a medical student being present at her consultation, we allow a single student to attend. If she does not want a medical student present we respect her wishes. This woman has agreed, and I am trying to show the medical student how to pass a speculum, an instrument which is inserted into the vagina to look at the neck of the womb; this is a task which requires some skill and about which the woman often feels quite embarrassed. The nurse returns and tells me that Dr Richards insists on speaking to me herself. I apologise to the woman lying on the consulting room couch, walk into the reception area, pick up the telephone and suggest Thursday. Jean replies: 'That's no good, because I am going to suspend your clinical contract tomorrow.'

I hear myself arranging to meet her at 6.30 p.m. the next day, walk past the clerks and the crowded waiting room, back to the consulting room and book an operation date for the patient. After she has dressed I explain, as if in a dream, what the operation involves. As she leaves, the registrar comes in for the operating diary. He takes one look at my face and asks me what is wrong. I do not tell him I am to be suspended. I've never heard of a doctor being suspended before, except for madness. On the verge of tears, I tell him only that I have heard from Jean Richards, the District Medical Officer, that my Professor of Obstetrics, Gedis Grudzinskas, has taken the case notes of some of my patients without my knowledge and these have been sent, with critical comments, to Gordon Bourne, the Regional Assessor for Maternal Mortality. His reply shocks me: 'I knew that Trevor Beedham [a fellow obstetrician] was gunning for you, but I didn't know about the professor.'

Elizabeth, the nurse, brings me coffee and I pull myself together and see the rest of the women booked for the clinic. There are moments when a woman's problems make me forget my own, but later I cannot recall who I have seen. For once, I finish the clinic on time.

As it happens, I already have an appointment with Mike Floyer, the Dean of the London Hospital Medical College, at one o'clock. I have asked to see him because last Friday I heard Jean Richards upsetting my secretary by demanding case notes of patients in my care. 'To send to Gordon Bourne,' she said, when I questioned her. I replied, 'Christ, Jean, if the professor thinks he's going to get rid of me I'll fight him every inch of the way.'

Driving through the back streets of London's East End to see the dean at the main hospital, I recall that Jean had mentioned Gordon Bourne's name a few months earlier, in September 1984, when an investigation was being considered into a case where I had allowed a woman whose baby was in the breech position to try a natural labour. But although I have seen Jean about every six weeks or so since then, she has never mentioned the matter again.

As I walk from the consultants' car park, past Queen Alexandra's statue in the garden of the hospital, I wonder what has been happening behind the scenes between September and April.

Along the corridor to the dean's office I notice, as I always notice, the rows of photographs of men who have taught medicine there. I remember the impact this phalanx of serious middle-aged faces had on me when I first came here twenty-eight years ago to be interviewed for entry to medical school. I sit, as I did then, on the hard leatherette sofa, and tell myself that I must keep calm; and above all I must not cry.

Mike is his usual friendly self. His gangling, rather vague appearance fits his reputation for 'patent honesty'. I find myself starting to speak before he offers me one of the low armchairs. 'I made this appointment because it's becoming impossible to work with the professor. But Jean Richards has just told me that she is going to suspend my Honorary Consultant contract tomorrow.' Mike, whom I had always trusted, shows no shock, surprise or sympathy. Calmly, he tells me that he was present at the meeting, five days ago, when the Chairman of Tower Hamlets Health Authority, its legal adviser, the District Medical Officer and the District Administrator decided to suspend me.

How can such a decision be taken without my knowledge? Mike replies, 'The professor should have told you. I rather thought he had... the college will go on paying you, but whether you carry on with your student teaching will depend on the professor. I don't know enough about obstetrics to argue about the decision.' I ask him what will happen to my patients while I am suspended. Mike says he supposes that the professor will look after them.

I drive to the GPs' surgery in St Stephen's Road for my antenatal clinic. It is a busy clinic. Between seeing the women I telephone lawyers and an administrator friend. During the clinic, Tony Jewell, a GP who is the TUC nominee on the District Health Authority, rings me. His wife is due to have her second baby under my care in three weeks' time. I tell him the news, swear him to silence and say that I hope I can get something done to stop this before tomorrow afternoon. After the clinic I return to Mile End to dictate the letters from the gynae clinic that morning. Usually I have all the details of the women in my mind and I merely have to glance at the folder in order to dictate the letter. But tonight

I have to read through all the notes before recalling each patient. I leave about half-past eight and eat with a friend. I feel dazed and am unable to taste the food.

Wednesday, 24 April 1985

At 4 a.m. I awake suddenly and completely. This is so unjust, so outrageous, there must be some way it can be stopped. I write a letter to the Medical Defence Union which, with the Medical Protection Society, is an organisation to which doctors must subscribe for the protection of their legal interests. Can we take out an injunction? In the early morning light I drive along the empty London streets to Harley Street and push the letter, marked URGENT, through the elegant door of the MDU in Devonshire Place.

After the morning antenatal clinic comes the ward and necessary excuses to the women in my care. One has been admitted several times with pelvic infection and is due to have a laparoscopy to see whether her tubes are damaged. I have to tell her that my registrar will do the operation. She looks disappointed and is surprised by my change of plan. It is not that the operation is hard to do, but I know her and she has trusted me through several difficult years, and I had promised to do the operation myself. We always organise our lists so that the doctor who sees the woman in outpatients does the operation. It makes so much difference to women when they already know the doctor who is to do the operation – it also makes mistakes less likely to occur. I almost break down as I sit on the bed to tell another woman who has lost two babies that I can no longer care for her.

I meet five of the junior staff in my office. In confidence I tell them about my suspension, now only minutes away; I ask them to look after the patients and we talk over the outstanding problems.

I drive numbly to the administrative headquarters in the main hospital at Whitechapel to keep the appointment with Jean Richards. The Medical Defence Union have arranged for a solicitor to meet me at the front door. He looks awfully young.

I tell the solicitor what has happened as we walk up the narrow stairs to the top floor where Jean has her office. Jean, a few years older than me, also trained at the London Hospital. Business-like, she hands me the papers relating to my suspension, explaining to the solicitor that I am being charged with professional incompetence. As I check the documents, we discuss things calmly, even amicably. I am more concerned with arrangements for the care of my patients. The solicitor says: 'You seem like old friends.' Jean replies, 'We are, we've known each other for twenty-five years.'

Thursday, 25 April 1985

Again, I wake at 4 a.m. Rereading the suspension documents, which cite five cases in which my management of labour is said to give rise to serious concern about the safety of patients in my care, I think: this isn't about competence, it's about attitudes, about a different approach to maternity care.

The strange thought that I am not to be allowed into theatre preoccupies me during the three mile drive from home to Mile End Hospital. Jean telephones me, reminding me that I must leave my office and offers transport to move my belongings. I begin to pack up my papers, make telephone calls, dictate letters. Just before two o'clock, the professor comes to see me. Jurgis (also known as Gedis) Grudzinskas is forty years old, with striking blue eyes. His fair hair is beginning to recede a little. Although Australian by upbringing, his accent is mid-Atlantic. His usual friendly manner is replaced by a hurried formality. In four minutes precisely, he tells me that he learned about my suspension that morning, is cancelling my lecture scheduled for the afternoon, that I must leave my academic office in his department too, and am to be withdrawn from teaching. He hands me a letter of confirmation. His action provokes a strange response in me. A cold rage prevents me from speaking. And, inexplicably, my anger is mixed with pity for him.

I spend the rest of the day making arrangements for other people to deal with outstanding clinical problems. I am surprised to find that someone has already told my junior staff that five cases are involved. I reassure them that those who have been involved in the care of the five women should not be damaged by battles between consultants.

Friday, 26 April 1985

It feels unreal to be barred from working and cut off from my professional life. The loss, the sense of powerlessness increases when, simultaneously, I find myself delivered into the hands of another set of professionals, with a completely different language and way of working – the lawyers.

The solicitors instructed on my behalf by the MDU, Hempsons, have their offices in Henrietta Street in Covent Garden. The heavy wooden door with its brass plate leads to a worn, wooden staircase. The small waiting room has Regency chairs, *The Times* and vases of flowers. I sit there with some impatience and trepidation. After ten minutes I am taken across the street to the third floor of a newly decorated cream and brown Gothic building which reminds me of an Oxbridge college.

I am expecting to see Mr Watt, with whom I have had dealings before, and am surprised to be greeted by another solicitor, who introduces himself as Mr Leigh. He is about thirty-five, good-looking, with a self-confident manner. As we size each other up I think: intelligent, quick to grasp the facts; but will he understand that I am not incompetent? This is a battle about the care of women, usually provided by men – and the law is dominated by men, too. I try to convince him that the situation will actually 'right itself' once the truth is known.

The press have already telephoned. I accept his advice not to make a public statement.

It is ten minutes past seven when I leave, grateful for having had the opportunity to talk. The usual office bustle has ceased and I walk rapidly to my car. As usual, I am a little behind schedule. I have to be at the medical students' dinner within an hour and must go home first. Threading my way through the tourists, I wryly think that I might manage to get to things on time in the next few months: I will no longer have to answer a telephone call as I leave the office for a meeting, or see the patients whose problems spill over from the morning to the afternoon clinic. As I unlock my front door, uncharacteristically thinking about what to wear that evening, it hits me. I don't have a working day any more. There will be no more calls in the middle of the night, no more driving through dark streets to see a labouring woman. I feel useless. All I can see is emptiness. Fortunately my sixteen-year-old son hears the key turning the lock. 'What's for supper? Are you being paid? So what's the problem?' I laugh and dash upstairs to change, wondering how I'm going to cope, facing all the people who know I am suspended, but won't know why.

Chapter 2

The Making of an Obstetrician

Women constitute half of the world's population, perform nearly two-thirds of its work hours, receive one-tenth of the world's income and own less than one hundredth of the world's property.

United Nations report, 1980

I did not start my medical career as a 'radical in the labour ward'. But my career as a doctor, like that of many women, has not followed an orthodox pattern. What I have learnt from being a doctor and a working mother in four continents, and what I have learnt from patients, is that women are individuals, and they should have control over their own fertility. Informed choice is a prerequisite for that control, and professional advisers who are prepared to share information and decision-making with the woman are essential.

I was born in 1935 and spent the first five years of my life in Norbury, a green and undistinguished suburb of South London. At the outbreak of the Second World War my father, who was working as a chartered surveyor, was called up and sent to Scotland. My mother and we children – I had a brother and sister by now – were evacuated to Horsham in Sussex.

When I was eight years old, my life changed completely. My mother died and we were sent to boarding school in Devon. After the war my father remarried. He bought a large Victorian house in Surrey cheaply, as the garden was pitted with bomb craters, and proceeded to rebuild the house and transform seven acres of a hawthorn and bramble wilderness into a beautiful garden. The idea that it was possible to change things physically and in an unorthodox way was firmly implanted in my mind as I sat on ladders to steady them while my father knocked down chimneys and walls, and dug out tons of chalk to create his garden.

I went to Croydon High School for Girls: a direct grant school, proud of its academic reputation, but also concerned to produce young women who were not just bluestockings but cared about people as well.

No one in my family had been to university. My father had left school at sixteen and educated himself at evening classes; so had his three sisters whose formal education finished even earlier, at thirteen or fourteen. He and one of my aunts had started their own businesses and all my aunts worked, two choosing not to have children.

I was not part of a class which accepted status and success as their due: my family was self-directing, hard-working and earned respect because of the quality of their work. I remember the feeling of independence when I got an exhibition to pay my fees in the sixth form and how privileged I felt to have the chance of a good education and, later, a profession. The example of my family's disciplined approach to work has remained a powerful influence in my own working life.

I went to Cambridge in 1953. There, for the first time in my life, I was discriminated against because of my sex. From the age of fourteen I had wanted to be a research chemist, but after a year of physics, chemistry, mineralogy and mathematics – and seeing how research chemists actually work – I decided I wanted more contact with people. One morning in the summer vacation I woke up knowing that I wanted to be a doctor.

Two men who had changed to medicine from classics and modem languages were allowed to learn three science subjects from scratch and complete their second MB, the initial stage of their medical degree, in three years. I had only to learn one new subject; but I had to wait a year for admission to the medical course because there was a quota for women students; my participation would have increased the number of women medical students by half a percent, to 10.5 per cent. So I had to spend a fourth year at Cambridge which I accepted philosophically; academically it was a fairly relaxed year. I took the opportunity to attend psychology and history of art lectures and hardly spoke to medical students because I was 'out of phase'. My father had not been pleased with my decision to do medicine and thought that three years of higher education was enough, so after I obtained my degree, my tutor found a grant for my fees.

I started clinical training at the London Hospital Medical College in the East End of London in October 1957, along with three other women and about fifty men. Not as upper class as St Thomas's, as intellectual as University College or quite so rugby-oriented as St Mary's, the London Hospital Medical College (founded in 1785, the first medical school in England) has always had a tradition of service to the local community. An unusually high number of graduates for a London college – about half – went into General Practice, and it was comparatively progressive in its attitude to women. In the fifties, other hospitals rarely appointed women even to the most junior posts, but at the London women had been known to become registrars! One of the three clinical professors was a woman, Dorothy Russell, a distinguished neuro-pathologist.

As students, we were divided into groups of between six and eight, and as we moved through the specialties in our second and third years, we were attached to the teams of doctors which made up a 'firm', and got to know each other well. I found the clinical work with patients absorbing and enjoyable, although in some specialties death was frighteningly close and the suffering of people hard to bear.

In those days, before the 'rationalisation' of the health service, the London Hospital was supported by a network of smaller hospitals in the area now known as the London Borough of Tower Hamlets. Most of our patients lived in Stepney, Bethnal Green, Bow, Poplar, Wapping, Spitalfields and the Isle of Dogs, although for the special departments they came from all over the East End of London and Essex.

As a port area, East London has been the traditional entry point of refugees, starting with the Huguenots who came to Spitalfields to escape religious persecution after the Revocation of the Edict-of Nantes in 1685. Since the Huguenots, successive waves of immigrants have come to the East End, migrating out as they became more prosperous. When I was a student, many of those living in the vicinity of the London Hospital had come from Russia and Poland at the turn of the century and still spoke only Yiddish. The shops in Brick Lane, now filled with Halal meat, exotic vegetables and spices, were then Kosher butchers, grocery stores with pickled herrings and lox, and, a rarity outside the Whitechapel area in those days, bakers selling bagels and good rye bread.

I lived, for the final year of my training, in a hospital house just behind the outpatients.

I could get out of bed at five to nine, dash downstairs and be sitting in outpatients for nine o' clock. Two of my teachers, Dr Archie Clark-Kennedy and Dr Donald Hunter, made a deep impression on me. Dr Clark-Kennedy emphasised that one must see the person as a whole and understand their place in the world, as part of a family and a community, not just a 'patient' in a hospital bed. And I can still remember the passion with which Donald Hunter, who founded the specialty of industrial medicine, spoke on our ward rounds about the exploitation of workers, and the callous disregard of employers for safety regulations. I remember, too, his distaste for the way that some doctors in private practice behaved towards patients. He often quoted the great Canadian physician, Osler: 'Listen to the patient; he is telling you the diagnosis.'

When I did my obstetric training in 1958, we still had quite a large number of home deliveries. The district midwives had a house behind the Medical College on Turner Street from which they would issue forth on their bicycles with their black 'midder' bags strapped on the backs. They and the students were ruled firmly by Sister Gladys, who never seemed to have any time off. During our first month of midwifery we were not supposed to leave the premises either and were called in turn to look after women in labour, with whom we sat until they were delivered either in hospital or at home.

My first delivery was in the district. I had never even seen a film of a baby being born. An Irish woman was having her fourth baby in a flat in Blackwall Buildings. The midwife helped me through the delivery. 'Now,' she said, pretending she was speaking to the patient, 'Doctor is going to put on her gloves. Now, Doctor is going to do a vaginal examination, and she will be feeling where the head is, and whether the neck of the womb is still there.' (I had never felt either a baby's head or the neck of a womb before.) The woman wanted to push, and I could see some dark hair as the baby's head became visible. Another push; and suddenly there was this baby crying on the bed. I was astounded. It seemed so easy. I'd been brought up on *Gone with the Wind* and had expected agony and writhing and sweating as the woman pulled on knotted sheets. I often wonder whether the fact that my first experience of birth was so natural and relaxed has influenced my approach to obstetrics. Perhaps a doctor whose first experience is of seeing a Caesarean section has his or her view of the process of childbirth set by that experience, so that surgical rather than natural delivery seems the normal way to have a baby.

One experience which I will never forget was attending a fifteen-year-old girl at East Mount Street. She had concealed the pregnancy and had delivered a stillborn baby lying on an iron bedstead among dirty sheets in a bleak, carpetless room. I felt a numbed horror. It made me incapable of speech or any kind of helpful gesture towards the pale, thin girl with her dead baby lying silent between her legs. I will never forget the feeling of emptiness, which was mirrored by the cold house, her unfriendly and uncommunicative mother and the bare room with the iron bed.

The same feeling of emptiness struck me again later that month at another stillbirth. The woman had a malignant melanoma (a cancer of the skin) and they ruptured her membranes (broke her waters) to speed up the birth. It was obvious that something was wrong when the liquor (the fluid round the baby) shot right across the room, hitting the registrar. The midwife leant down to listen for the baby's heart beat, and I could tell from her face that it wasn't there. The liquor had come out too rapidly and the pressure changes had caused the placenta to separate from the uterine wall, cutting off the baby's oxygen supply. Suddenly, again, there was this awful feeling of emptiness in the room. Nobody said anything. But I knew, strongly and instinctively, that it was wrong not to tell the woman.

Obstetrics and Emotion

Those two stillbirths made a deep impression on me and have influenced my thinking on the way that doctors' own feelings, if unacknowledged, can block their ability to be of help to the patient.

Even today, despite a reduction in the perinatal mortality rate – death of babies between the seventh month of pregnancy and the first week of life – one woman in a hundred leaves hospital without a live baby, and in a unit delivering 3000 women a year, a perinatal death will occur every fortnight. But doctors still have difficulty in dealing with their own feelings about stillbirth. In 1970, an obstetrician named Pat Giles, a professor in Perth, Australia, studied forty women who had lost babies in the first week of life or as stillbirths, and said, 'Although doctors treated the women's physical symptoms and prescribed sedatives liberally, in about half the cases they avoided discussing the death of the baby.'

Later in my career, I began to note how women who had not delivered a live baby, or whose babies had died, were given a separate room, to spare their feelings, but often these rooms were missed out of the ward round. Students were not allocated to these women. They were discharged home as soon as medically possible, and if they failed to keep their postnatal appointment, there was a tendency to leave it at that. I had no idea what happened to the babies and apart from signing the stillbirth certificate and requesting a post-mortem, the doctor was not involved in thinking about the disposal of the body.

I remember vividly the first time (after nine years of obstetrics and over 100 perinatal deaths) that I asked a woman if she wanted to see her dead baby. The baby's skin was just beginning to peel and he had a forceps mark on one cheek. But I wrapped him up and carried him to his mother. 'Oh,' she said, 'isn't he beautiful.' The midwives had wanted to stop me, but they too realised, when they saw how naturally the woman held him, that what they had been taught needed to be changed.

Doctors have very little training, either formal or informal, in dealing with their own feelings of pain and sadness. Those who choose obstetrics enjoy their work because of the rewards of delivering women of healthy babies, and often feel a sense of failure when they cannot achieve this. In most British hospitals there is no support group for the house staff where they can discuss and explore their feelings. This will depend on the relationships between individual doctors and consultants which are hampered, often, by the hierarchical nature of the profession and the need for references within the career structure, so that it can be very difficult for a young doctor to openly admit what he or she is going through.

Doctors experience all the classic symptoms of grief – shock, denial, guilt and anger, but these are often only expressed in ways which make the death harder for the baby's mother to bear. Shocked, the doctor may appear callous as he blocks off his feelings in order to control the situation. Denial may be expressed by his or her inability to say plainly that the baby is dead, and by the use of artificial aids which hopelessly extend the 'life' of the baby in the intensive care unit. The pain and sadness is banished by discharging the woman early, and even by arranging for the postnatal examination to be done by her general practitioner. Anger and hostility may even extend to the woman herself, whose lack of antenatal attendance and failure to submit herself to tests may be censured.

If a doctor has made a mistake, his or her feeling of guilt may be overwhelming, and shame makes it difficult to admit errors. The lack of a suitable framework in most hospitals for doctors to admit these feelings and understand what is happening to themselves is, I think, responsible for the seemingly uncaring attitudes which some doctors develop.

The Birth of My Own Children

Most obstetricians see more abnormal deliveries than normal deliveries because normal deliveries will be dealt with almost entirely by the midwives. During the two months of my student obstetric training I did eighty-seven deliveries altogether, the largest cluster of normal deliveries with which I have been involved. It is still true today that the only time a doctor will see and spend time with straightforward deliveries is when he or she is a student.

Just after my finals I married and I had Yewande, my first baby, in the middle of my pre-registration year. I knew my husband Mike wanted to take a job abroad and that if I wanted to get registered before we left I had to get the time in, so after medical posts in Christchurch and Exeter, I offered my services to the London Hospital without pay. They made me stop work when I was thirty-six weeks pregnant, four weeks before the baby was due; then, of course, I was two weeks overdue! I was full of energy, and used the time to decorate the house. When my baby was five weeks old I got a paid job in the Receiving Room (Casualty), which was really the only possible post at the London for a woman with a baby in those days, when everyone worked through the weekends and every night and lived a (fairly) monastic life in the doctors' mess. In the RR we worked a shift system. We had one day a week off and worked nights, 11 p.m. to 9 a.m., for seven days every six weeks or so. I used to go home and breastfeed Yandy at lunchtime and she slept behind the RR in the doctors' room when I was on nights. The next year, pregnant again, I did a locum in general practice and worked until my estimated date of delivery, but again I was overdue and was induced at forty-two weeks by John Hartgill, then the middle registrar at the London Hospital and now the senior consultant there.

When my second daughter, Wendy, was three weeks old, we went to the United States. Mike had got a job in educational research in Boston, working out ways of teaching science to primary school children. There I got a job as a research assistant with Professor Ed Kass at Boston City Hospital, situated in one of the poorest parts of the city. It was an intellectually stimulating and happy department and I enjoyed learning about epidemiology and infectious disease.

Pregnant for the third time, I didn't fancy the epidural and forceps package then fashionable in the States and found an obstetrician who believed in normal delivery. Nicholas took five hours to be born, and I was sitting up and drinking coffee ten minutes later. The obstetrician turned to the nurses who had never seen a woman give birth without forceps before. 'That's natural childbirth,' he said.

Mike's job then took us to Nigeria, to Awo-omamma, a village in the east, where, in a small local hospital, I learnt surgery and obstetrics from an excellent Italian surgeon, Dr Angelo Caroli. When he went on a much needed holiday I found myself in charge, single-handed, of the small independent hospital. I quickly learned about management and finance, as well as how to face up to frightening uncertainty about the vast range of clinical conditions provided by the seventy-five patients.

We next moved to Enugu, the capital of the eastern region of Nigeria, where I learned that women will risk death to rid themselves of an unwanted pregnancy. I was forcibly hit by the injustice of a health system where money is the key to living or dying: where women died needlessly, and in agony, because they could not afford to pay for surgery.

Women also died for other reasons. Anaemia was common and of 1200 women who gave birth in 1964, sixty-nine died during labour because blood transfusions were not available. I set up a blood bank, with the help of a peace corps volunteer who had been 'laid off' by the Eastern Nigerian Broadcasting Corporation after the coup which preceded the Biafran civil war. In the following six months only five women died. The figure was down to three in the next five months, but I had to leave the hospital. We had planned to move to Kenya, but with the outbreak of the Biafran civil war, I was evacuated with the children to England. We later rejoined Mike in Kenya.

A Woman's Right to Choose

In my training as a doctor, I was taught that abortion was wrong. It should only be performed if the woman's life was threatened by the continuance of the pregnancy. The first time I questioned this teaching was as a medical student when I saw a married woman, in her thirties with three children, die slowly from renal failure. She had syringed her uterus in an attempt to abort herself because she felt she could not cope with another child.

Her husband visited her every night and the love between them was obvious. She seemed no different from many women I have seen in the gynaecological wards or having babies. She was an ordinary housewife who had taken this desperate measure on her own and had died in the attempt. Nobody discussed with me the reasons for her death. It was accepted in silence. The 'finality' of her action was ignored.

I moved on as a medical student, with this experience buried and half-forgotten, through finals and marriage, house jobs and three babies in just over three years, until in Enugu I saw four young women die from attempts to induce abortion with a 'native' medicine. In Kenya I decided to specialise in obstetrics and gynaecology, and during my eighteen months in Nairobi I saw the effects of septic abortions daily. Every night we had an abortion list which included at least ten women with incomplete abortions which we had to complete.

On one occasion I was told that there was no legal way we could terminate the pregnancy of a young girl, only just eleven. She later returned to us, having had an illegal abortion, with a severe infection of the womb. I felt I should not have allowed this to happen. But I could see no way to perform an abortion. I did not know how; and if I had known, I did not know where I could have carried it out.

The questions which now began to worry me were: how could we as doctors refuse to help women who did not want to be pregnant? Was it ethical to refuse this help when the woman's only alternative was dangerous and unskilled assistance? Why did some of my medical colleagues – trained in Britain, members of the Royal College of Obstetricians and Gynaecologists (RCOG), and subscribing to the British medical code – lie to me about their illegal abortion activities, and appear to forget medical ethics when money was involved?

When, having returned to England in 1969, I had passed my exam for membership of the RCOG, the first step towards a consultant post, I decided to do some work in areas which I felt were neglected in orthodox NHS training. I studied family planning and venereal disease, and took psychosexual training. During this time I worked for a year with the Pregnancy Advisory Service, for the first month as a counselling doctor, and then as a gynaecologist, both seeing women before the operation and operating on them.

In these twelve months, there were only two women (out of 750) whose decision to request an abortion I felt to be wrong. I spent a long time advising both of them about a way round their problems. In both cases I delayed the operation for a week to give them time to reconsider. But both returned unconvinced and the abortions were carried out.

From the experience of talking to these 750 women, I learnt that it was impossible to pick out those who were so desperate that they would go anywhere to get an abortion from those who, given different laws, would accept the pregnancy. You had no choice but to believe what the woman told you as the doctor.

I learnt that some women have to know whether they can have an abortion before they can fully grasp their situation and be quite sure that is what they want. I quite quickly learnt to recognise those women who were ambivalent and needed more time to decide. And I learnt to spot those who were being pressured by their parents or partners into an unwanted abortion.

To me, the death of even one woman by illegal means, who could have had a legal safe abortion, is an unnecessary tragedy. But all doctors reach their positions on abortion by a different route. They all have their view of the gestational stage where they feel that the rights of the fetus take precedence over the mother's. Where that limit should be will continue to be debated hotly, but I would not like the law to be changed because it is now possible to keep alive a fetus of twenty-six weeks if superlative neonatal intensive care is available. I have interpreted 'viability' as natural viability, and I am still prepared, if really necessary, to do an abortion at twenty-six weeks. Very occasionally there are cases where women, usually young teenagers, do not reach the gynaecologist until over twenty-four weeks, the time limit that the DHSS have made the abortion charities accept 'voluntarily', and which most doctors would accept today. But I believe that it is the mother's view that should count. I have learnt from bitter experience that women will take the law into their own hands.

I can understand that people who have not seen women die from self-induced abortion may find it difficult to understand my own view. But such tragedies were not rare in England before the 1967 Abortion Act, although they were not as common as in Africa. Today the wards are no longer filled with women with infected abortions, and it is now rare to have women coming in with the haemorrhage once associated with 'spontaneous' abortion.

Doctors need to accept that ultimately the woman does make her decision, whatever the law says, and whatever her doctors think.

In July 1973, now a divorced mother of four, I took my young family to Gisborne, New Zealand. My post, newly created, was as a specialist in obstetrics, gynaecology, venereology and family planning. In Gisborne I found a 30 per cent extra-nuptial pregnancy rate and virtually no family planning service.

The abortion law was restrictive – much the same as in England prior to the 1967 Act – but, with the support of a progressive medical superintendent and a consultant psychiatrist, we established an abortion service. We also set up open-access family planning and venereology clinics and a regular review of the maternity service (80 per cent of women were looked after by their GPs and hospital midwives). During my three years in Gisborne, the perinatal mortality rate fell from twenty-nine per thousand deliveries to ten.

Chapter 3

Return to the London

The London Hospital, Mile End

Signs outside warn 'beware of falling masonry'. This is a small, very friendly, but old and tatty hospital. Though externally a 'dump', it is surprisingly progressive. Caring, considerate staff who treat women as individuals with minds of their own, although there are variations in practice and attitudes between different consultants... student midwives and medical students present at the birth 'are not obtrusive'.

The New Good Birth Guide, 1983

Although my ideas were changing during my years abroad, it was not until working as a locum senior registrar at the West London Hospital, in 1976, shortly after my return to England, that I seriously reconsidered the conventional approach I had absorbed – and taught.

Watching a woman labouring to give birth to her first child, I thought that she needed some pain relief, and when she questioned my advice, I said, 'I've seen far more women in labour than you have.' The next day she told me that I had been quite wrong: she had felt she was doing well and the pethidine injection – and my dismissive advice – had upset her inner feelings and rhythm even though she had had a normal delivery. I realised that my interference had nearly ruined her feelings about the birth; I had interfered with her perceptions, marred her achievement.

I remembered this incident when, six months later, in November 1976, I went to work at Mile End Hospital as locum lecturer/honorary senior registrar to Professor Peter Huntingford. On our first visit to the labour ward we saw a woman pushing ineffectively in the second stage of labour. Outside I asked Peter why she had not been offered a forceps delivery which I thought she needed. He replied, 'Why interfere? The baby is all right, so is she. She is not ready to give up yet.'

These two experiences finally made me change my approach to childbirth. I was lucky to find myself working with Peter Huntingford at this relatively late stage in my career. His attitudes towards women, combined with his intelligently informed experience, made him an excellent teacher.

Peter had had a brilliant academic career. He had been an editor of the *British Journal of Obstetrics and Gynaecology* and a professor at the early age of thirty-four. As clinical professor, he was based at the London. He had done a lot of research and was convinced that obstetric care in this country was going the wrong way. He felt that the rate of technological intervention was increasing too fast, without proper research to show whether it was actually improving birth for either the baby or the mother; and that doctors should be more sensitive in their attitude to women, involving them in a partnership where decisions were jointly made after the woman had been given the fullest information. He also thought that students, if they were to make worthwhile doctors, needed to observe good practice in action.

Peter took the chair on condition that his priority would not be academic research, but to establish a first-class service for women in Tower Hamlets.

Tower Hamlets was the name given in the 1960s to the new borough created out of the East End districts of Whitechapel, Bethnal Green, Stepney, Bow, Spitalfields, Poplar, Wapping and the Isle of Dogs. It is one of the most deprived areas in the country. Half of all households live below the official poverty line established by the Diamond Royal Commission in 1982, and the borough has the highest proportion of council housing in London. Of the sixteen districts covered by the North East Thames Regional Health Authority, Tower Hamlets has the highest proportion of single old people, of children in care, the highest rate of tuberculosis and of infant mortality.

In 1976, Peter moved the academic department away from the Whitechapel branch of the London Hospital and the Medical College to its less prestigious branch, the Mile End Hospital, because he hoped that with the proposed merger of Bart's, the London, and Queen Mary College, 'a major clinical academic presence at Mile End would be useful'. He set up an obstetric and gynaecological service where women were offered choice and treated as intelligent, thinking people. Although I had been a consultant for three years by now and was used to teaching, Peter's extensive theoretical and practical experience made ward rounds and seminar sessions fascinating.

I had always tried to inform people clearly so that they could make proper choices about their lives. But I learnt from Peter to cut out the unnecessary adjectives – 'just a *small* cut', 'only a *tiny* prick' – which at best confuse people, and at worst, as they reel from the unpleasantness of a painful penicillin injection, destroy their trust in the doctor.

During my medical training at the London Hospital in the fifties, the gynaecology clinic at Whitechapel had made a deep impression on me. It seemed to embrace everything that was wrong about the way women were treated by the health service. The women sat in skimpy gowns, on rows of hard seats only a couple of feet from examination cubicles in which incomplete plywood partitions were closed front and back by curtains. There was no privacy – a doctor commonly walked through, whisking aside the curtain to see who was lying on the bed, or not drawing the curtains fully before examining a woman. The voices of the doctors asking the most intimate questions could be heard clearly by those waiting their turn, but I doubt if any of the doctors wondered why the women whispered their replies.

It was the archetypal cattle market. No wonder students hated gynae – we 'clerked' women (took their medical histories) in an outer corridor, writing on boards projecting from the wall, with another group of women only a few feet away. It was pure chance if the registrar called you to see the same woman you had clerked, and there were so many patients that teaching was a very hit-and-miss affair.

When I returned to the London Hospital twenty years later, the only change which had taken place in that clinic was that students taking histories for patients were separated by small perspex screens. I quite understood why Peter Huntingford had moved to the Mile End site where the consulting rooms, though old, were at least solidly built, had changing cubicles and enabled women to speak about their problems without fear of being overheard.

In August 1977, when I was appointed senior lecturer, Peter put me in overall charge of all student teaching. At Mile End, we had organised the clinics so that a woman who agreed to being seen by a student had her history taken in a private room and was present, fully dressed, to comment on the student's interpretation of what she had said when the history was presented to the consultant. The student then examined the woman with a consultant or registrar.

At the end of each two month attachment I gave the students a questionnaire about the course. Consistently they said they preferred the experience gained in the Mile End clinic.

In the gynaecological clinics, I found that many of our patients came from the same kind of community as they had twenty years earlier – large, extended families, not given to complaining despite the adversity they often faced. Women often saw their mothers and sisters every day; family life, birth and death were very important. They appreciated the 'local' service we provided, which tried to meet the needs of the community.

There had been some changes in the local area during my years abroad and which I saw in the antenatal clinics: among the newer residents were Cypriot, West Indian, Somali, and Chinese families; Vietnamese 'boat people'; Sikhs from the Punjab; and Gujeratis from East Africa. But their numbers were small compared with the large community of Bengalis from Sylhet in Bangladesh. By 1985 the Bengali population accounted for almost half the births annually in Tower Hamlets. Although the paediatricians, supported by the obstetricians and a community physician, managed to get two interpreter posts funded by 1981, this was insufficient for our needs, and we had to continue to use husbands as interpreters which in obstetrics and gynaecology has considerable limitations.

Only a few women were so deeply religious that they would rather die than see a male doctor. But we knew that all of them preferred to see a woman. This was difficult for us, as a department, to arrange. It often leads to a heavy workload for women doctors, but it is a pressure which is hard to resist.

The Day Care Abortion Service

In 1977 Peter Huntingford won his battle to get funds to start a day care abortion service at Mile End, using the outpatient department. Partly as a result of his research into fetal monitoring, Peter had been a founder member of the anti-abortion organisation, the Society for the Protection of the Unborn Child. But he had completely changed his mind on the issue as he listened to women seeking abortion after the law was changed in 1967. Through our different backgrounds we both realised that the only person who could make the abortion decision was the woman herself. We felt that the service was crucial to the women of Tower Hamlets; that it was quite wrong that these women, from one of the poorest districts in the country, should have to pay for an abortion or continue with a pregnancy which they *knew* they could not cope with, physically, emotionally or financially.

Using non-medical counsellors, we provided an out-patient abortion service to women who were healthy and less than thirteen weeks pregnant. As the service became known to local GPs they began to refer all their patients who needed abortions to us. Cheap to run, the day care service at Mile End dealt with half the women needing abortions in the District as outpatients, and most of the rest were operated on as day cases in the ward.

Although the day care service freed gynaecological beds at Whitechapel, which should have shortened the waiting lists there, our colleagues were not altogether happy with the service. When I was suspended, Jean Richards told me that some of my colleagues' opposition towards me stemmed from the day care abortion service which 'had turned Tower Hamlets into the abortion capital of London'. In 1983, Jean Richards commissioned a study of the clients of our service for the District Health Authority. It remained 'confidential' and was never presented to the Health Authority – perhaps because it did not bear out the accusations that women from outside the borough were being accepted, nor the rumour that we were doing more late abortions than before. In fact, in 1983 only 3 per cent of women were more than seventeen weeks pregnant when they had abortions at the London, compared with 9 per cent in 1975.

Choice in Childbirth

We tried to offer women a choice of services in childbirth by sharing antenatal care with GPs who were interested in cooperating with us and by encouraging the midwives to regain their autonomy and take on home deliveries (providing telephone back-up during labour and hospital support if necessary). In 1975 Peter unsuccessfully tried to persuade the NHS consultants to allocate a few beds to GPs so that family doctors could have their own delivery unit in the London Hospital. He offered the GPs the use of his own beds at Mile End, and as an alternative, started a 'domino' ('domiciliary in-and-out') scheme where women with normal pregnancies are looked after by their own doctor and community midwives throughout the pregnancy and labour, and return home after only six hours in hospital.

GPs had the choice of seeing the woman throughout the pregnancy and labour or sharing the decision about the type of care with us. Naturally, if there were complications, they would refer the woman for a second opinion. What our colleagues appeared to dislike most is that we offered the GPs choice. They felt that the consultant should take the decision about the woman's delivery. Fundamentally, the issue was power.

In spite of his academic and clinical experience, Peter had found the position of professor difficult. The lack of funds to do the things necessary to upgrade the fabric of the department and set up a modem service contributed to the difficulty in creating a united department. And although Peter's hard work and dedication – both to the National Health Service and to the students – was not in doubt, there was unspoken animosity within the Division of Obstetrics and Gynaecology about the kind of services we were providing.

Peter gave up the Chair of Obstetrics and Gynaecology in 1981, moving to Maidstone to work as an NHS consultant. After he had left, a senior professor remarked that the only thing Peter gave the London Hospital was a 'certain dubious notoriety'. In retrospect, I see that he probably included me in the same category.

I was happy at Mile End, away from the medical politicking at Whitechapel, and I wanted to continue the work we had started in the Academic Unit. But my position was weakened by Peter's departure. A battle began in the Division of Obstetrics and Gynaecology where I was always outnumbered by four voices to one.

The Balance of Power Shifts

It was to be two years before the new professor took up his post and in the 'interregnum' many of the positive achievements brought about by Peter were quietly undermined and eroded. The balance of power and status began to shift back towards Whitechapel with the appointment of Trevor Beedham as consultant, previously one of our two senior registrars, in July 1981. Although Peter had written seven clinical and operating sessions at Mile End into the job description for this post, I found that after Trevor Beedham was appointed he was allowed to rewrite his timetable, transferring the major part of his input and half his workload to Whitechapel and joining their on-call rota.

I also found myself outmanoeuvred over the appointment of a locum senior lecturer, to tide us over the interim before a new professor took up his post. At less than twenty-four hours notice, I was summoned to an impromptu appointments committee of four – the then Dean of the London Hospital Medical College, Professor David Ritchie; the Chairman of the Academic Division of Surgery, Professor John Blandy; the Chairman of the Division of Obstetrics and Gynaecology, Leonard Easton (who was shortly to retire); and me, representing the Academic Unit of O and G.

Leonard Easton suggested that we promote our senior registrar to the locum post, and I proposed that the post be advertised, as we had seen some excellent candidates when interviewing Trevor Beedham, earlier in the year. As an example, I suggested that the Australian woman who had performed well at the earlier interview, had more experience than any of our senior registrars and was currently conducting a substantial research project, might respond to an advertised post.

After some discussion Professor Ritchie seemed to be in favour of advertising when Professor Blandy weighed in with a vote 'for the chap we know'. It was then that one of the panel mounted an amazing attack on the Australian woman, repeating gossip that she was a difficult woman to work with, continuing with innuendo about her personal life which it would be wrong to repeat. I was disgusted by this behaviour and so angry that I could hardly express my disapproval. I left the room abruptly.

I felt like handing in my resignation to protest at this method of filling a post, but a senior professor, Sidney Watkins, calmed me down. I was powerless; I had to accept the committee's decision to appoint the existing senior registrar as Peter's temporary replacement. But I knew that as a senior registrar, he would, at some stage, rely on the support of the other consultant obstetricians for promotion to a consultant post himself. Because of this he would be unlikely to support me in any discussion over the services to women in Tower Hamlets.

These two appointments were crucial to reducing the workload of the obstetric unit at Mile End Hospital. Instead, I found my workload increasing. After Peter left, GPs tended to send women with more difficult social and psychological problems to me, and the referrals to the day care abortion unit rose to 1000 a year, nearly twice as many as our sessions allowed for. By 1982 I found that my share of the obstetric work at Mile End hospital had increased to the point where, even if we started at 8.30 a.m. and had a midwife do the bookings, I could no longer manage with one antenatal clinic a week.

Community Antenatal Care

For some time, I had been impressed by the work of Ken Boddy in Sighthill, and Ron

Taylor and Luke Zander in Lambeth. They had extended the concept of 'shared care', the system of giving GPs some of the responsibility for women's antenatal care, to completely community-based schemes where women did not have to visit the hospital at all, even if they suffered from high-risk conditions like diabetes.

In the sixties and early seventies, antenatal care was almost entirely hospital-based. Women began to object that they were being treated like cattle, block-booked into impersonal hospital antenatal care units where there was nowhere for their children to play, and where they had to wait for hours to see a different doctor each time. The doctor they saw was often hurried and harassed, didn't explain things to them properly and they felt treated them as a walking incubator. The lack of continuity of care from both doctors and nurses in the hospital clinic could lead to missed test results, forgotten prescriptions, confusing advice, and lack of encouragement to ask questions.

Ken Boddy pioneered a community obstetric scheme at Sighthill Health Centre, on a housing estate in Edinburgh, in 1978. Luke Zander, Senior Lecturer in General Practice, and Professor Ronald Taylor, both of St Thomas's Hospital in Lambeth, extended this scheme so that in their area a hospital consultant visits local practices weekly to advise GPs and carry out joint consultations with patients.

After visiting their practice, I thought the best solution to the increased workload at Mile End was to hold such antenatal clinics in GPs' surgeries, involving the family doctors and community midwives in sharing the care. I was already meeting regularly with some of the newer, younger, vocationally trained GPs who were replacing the older family doctors, and in September 1982 I started the scheme with three group practices. I enjoyed the more informal contact with the women, got to know more of the community midwives and, as the GPs took on community obstetric care, began to meet with the midwives every Monday morning to make sure they had the advice and support they needed. This move increased the proportion of women I saw personally, and enabled the GPs to develop their obstetric skills.

I mentioned the scheme to my colleagues, who expressed neither interest nor disapproval. It was not until 1985, after a district report on perinatal mortality had commended this initiative, that Professor Grudzinskas, who had never before discussed the overall scheme with me, attacked my participation in it in front of my colleagues, two of whom nodded in agreement with him. In their view, it was a 'misuse of medical college funds' for a teaching consultant like myself to make antenatal visits to GPs' surgeries.

Hospital divisions are supposed to work by consensus, and doctors have to be tolerant of each other's practice. However, there is always a struggle over the allocation of beds, junior staff and operating sessions, which seems to me to be about power and status rather than how to provide the best patient care or student teaching. I was interested in providing a good service for the women and jointly planning how to do this in a deprived, working-class district with shrinking resources. When I found that the booking system of my colleagues at Whitechapel apparently favoured middle-class women from outside the area, I was frustrated when they refused to consider ideas for reworking the system or to examine data which would tell us how many of these women needed the specialised services of a teaching hospital.

In the summer of 1981 I talked with Professor Kass, with whom I had worked nearly twenty years earlier in Boston, telling him of the problems facing the department and the difficulty in getting unity and a sense of direction within the division. Senior registrar accreditation had been withdrawn by the RCOG – a vote of no-confidence in our training programme which damaged recruitment at both senior and junior registrar level just as we lost the experience and dedication of Peter Huntingford.

Professor Kass's advice was simple: 'Keep your head down, your mouth shut and get on with the work. Don't waste time in arguments but use data to make your points.' I took his advice. I worked hard with the students, enjoying the challenge of organising the final examinations, and was pleased and relieved when the students did well. I was left alone at Mile End and rarely saw my colleagues, except at the increasingly lengthy and acrimonious meetings of the Division of Obstetrics and Gynaecology, where even relatively minor and uncontentious matters about the delivery of care to women in Tower Hamlets seemed to take increasingly more time to resolve.

The Attack on the Day Care Abortion Service

The position of Chair of the Division of Obstetrics and Gynaecology rotates, by election, among the five consultants in the division. In November 1982, the chairman was John Hartgill. A New Zealander, John had been appointed as a consultant twenty-five years earlier, having trained at the London with Peter Huntingford. John looks younger than his sixty years and cultivates a charming 'I'm just a simple chap' manner.

While I was abroad on study leave that November, John circulated a document which had caused great argument in the division. He wrote that women over twelve weeks pregnant, or with medical problems (those in my opinion with most need of counselling), should go not to the day care abortion clinic where counselling was available, but directly to the consultants' gynaecology clinics, where there were no lay women counsellors and where many of our junior staff, as in other units, had a conscientious objection to abortion.

Fortunately he added a paragraph which said that GPs and women could choose their own consultant, so the G Ps continued to refer to me and the circular made no difference to the working of the day care unit. Before Peter left he had warned me that John had opposed my re-appointment as senior lecturer in 1980, and although by 1982 John's dislike was apparent, I thought this was due to philosophical and practical differences in our approach to obstetrics and gynaecology, rather than to any personal antagonism or doubts about my competence.

The New Professor Arrives

By January 1983 we had a new professor. The Chair of Obstetrics and Gynaecology at the London Hospital and St Bartholomew's Medical Colleges had finally been advertised in the spring of 1982, nearly a year after Peter Huntingford left. I applied, somewhat unrealistically, as I knew that having had a female career pathway – juggling children, jobs and several moves to different countries – my CV was not that of the successful academic. I was not shortlisted, but, in conversation with the dean, David Ritchie, I expressed my view that we needed someone with the experience to deal with the conflict within the division.

The dean did not tell me who the candidates were. Nor did anyone else. It seemed extraordinary to me then – and still does – that the applicants were spirited round Mile End Hospital without meeting me and yet I would be the person to work most closely with the new professor. I was completely excluded from the appointment, and only learned who the candidates were because a registrar told me, having heard one of my consultant colleagues discuss them with his anaesthetist during an operation.

The appointments committee included, on the NHS side, John Hartgill, as Chairman of the Division, and Gordon Bourne, representing our sister hospital, Bart's, with whom we shared the joint professorship. Professor Ritchie and Professor Blandy represented the Medical College, while Professor Tim Chard represented St Bartholomew's Medical School. There were two university external assessors.

There were four older and more experienced candidates but the committee chose a relatively young man, who had got his MD in Professor Chard's department and worked for Gordon Bourne at Bart's. Gedis Grudzinskas was then thirty-eight years old. My initial impression was favourable. I remembered him as the only lecturer from Bart's who turned up to teach students without having to be reminded several times about the commitment. His research into placental proteins was laboratory-based – something we lacked. A fellow lecturer told me that he was a good politician. He had left Bart's and returned to Sydney as Senior Lecturer at the North Shore Hospital eighteen months earlier. In the summer of 1982, before he took up his appointment, he came over to England to visit the department. Over dinner he seemed friendly and enthusiastic. I met him again in October, when, although the dean had recommended me as the college representative on an appointments committee for a consultant post (Mr Easton's replacement), my consultant colleagues objected to my participation and insisted that Gedis Grudzinskas was brought over from Australia. During this visit I introduced him to all the staff at Mile End Hospital and sought his advice on how to respond to the attack on the day care abortion service. Over the next two months we had several telephone conversations, and when he took up his appointment in January 1983, I was hopeful that his pure science interests and my psychosocially orientated research would complement each other to produce a well-rounded academic department.

Different Approaches

During the first year of his appointment Gedis and I had several discussions about improving teaching for the students and training for the registrars. There were already indications that our clinical approach was very different. On two occasions Gedis expressed 'concern' about my clinical practice. The first time, he seemed worried about the use of prostaglandin pessaries for induction, which he called a 'research procedure'. I was puzzled by his use of the term 'research procedure' and quoted some published papers about the use of prostaglandins with which he appeared to be unfamiliar. The second time, the issue was abortion – he was unhappy about my decision to terminate the advanced pregnancy of a twelve-year-old girl. She had been referred to me by her GP when already twenty-five weeks pregnant. Recent improvements in intensive neonatal care mean that it is just possible for babies of this gestational age to survive. However, without such technology their lungs are too immature to support life, and in my opinion this child was too young to continue with the pregnancy, cope with a baby, or go through the trauma of giving a baby up for adoption. So without delay I arranged to start her 'labour', using an epidural to relieve pain. During our conversation about this, Gedis told me he needed a summary of the case so that he could protect me from the criticism of my NHS colleagues. At the time, I believed him.

As an academic and senior lecturer in the professorial department, I was answerable to the professor for my research and teaching. However, as holder of an honorary NHS consultant contract (I was paid by the college but worked for the Health District), I was a consultant in my own right and neither the professor, nor any other doctor, could direct my clinical decisions as long as they were within the bounds of acceptable medical practice. I was, therefore, surprised by this interference from a man who, although my senior in the academic hierarchy, had considerably less clinical experience than I did. I thought his behaviour could perhaps be attributed to a lack of administrative experience and initial difficulties in managing the delicate balance between the NHS input into the division and our academic unit. It was not until December, at the end of Gedis' first year, that hopes of a creative and friendly working partnership were dashed completely.

The First Major Dispute

The first substantial point of conflict concerned our response to the District Strategic Plan, which forecast less money and fewer beds for Tower Hamlets. We discussed the issue within the Division of Obstetrics and Gynaecology, where John Hartgill (then the Chairman) and Gedis Grudzinskas drew up a plan which meant losing twenty beds, two operating sessions and two junior staff, in order to achieve centralisation on the Whitechapel site. At the October division we reached a compromise but the following day, without consulting me first, they presented a changed plan to the District Administrator leaving out the safeguards I had negotiated and in addition cutting another ten beds. In the November division I expressed my disapproval of their action (i.e. changing our agreed position without consultation) but reiterated my support for centralisation of services. However when the plan was presented to the District Health Authority in December, by John and Gedis, the way the case was made deeply concerned me. I told the Professor that I thought the plan could lead to an inadequate service for the women of Tower Hamlets and that the option of centralisation on the Mile End site had not been adequately costed or considered. I could no longer keep silent.

The professor ordered me not to make a move that was contrary to the division's plan. I reminded him that, as this was a National Health Service rather than an academic matter, he could not direct my actions. It seemed to me there were two options. Either I went secretly to the District Health Authority members and told them my anxieties, pointing out how the case presented to them had been poorly researched and costed and, in my view, distorted to make the case which suited my colleagues; or I could use the medical advisory system to present a paper arguing my own position. I decided that the second way was the more honest, and I duly wrote a paper which included perinatal and maternal mortality figures to counter allegations the professor had made that obstetrics at Mile End was not safe. I addressed the paper to the Final Medical Committee, the body which is composed of the Chairs of all the Divisions in the hospital, and concerns itself with questions of policy, staffing and the provision of services. It also puts forward the consensus view of all the consultants about matters of district policy, via a representative on the District Health Authority. My paper was, however, not discussed, and they agreed to support the division's plan.

The Division of Obstetrics and Gynaecology passed a motion censuring my action in presenting my dissenting paper to the Final Medical Committee. They referred this motion to the FMC who declined to discuss the matter further. But later its chairman, Professor Sidney Watkins, remarked to me, 'It seems to be a crime to express a contrary opinion in the Division of O and G.'

I then received a letter from the professor:

20 February 1984. Professor Gedis Grudzinskas to Wendy Savage:

Further to our discussion on 12 January 1984 and I 7 February 1984, I wish to confirm that, having considered at length your activities as senior lecturer since my appointment over twelve months ago, I am concerned about their counterproductive nature, which is detrimental to your position and the interests of the Academic Unit and the Medical College.

Despite repeated verbal warnings, you continue to fail to coordinate your activities with those of your colleagues in the Academic Unit, and the College and Hospital Divisions.

As head of your department, I have, over the past year, and after many discussions with you and our other colleagues in the Hospital Division, secured agreements which should allow us to offer better clinical service as well as to improve the standard of teaching and research. To deliberately, and in my absence, take active steps to undermine these agreed plans (to which you were a party) is unacceptable to me as head of your department. In addition you have refrained repeatedly from acting in accordance with directions aimed at the rational deployment of the Academic Unit resources for the purposes of enhancing our teaching and research potential within the context of our clinical service commitments, conducted jointly with our NHS colleagues. This behaviour is not only disloyal to me personally, and to your colleagues, but it has compromised your position in the Academic Unit, the College and Divisions, at a critical time in the history of this unit.

These matters are raised in detail with you formally, in order to emphasise the seriousness with which I view this subject. From a senior member of the unit, I consider that respect for the position held, loyalty to the Head of the Unit, action in accordance with the head's directions on teaching and research, and the relationship of the Unit to our NHS colleagues are reasonable expectations.

It is of prime importance that you consider your responsibilities to the aspirations and agreed strategy of the unit a major priority. Furthermore, if you continue to act in this inappropriate manner without any significant change in your activities, I shall be forced to advise the review of your own employment positions. It is only fair to warn you that in these circumstances this may lead to termination of your employment.

The professor had sent copies of this letter to Professor Mike Floyer, the new Dean of the Medical College, Professor John Blandy, Chairman of the Academic Division of Surgery, and Professor Tim Chard, who represented St Bartholomew's Hospital on the Academic Unit.

Shocked by this turn of events, I went to see the professor in his office. At our meeting, Professor Grudzinskas told me that I was not doing enough research (although I had two grants and three research assistants in post) and was doing too much clinical work. I agreed that I was doing more clinical work than the six sessions which my job description allocated to me, and I explained that I could cut this down if there was more input at Mile End from the senior registrar, who was increasingly spending most of his time at Whitechapel.

Giving me no specific example, the professor then said that people were 'sniggering and laughing at me', that my colleagues did not like my clothes, my politics or my style, that I had harassed a lecturer, that my standing in the Division of O and G had fallen, and that I was 'disruptive'.

I went to see Mike Floyer, who was supportive and listened to my explanations about the dispute. He told me that he had reminded Professor Grudzinskas that without me the student teaching would have collapsed after Peter Huntingford had left. He offered to see us together, and I thanked him and said that perhaps we could sort it out between ourselves.

I thought it wise, as my job was at stake, to seek legal advice about the terms in which I should reply to the professor's letter.

5 March 1984. Wendy Savage to Professor Gedis Grudzinskas:

I appreciate the full and frank discussions that I have had with you and separately with the Dean, since receiving your letter of 20.2.84. These have clarified for me some of your anxieties about the Academic Unit and I hope I have reassured you that I have not been disloyal to you either personally or as head of the unit.

I was sorry that after the meeting we had on 2.3.84 you did not feel able to withdraw the letter, as I had asked you to, which leaves me no alternative but to reply to you in legalistic terms.

Your letter of the 20.2.84 purports to be a formal warning which may lead to termination of my employment. I must tell you that I reject totally your view that any such warning is justified, because your allegations in the first three paragraphs are untrue. In particular I have not undermined agreed plans but have merely exercised my right to express my opinion about those plans to the Final Medical Committee. In any case, I believe you have seriously overemphasised the impact that my representation had on hospital and college staff outside the Division of Obstetrics and Gynaecology.

I am able to state quite categorically that your allegations are untrue because I know that I have fulfilled my job description to the best of my ability. It is significant that you have not in your letter given any details of a single occasion when I have failed to carry out any proper direction or have failed to co-ordinate my activities with those of my colleagues. You claim to have raised matters in detail in your letter, but have not done so. If you have any specific complaints, please let me know what they are so that I may have the opportunity to revise them.

However, I hope that, avoiding further recriminations about the past, we as members of the Academic Unit can sit down with the other members of the Division of Obstetrics and

Gynaecology and jointly find a way forward. As no individual acting alone can be expected to heal the wounds that have been incurred in the past, I wonder if the help of some arbitrator or negotiating body should be sought? If all five of us could sit down and together resolve some of the deep-seated, but unexpressed differences which divide us, perhaps with the help of the 'Three Wise Persons' or someone from outside the London Hospital, we could reconcile our viewpoints and find a way of working productively in the future.

Within the Medical College, might not the problems associated with both of us having too much to do, be solved by asking the District Health Authority to pay for enough of our sessions to fund another Senior Lecturer, perhaps with a more research orientated role to strengthen our small department?

As I said to you on 17.2.84 I remain confident that together we can build a good department, and whatever the difficulties that have occurred in the past year I will support and have supported you in that aim.

My reference to the 'Three Wise Persons' was to the special professional panel, colloquially known as the 'Three Wise Men' to whom doctors can in confidence refer colleagues whose behaviour, they consider, because of illness, drug or alcohol abuse, is putting patients at risk. I had briefly discussed this possibility with the Professor of Psychiatry, who was a member of the panel, and he thought they could be used in the way I suggested.

The professor briefly acknowledged this letter on the seventh of March, together with his arrangements for 'cover' during his leave. They did not include me, in spite of my official responsibility to deputise clinically and academically for the professor in his absence. On his return from holiday he wrote to me again:

19 March 1984. Professor Gedis Grudzinskas to Wendy Savage:

Thank you for your letter of the 5 March 1984 which, in addition to other matters, requests clarification of my expectations of the Senior Lecturer position outlined in my letter of 2 February 1984. From your reply it seems that you have not fully understood or appreciated the points I raised in relation to your role and responsibilities as a senior member of the department.

As you are aware, it is the duty of the academic clinical staff at all levels to undertake teaching and research, in addition to clinical service duties under the direction of the Head of Department. My expectations are, therefore, firstly that you conduct your clinical service duties within the six clinical sessions stated in your contract; secondly that you participate in other clinical activities only if the major implications of your involvement are teaching and research. Proposed involvement in such extra clinical duties is to be approved by the Head of Department, and finally to promote by teaching, supervision and research, the advancement of obstetrics and gynaecology in the remaining five sessions.

...The issue is your failure to comply with my directions and the agreed plans of the division. In these circumstances it would not be appropriate to involve a third party. It is important therefore that I refer you back to my original letter of 20 February 1984 and reiterate that you consider your responsibilities to the aspirations and agreed strategy of the division as your first priority.

6 April 1984. Wendy Savage to Professor Gedis Grudzinskas:

Thank you for your letter of 19 March 1984. It is perfectly true that I did not understand the points that you raised in your letter of 20.2.84. That is why I asked you for clarification but your latest letter does not provide this. You have given no instance in which I have failed to comply with the duties set out in my job description and I do not find your statement of your expectations helpful, because it is almost entirely negative: apart from reminding me of my obligation to conduct six clinical sessions and five teaching and research sessions, you merely tell me that I must not participate in other clinical activities without your approval. Could you please tell me what you wish me to do. I will then do my best to fulfil your proper and reasonable expectations. I would like to repeat that I cannot accept that my expressions of opinion on the District Strategic Plan are in conflict with the duties of my position or can be properly restrained by your directions. This view has been confirmed by legal advice. I would ask you to read again my letter of 6 March, 1984, which was written in a spirit of friendship and in the hope that we can build an active, modern department of obstetrics and gynaecology.

18 May 1984. Professor Gedis Grudzinskas to Wendy Savage:

I have considered at length your letter of 6 April 1984. I must conclude from your correspondence that you have demonstrated a lack of insight into the problems I have raised in my letters, and the manner in which I should like you to deal with them. I would, therefore, like to terminate this correspondence.

I believe that the contents of my letters have been quite explicit concerning my requirements ofa senior member of this department, and I shall review your performance over the next few months to determine whether there has been compliance with my directions. If this turns out not to be the case, I shall be forced once again to raise the subject of termination of your employment.

29 May 1984. Wendy Savage to Gedis Grudzinskas:

Your letter of the 18 May 1984 leaves me no alternative but to ask the dean to meet with us on his return from holiday, so that you can tell me in his presence, in what way you consider that I am failing in my duties, so that I know what to do to meet your wishes.

I must make it clear once again that you have not specified hitherto where you consider me at fault: clearly I cannot take any steps to resolve the situation until I know this.

The professor refused the three-way meeting I had asked for, and the issue of my protest at the way the plans had been put before the District Health Authority was not discussed again. But although I did not know it, the professor had already taken steps to secure an investigation into my clinical practice, which led to my suspension in April 1985.

Chapter 4

The Hidden Agenda

In this age of liberty, no man has the right to defame the character of another, merely because he holds a different opinion.

Letter to the Lancet 27 September 1830, from 38 medical students from the London in defence of one of their 'chiefs'.

In April 1984, a young Bangladeshi woman, Mrs U, had her second baby at the London Hospital (Mile End) under my care. Her first baby had been delivered by Caesarean section, and now this second baby had turned late in the pregnancy to a breech position (bottom first).

It seemed likely that she would need a Caesarean again, but I decided to allow her a 'trial of labour' first. I have come to understand that it is important for some women to feel that they have tried to deliver a baby vaginally even if, at the end of the trial of labour, they end up having a Caesarean section. Ten years ago I would not have understood that, and would have thought that there was no point in a woman labouring in vain. I have learnt since then that some women need to know, through their own bodies, that the baby is not going to deliver vaginally.

When Mrs U was transferred to the labour ward, the duty registrar, Toby Fay, confirmed with her and her husband that they wanted to try a normal labour, even though the baby was in the breech position.

In a normal, straightforward delivery, the birth is handled entirely by the midwives. In the case of a delivery which may be complicated by, for example, a breech presentation, the duty registrar will oversee the birth, following a plan of management laid down for this labour by the consultant. If anything arises during the labour which this registrar cannot deal with, he or she contacts the consultant to confer, seek approval or confirm changes in the plan for delivery. If a labour is not straightforward, I like the registrar to keep in touch with me throughout; this differs from the practice of some consultants, who lay down a set of 'protocols' for the members of their team to refer to. But I believe it allows for more flexibility to manage each woman's labour individually, and is a better way of helping junior staff to develop their skills.

Because Dr Fay was due to take his membership examination for the Royal College of Obstetricians and Gynaecologists, the MRCOG, we had discussed the ways in which my plan of management for Mrs U's delivery would differ from the 'textbook' management of this kind of case. I had explained to him, the two reasons why I thought it important to let a woman feel some contractions if she wanted to, even though a Caesarean section was likely. The first was that women accepted the need for and the discomfort of a Caesarean section more easily if they had felt physically that they were going to be unable to deliver normally. The second was that if they were not convinced of its necessity, they might try and deliver at home the next time they became pregnant.

In England with good roads and ambulances this was not as dangerous as in the Third World. My experience in Africa had shown me however (and there was always a possibility that the Us might return to Bangladesh) that there was a high risk of the mother and baby dying if the scarred uterus ruptured miles from the hospital.

Three successive registrars looked after Mrs U during her labour, which was not carried out exactly as I had planned. The baby, a boy, was eventually born by Caesarean section and was well at his birth. Unexpectedly, he became ill forty-eight hours later and, despite excellent and energetic treatment by the paediatricians, he died on 4 May, the following week.

I suggested to the baby's parents that if we did a post-mortem, it would enable us to find out exactly why their baby had died. They discussed it with their Imam, who said that it would be against their religion, and, respecting their wishes, a post-mortem was not carried out.

On Monday May 13, Trevor Beedham, now the new Chairman of the Division of Obstetrics and Gynaecology, came to tell me that Professor Grudzinskas had asked him to set up an investigation into my handling of Mrs U's delivery. I felt some sympathy for his obvious embarrassment at having to relay the professor's decision, but I was disturbed that he apparently did not know what kind of an enquiry the professor had in mind.

The paediatricians (doctors who specialise in the care of children) had suggested that the reason the baby had suddenly become ill two days after his birth was because the delivery had produced a tentorial tear, which is a split in the delicate membrane between parts of the brain. If a baby's head is subjected to either a lot of moulding (squashing the head out of shape in the bony pelvis) or sudden changes of pressure (for example, if forceps are used high in the pelvis, or if the baby's head passes very quickly through the pelvis in a vaginal breech delivery), the tear may reach a large blood vessel in this membrane and cause bleeding inside the skull. This causes pressure on the brain and the baby usually dies shortly after birth.

I was doubtful whether this had happened in this case. In my experience, babies with this kind of bleeding were unwell from the time they were born, although symptoms of pressure on the brain, such as jitteriness and fits, or paleness due to loss of blood, might be revealed as much as six or twelve hours later. This baby was not unwell when he was born, and fed well for at least a day. I thought it more likely that the intracranial bleeding (inside the skull) was a result of the blood clotting problem which had also been diagnosed when he became ill.

Although Mrs U's labour was not successful, Hani Youssef, my registrar, who had carried out the Caesarean, had told me that the delivery of the baby was uneventful. I told Trevor that there was no evidence in the case notes to suggest that my registrar had delivered the baby badly, producing a tentorial tear, and I did not think that the baby's death was due to the labour or delivery.

As we parted I remarked that I thought that whatever worries the professor had about this delivery would be answered by a full discussion at the perinatal mortality meeting, which was due to review the U case the following day.

Tuesday, 14 May 1984

I arrived at Whitechapel before 8 a.m., slightly earlier than usual, to see a young woman whose heart had stopped in the anaesthetic room the previous Saturday. Despite the doctors taking the correct action immediately she had suffered severe brain damage, and it was already clear to me that there was no hope when I saw her and her family on Sunday. This morning her condition was unchanged and the nurses told me that test results for brain death would be ready after my gynae clinic and teaching session. I spoke to the woman's mother and husband briefly, arranging the harrowing interview for the afternoon when the results would be known.

It took place in the hostel where relatives stay when patients are very ill or live far away: a dark and gloomy place, in spite of attempts to cheer it up with bright curtains and modern furniture. On this day the small room was crowded, silent and filled with cigarette smoke. I broke the news as gently as I could.

It was 5.15 p.m. when I left the family for the perinatal mortality meeting where Mrs U's case was to be discussed. I hurried through the hospital garden, deeply saddened by this tragedy – a young woman, suffering a cardiac arrest while her first pregnancy miscarried. I did not feel like arguing when Trevor, who was waiting outside the lecture theatre where the meeting was to be held, told me that Mrs U's case would not be discussed. I thought we would discuss it the following month. It did not cross my mind that Professor Grudzinskas would then postpone the case discussion for the June, July and August meetings.

Although I did not know it, Trevor had already acquired and summarised the case notes of Mrs U and discussed the matter with Sotiris Argyrou, the District Administrator, Professor Watkins, the Chairman of the Medical Council, and the Medical Protection Society.

Nearly two years later, Trevor Beedham told the enquiry panel that he had been advised by the Medical Protection Society not to discuss the case at the perinatal mortality meeting; to consider the implications of pursuing an enquiry; and to follow his conscience. However, it emerged that this was only part of the advice given to him. When Professor Watkins, whom he had also consulted, learned of Trevor's evidence to the enquiry, he wrote a letter to my solicitor, a copy of which was sent to the enquiry chairman.

6 March 1986. Professor Sidney Watkins to Brian Raymond:

> …Mr Beedham and I agree, that the content of the discussion in question (May 1984) went as follows: ...[I] said to him that it was extremely difficult ever to prove incompetence. I read to him the requirements, quoted in a legal case in which I had been involved, that have to be established as facts to prove an allegation of deviation from normal practice. At this stage I said that if I was in his position I would have nothing to do with an enquiry, 'I wouldn't touch it with a barge pole.' My final statement was that, 'I would not wish to see the lid taken off the Pandora's Box of incompetence, as the effects would be widespread and damaging and one could not predict where the damage would stop.'

In spite of Professor Watkins' advice, the move for an enquiry pressed ahead. Trevor, in his capacity as Chairman of the Division of Obstetrics and Gynaecology, circulated a letter to my colleagues and administrators which, while passing the ball back to Professor

Grudzinskas' court, also served as the formal request for an enquiry to Sotiris Argyrou. (In fact Argyrou had already been informally consulted.) The letter was not marked private or confidential and fuelled gossip within the London Hospital and wider medical circles. It was tantamount to issuing a public statement that I was incompetent and not fit to be allowed near patients. However, as Trevor Beedham was to admit at the enquiry, many of the 'facts' within it were incorrect and misleading.

21 May 1984. Trevor Beedham to Professor Gedis Grudzinskas:

> I have now had time to assess the request made by yourself, the Director of Midwifery, Mr Oram and Mr Hartgill for an enquiry into the management and delivery of Mrs A... U..., hospital number .... She was booked under the care of Mrs W. D. Savage, the Senior Lecturer, who personally supervised her.
>
> When I discussed Mrs U with Mrs Savage on the 13th May 1984, she described her management as 'controversial' and thought it unlikely that anyone else in London would have managed that case in that way. She was not absolutely sure that Mrs U and her husband clearly understood the controversial aspects of her management and certainly there was no written agreement for a research procedure. During the course of the labour, and over some hours, whilst Mrs Savage continued to direct events personally, the duty medical staff became so fearful of the outcome that they telephoned Mr Oram, yourself and Mr Hartgill.
>
> Since the discussion with Mrs Savage, I have taken further advice about Mrs U's care and have been told that further public discussion should be postponed. In consequence the case was not presented at the Perinatal Meeting on 14 May 1984.
>
> I am concerned about the effects of such 'controversial' management (which is not a recognised research procedure) on our junior staff and midwives, and about their ability to maintain the best standards of patient care in such circumstances. The anxieties of the junior staff appear to be reflected by the consultants who support the request for an enquiry and who, for some time, have not been prepared to invite the Senior Lecturer to cross-cover for them. In view of the gravity of this problem, I think that initially the solution must be sought within the Academic Unit, but because of its wider implications I am sending copies of this letter to the District Administrator, the Chairman of the Medical Council and the Secretary of Mile End Hospital.

It was only at the enquiry, one year and nine months later, that five damaging statements in this letter were publicly shown to be untrue:

Firstly, Trevor Beedham had stated that the call for an enquiry into my practice came from the Professor of Obstetrics, Gedis Grudzinskas, the Director of Midwifery, and my consultant colleagues, David Oram and John Hartgill. But the enquiry panel was later to examine a letter which the Director of Midwifery wrote to Trevor Beedham in June 1985, denying that she had asked for a special enquiry in the U case, David Oram was to tell the panel: 'I do not recall putting my hand up and initiating things'; and John Hartgill's written statement, prepared for the enquiry, was to be completely silent on this point.

Professor Grudzinskas, on the other hand, was to recall that he had asked for the initial enquiry into the U case, and that he spoke with Trevor Beedham in his capacity as Chairman of the Division of O and G. The impression created in the letter, however, was that all the other consultants and the midwives were united in their anxieties about my practice and its effect on patients.

Secondly, in his evidence to the enquiry, Trevor Beedham was to concede that I had not described my management of Mrs U's case as controversial. Nor, as he agreed under cross-examination, had I suggested that it was a 'research procedure'. This was a very damaging allegation, suggesting that I was experimenting on my patients without their knowledge or consent – using women as guinea pigs.

Thirdly, Trevor Beedham's letter claimed that over some hours during the course of the labour, duty medical staff became so fearful of the outcome that they telephoned David Oram, John Hartgill and the professor for advice. But the enquiry revealed that only one person had telephoned for advice, making two calls within one hour before labour commenced. Toby Fay, David Oram's registrar, telephoned David, and then the professor (but not John Hartgill) because he wanted advice on how he should react if he was asked to carry out a plan of management with which he disagreed.

Fourthly, the other consultants had never told me that they were unhappy for me to cover for them during holidays or illness. David Oram told the enquiry that he had no anxieties about my clinical ability to cover his practice; the only reason he did not ask me to cross-cover with him was that it was administratively easier to share with Trevor Beedham, who worked, as he did, on both sites whereas I worked almost exclusively at Mile End.

Soon after the professor's arrival in 1983, a new duty rota was circulated in which one month I was covering at Mile End paired with John Hartgill at Whitechapel, while for the other three months the younger consultants were on call for both sites. When I protested about this change, never discussed at the divisional meeting, which could be seen as a lowering of my status, and which I felt was an attempt to isolate me, the professor implied that this was John Hartgill's idea, and that the situation would be resolved when obstetrics was centralised. There was never, at any time, an implication that there was any question about my competence.

At this time Professor Watkins was in his third year as Chairman of the Final Medical Committee and Medical Council. The paths of obstetricians and neurosurgeons rarely cross, but in 1980 I had referred a young woman dying of cervical cancer for treatment of her intractable pain to Professor Watkins. Early the next year he had referred me a patient who was twenty-nine weeks pregnant when she was admitted unconscious with a brain tumour. I advised against doing an elective Caesarean section prior to the long operation he planned to remove her brain tumour. But because of the risk of haemorrhage or raising the pressure in the brain during the second stage of labour, Professor Watkins asked me to do an elective Caesarean at forty weeks and she had a healthy 8lb baby who has done well.

During this time I got to know Sid Watkins – the only person at the London who makes me laugh! When I got Trevor Beedham's letter on 22 May 1984, I was extremely upset, and rang Sid for advice. He asked if my visit was official or unofficial. Somewhat startled, I replied 'official' because it was in his capacity as Chairman of the Medical Council (see chapter 5, p. 63) that I wanted his help. I told him what had happened in the U case, and as a neurosurgeon he agreed that bleeding into the head was more likely to happen following a blood-clotting disorder than the other way round. He told me that Trevor Beedham, as Chairman of the Division, had sought his advice formally and that he had told him to have nothing whatsoever to do with setting up an enquiry, and that he had also advised him that incompetence was almost impossible to prove.

Sid knew what problems I had faced in the Division of O and G and also had little expectation that the dean would support me. I had told him how inaccurate and damaging Trevor Beedham's letter was but when I went to see him he had not yet received his copy of the letter. It was not until August of 1985 that I learned that he had never received it. In retrospect that was very important in understanding why I was not more anxious. I knew that he met Sotiris Argyrou, the District Administrator, every week and assumed that Sid had given him the same advice as he had given to Trevor Beedham.

Thursday, 12 July 1984

Acting on the advice of Hempsons, the solicitors allocated to me by the Medical Defence Union, I complied with Professor Grudzinskas' requests for a report on the handling of Mrs U's case – despite the fact that he had no clinical (as opposed to academic) authority over me, and was not, strictly speaking, entitled to make such a request. I sent the report with a covering note, pointing out the inaccuracies in Trevor's letter. I wanted to circulate copies of this note because so many people had seen the letter, but Hempsons advised me 'not to send copies to anyone else for the time being'. With hindsight, I think this was an error. It allowed the secret manoeuvres to continue.

The proposed discussion of the U case was postponed once more at the June perinatal mortality meeting, and again in July, at Professor Grudzinskas' request.

I had promised Mr and Mrs U that I would have a full discussion of their child's death with them after the meeting. Because of the postponements I had to write to them in June, and again in July, to explain that it had not yet been discussed within the hospital.

Tuesday, 5 August 1984

After cancelling the perinatal mortality review for the *fourth* time, the professor talked over Mrs U's case with me when he called at my office to borrow my dictating machine. I asked if this was the formal discussion of the case which he had proposed, but he replied that it wasn't, as he didn't yet have the X-rays and the cardio-tocographic (CTG) strips which are the recordings of the baby's heart beat. (They were found and sent to the professor in early October.)

I wrote again to Mr and Mrs U, explaining that their case would not be discussed at the August meeting either. Although I was not, at the time, aware of the reasons for the repeated postponement of the U perinatal mortality discussion, it was nonetheless a source of concern to me, because it denied the Us a proper, formal consideration of the circumstances surrounding the death of their baby and made them feel that the hospital, and its doctors, were not giving them a straightforward, honest explanation. If the normal discussion had taken place, however, it would have been necessary for Professor Grudzinskas and Trevor Beedham to inform me openly that the handling of the case was being taken up with the administrators. As it happened it was not until my suspension in April 1985 that I really knew what was going on.

In early July the Us consulted the Community Health Council. However, they did not at that time wish to press a formal complaint. They went back to the CHC in August, the CHC wrote to Mr Argyrou, who forwarded the letter to me. I arranged to meet them with the paediatrician who had cared for the baby on 24 September. It was at this meeting that I realised for the first time quite how the case had been presented to the parents. I told the Us that as there had been no post-mortem the cause of death could only be a 'guess' and that, even if it were true, which I doubted, that the baby had suffered a tentorial tear, then an earlier Caesarean section would have made no difference.

Since my explanation was accepted in front of the secretary of the Community Health Council who was advising the parents, and as this complaint had come through the District Administrator, I thought the matter was closed.

In addition, as I heard nothing further from the professor, I assumed my report to him had been satisfactory. After October, neither the professor, nor Trevor Beedham, nor any other person, spoke to me about Mrs U's case again, until after my suspension.

The formal action had actually begun in the summer of 1984 when, without my knowledge, the U case was considered by the district team of officers (the medical, nursing and administrative officers responsible for the running of the health service in each district).

The team of officers could have dealt with the matter in several ways: they could have considered the case report I had prepared for the professor; they could have used the obstetric databank – one of the most extensive in the country – to see whether there was any evidence of higher mortality or morbidity (death or complications) in my practice, to put this isolated case in context; in view of the conflict between me and my colleagues within the Division of Obstetrics and Gynaecology, they could have reasonably sought an informal, independent opinion. They could have sought the advice of the RCOG or discussed the situation with the Chairman of the Medical Council of the London Hospital. And they could have asked me for my views.

The team of officers did none of these things. Instead, they took an extraordinary step: they asked my two younger and less experienced colleagues, Trevor Beedham and Gedis Grudzinskas, the men who had originally asked for an enquiry into the case, to comment on my management and my fitness to carry out my duties.

At this stage the only evidence before the district team of officers that my conduct was questionable was that in the opinions of Professor Grudzinskas and Trevor Beedham this was so. But instead of seeking confirmation from others of the 764 consultant obstetricians in England and Wales, they returned to these two for further information.

Wednesday, 15 August 1984. Dr Jean Richards to Professor J. G. Grudzinskas/Trevor Beedham:

> It was agreed to formally ask you to present two reports as follows:
>
> 1. A report on the particular incident involving the death of the baby. They need to know whether any departmental policies need to be reviewed in the light of this incident, etc. and the opinion on the clinical management of the case.
>
> 2. We need a report on the competence of the consultant concerned to carry on in clinical obstetric care. The initial reports we had from Mr Beedham indicated that there was

> considerable doubt on this matter. The authority needs to be assured that the clinician is safe to continue managing obstetric patients.

The first of these queries is standard management practice, but the second is most unusual. If competence is questioned, the Regional Medical Officer usually seeks an independent opinion via the RCOG or their regional legal department, using doctors skilled in dealing with medical negligence claims.

Thursday, 20 September 1984. Trevor Beedham to Dr Jean Richards:

> ...My enquiries at the time indicated that the duty staff made every effort (including contacting three of my colleagues) to change the management which they regarded as having a predictably morbid outcome. Once these circumstances became known to me I was informally advised by my defence organisation (in a situation which they regarded as indefensible) to inform the officers of the Health Authority in the interests of patient care, and to refute complicity... I have been advised not to comment about the ability of the consultant concerned to carry on clinical obstetric care, thus I cannot give the Authority the assurance it seeks.

Trevor Beedham wrote his initial letter in May, some eight days after he had spoken to me, but by September when he replied to the formal request from the District Medical Officer to comment on my competence, he had had ample time to confirm whether his initial understanding of the situation was correct. His use of the privileged 'informal' advice given to him by the Medical Protection Society also strengthened the case against me.

A day earlier Professor Grudzinskas had also written to Dr Richards, sending a copy of his letter to the dean and Trevor Beedham.

Wednesday, 19 September 1984. Professor Gedis Grudzinskas to Dr Jean Richards:

> I regret that I am unable to give the Authority the assurance that the clinician is safe to continue managing obstetric patients. Firstly, I have received legal advice that such a judgement should not be made by an immediate colleague such as myself, and secondly, I am currently enquiring into at least three additional obstetric and gynaecological incidents involving this consultant.

At the enquiry Trevor Beedham was to agree that he knew about and had seen this letter, although he couldn't recall the last sentence.

Tuesday, 27 September 1984

I knew nothing of the new investigation into 'at least three additional cases', but there was an indication that the informal enquiry into the U case was continuing. Dr Jean Richards mentioned to me on the telephone that she was looking for the case notes as she was thinking of sending them to Gordon Bourne, the Regional Assessor, because the Division of Obstetrics and Gynaecology had asked her to set up an enquiry under the terms of DHSS circular HM(61)112.

I had never heard of HM(61)112, but I remember responding sharply to the suggestion that the Division of Obstetrics and Gynaecology had asked for an enquiry, as we had never discussed the case (and there is no record of any discussion in the minutes of the meetings of the division). In fact, when Jean telephoned me on 27 September, Gordon Bourne had already formally agreed to assess the case.

Monday, 26 September 1984. Dr Jean Richards to Gordon Bourne:

> Mr Cumberlege [the Chairman of Tower Hamlets Health Authority] has asked me to say how grateful he is that you have agreed to assess the papers relating to this case and advise him whether there is a *prima facie* case for suspension. The case notes are in my office if you wish to peruse them.

From the correspondence introduced at the enquiry, it is clear that some verbal discussion had taken place between Mr Bourne and someone from Tower Hamlets Health Authority before 26 September, and looking at the evidence of Gordon Bourne at the enquiry, the possibility that this person was Professor Grudzinskas cannot be discounted.

It is interesting that suspension was mentioned at this early stage. HM(61)112 is the circular which sets out how the Health Authority should proceed if a doctor's competence is questioned. It requires the District or Regional Health Officer to collect evidence and present a case to the Chairman of the Health Authority. If, having taken all appropriate advice, he then decides there is a prima facie case of incompetence, he must then present the case to the doctor for his or her comments.

Suspension, on the other hand, is normally used only as an emergency procedure when a doctor suddenly becomes dangerous to patients, because of mental illness or addiction to drugs or alcohol. The mention of this step in Jean Richards' letter indicates that the possibility was in the minds of both herself and the chairman from an early stage.

The role of the regional assessor

There are fourteen regional assessors, appointed by the DHSS to examine the case histories of women who die during pregnancy, labour or the puerperium (the period immediately following childbirth).

Every three years, these men produce reports called Confidential Enquiries into Maternal Mortality, a successful attempt by obstetricians to look at their practice and improve services for women. The regional assessor's role in deciding whether there was a *prima facie* case for an enquiry under HM(61)112 would be pivotal. His report would be the sole basis for my suspension. It was, therefore, crucial to ensure that the person who performed the task of assessing my management of the five cases could not possibly be influenced (even unconsciously) by bias and that he was representative of 'mainstream' views in the obstetric field.

Gordon Bourne was a senior consultant at St Bartholomew's Hospital. Francis Cumberlege, in his affidavit sworn in August 1985, describes him as 'a man of very great experience and distinction in obstetrics, indeed he is of world reputation. By reason of his position as regional assessor, he appeared then, and appears to me now the proper choice to advise the Health Authority.'

Gordon Bourne has a large private practice in Harley Street, and is best known for his popular book on pregnancy. The *Observer* was to describe him later, in an article about the enquiry, as 'a well-known exponent of the father knows best school'; and a senior member of the RCOG has described him as 'an arch conservative' in obstetric practice.

Gordon Bourne was indeed well known, and perhaps particularly for his views on that aspect of maternity care which formed the crux of the allegations against me – the circumstances in which a Caesarean section should be performed. His conservative approach put him at one end of the medical spectrum on the delivery of breech births – he believed they should be dealt with surgically.

I pointed out to Jean the reasons why Gordon Bourne was not the most suitable person to give an independent assessment. It is strange that the health authority should have viewed Gordon Bourne as an impartial assessor. We shared a joint obstetric department with his at Bart's, and he knew both the professor, whom he had helped to train and whose approach to obstetrics he favoured more than mine, and myself. One could argue that although his job was to arbitrate between us, it would be difficult for him to be impartial.

Thursday, 4 October 1984

After Jean Richards had mentioned to me in passing that she was looking for the case notes of Baby U and was thinking of sending them to Gordon Bourne, I made an appointment to see her. She cancelled, on the grounds that the papers (on Mrs U) were not ready. Feeling very anxious, I went to see Mike Floyer and expressed my disquiet. He was friendly and reassuring, and said that he would be able to tell me more the following week.

But that same day Mike formally met Francis Cumberlege, Jean Richards, Sotiris Argyrou and Terry Dibley (Regional Legal Adviser) to discuss whether the U case provided *prima facie* evidence for proceeding to an HM(61)112 enquiry. The decision to send Professor Grudzinskas' reports to Gordon Bourne was taken at that meeting.

Friday, 12 October 1984

The dean reassured me again, saying that 'one case was not enough for a 112', but later in the conversation he mentioned in passing that there were 'others in the pipeline'. By this time I had asked a senior manager in the health service – a former Tower Hamlets district administrator – about the HM(61)112 procedure. He said that even if a doctor was not competent, it was almost impossible to 'get' him; and since I clearly was competent, I had nothing to worry about.

During the summer, the professor had asked me for case reports on two more women. Professor Grudzinskas told me he needed the first report, on a woman named Linda Ganderson, to defend me against 'gossip' amongst my colleagues. The second case, that of Denise Lewis, was apparently needed because of criticisms of my administrative arrangements for study leave. The professor said my registrar had not known where I was or what to do, and that David Oram had not known he was standing in for me. I provided the professor with a case report detailing the comprehensive verbal and written arrangements which I had made for the study leave. In conversation I told him of the daily telephone calls with my staff during the period I was away and the case notes showed that I was in constant touch with the staff. Both these cases were, I thought, satisfactorily dealt with before August.

As well as this succession of demands for case reports (which were not within the professor's remit as my academic, but not clinical, superior) I had weekly letters from him about teaching, research, staff, the contingency fund, and the abortion service. Whatever the intention behind them, I saw these together as continuing the pressure on me which had begun with the letters threatening my dismissal.

I knew that I was not incompetent, and that my differences with my colleagues stemmed from a difference in approach and attitude. Although I was determined to continue providing what I believed were the right sort of obstetric services for women, I felt that in time, once the centralisation of obstetrics took place, we would all learn to work together. Hempsons, who had seen the three case reports I had produced for the professor, told me that these things were always happening and they blew over.

Looking back, now that I have all the letters assembled, and the time to study them in depth, it seems almost unbelievable that I could not have understood what was going on. I think this is partly because, having worked in five countries with three different professors, I had never come across a situation like this before. I was also very busy and I tended to write my letters to the MDU or Hempsons late at night when I had finished what I considered to be my real work – looking after patients and teaching students.

Monday, 15 October 1984. Dr Jean Richards to Gordon Bourne:

> 1. Mr Dibley [legal adviser] felt that you ought to be warned that the opinion which we have asked you to produce for the Chairman may be shown to Mrs Savage if the Chairman, as a result of that opinion, decides that there is a *prima facie* case for which an enquiry should proceed.
>
> 2. Professor Grudzinskas is investigating 3 further cases about which there is some concern. It is felt that you may wish to wait until you receive details of those before you produce your final letter for the Chairman.
>
> I have been advised by Mr Dibley that Mrs Savage does not need to see any of the documentation so far until the Chairman makes the decision as to the existence or not of the *prima facie* case. I am, therefore, seeing her, but not showing her any of the letters which you have already received.
>
> Thank you so much for your help.

Jean Richards never did see me, having cancelled the appointment I made in early October. The first time I saw this letter was when it was exhibited at the enquiry.

Tuesday, 30 October 1984. Professor Gedis Grudzinskas to Dr Jean Richards:

> ...I enclose my comments on three cases, in addition to another, which has been brought to my attention, for your information. Regretfully, I am currently conducting an investigation into another case.

This case was Carol Lefevre, another woman whom I had allowed a trial of labour. Presumably he accepted my clinical judgement in this case as no report went on to Mr Bourne about her. Her healthy twins have appeared on many demonstrations and in newspapers since my suspension. She was delighted to have been allowed to have a trial of labour, even though she had a Caesarean section in the end.

Wednesday, 21 November 1984

I wrote to Hempsons, having learnt that the professor had acquired the notes of some of my patients, none of whom had complained about my care, before I'd even had the chance to do the reports he'd requested. I was advised to cooperate with the professor's requests and to deal with him by 'telephone rather than letter'.

Wednesday, 14 December 1984

Another request from the professor for me to provide detailed reports, this time of my handling of gynaecological cases. Producing these reports was extraordinarily time-consuming, and then and in subsequent months I expressed my exasperation to Mike Floyer at this waste of my time. I was astonished when a casual conversation with him revealed that, having spoken with Professor Grudzinskas, he had the (false) impression that the uterus of one of my patients had been perforated during an operation. I reported this to Hempsons, saying that I thought this was damaging to me.

My main concerns during this period were the continuing disagreements about the future of services for women within the department of obstetrics, my clinical work, which had continued to increase as GPs referred more women to me (between 1981 and 1984 the number of pregnant women in my care rose from 500 to 740 per annum), and my teaching and research commitments.

The reorganisation of the health service in 1982 and the cuts had added to the usual pressures, having a particularly severe effect on secretarial services. Poorly paid full-time posts were increasingly filled by temporary staff from agencies. During 1984 I had seven temporary secretaries. This meant I could never be sure that notes would be chased, results followed up and summaries prepared, unless I checked these details personally. It wasn't until I was suspended that I had time to realise that I had been routinely working eighty hours a week in order to deal properly with my clinical and academic work, committees outside the London Hospital, and the increasingly burdensome correspondence with the MDU.

My fellow consultants continued to work with me. There was no attempt to prevent me carrying on with teaching, treating patients and operating. No formal warning had been issued to this 'dangerous' clinician in the six months since baby U died. I was still unaware of the nature or extent of Gordon Bourne's investigation. (By now, he was examining five cases.) It would be another five months before I was suspended, and until then I remained in ignorance of the case being prepared against me.

In the first three months of 1985 both the District Medical Officer and the Chairman of the Health Authority urged Mr Bourne to produce his report on my management.

Tuesday, 15 January 1985. Francis Cumberlege to Gordon Bourne:

> You will, of course, know the routine that the first task is for me, as Chairman, to establish that there is a *prima facie* case. Your report on the cases referred to would help me in reaching my conclusion... I wondered when I could expect your report.

As an experienced chairman one would have expected him to say 'to establish whether or not there is a *prima facie* case', particularly as he must have realised the importance of taking a scrupulously impartial and objective approach.

Wednesday, 27 March 1985. Dr Jean Richards to Gordon Bourne:

> [Are you] yet in a position to submit your report... the chairman is most anxious for progress to be made in this matter as soon as possible.

In fact, in February 1985, Gordon Bourne had produced a draft report on the five cases. He later told the enquiry that he had meant to send the draft report to the Medical Defence Union, but his secretary had sent it to Dr Richards by mistake. What happened to the draft report in the next few weeks is a mystery. Gordon Bourne told the enquiry panel that he did not have all the correspondence as his filing cabinet had been cleared out when he retired from Bart's. From her letter to Gordon Bourne of 27 March, Dr Richards appeared to be unaware of the existence of the report.

Wednesday, 3 April 1985. Francis Cumberlege to Gordon Bourne:

> Months go by without a decision about Mrs Savage and I feel that further delay is damaging. I wondered if you are now in a position to let me have your report.

Damaging to whom? The patients were not complaining.

Perhaps he meant that the credibility of the case for suspension would be damaged if a whole year had elapsed between the 'dangerous' event and any action being taken.

Gordon Bourne Sends his Final Reports to Dr J. Richards

At the enquiry, it was possible to compare Gordon Bourne's draft reports on 11 February with the final versions which were produced in April. Although most of the material and the main recommendations are identical, it appears from internal evidence that the February reports were compiled largely on the basis of summaries of each case prepared by Professor Grudzinskas rather than from the case notes themselves. At the enquiry Mr Bourne was to state that he had partial photocopies of the case notes when he wrote the first draft of his reports, but had not seen the original notes. My secretary was asked to provide three of the relevant case records, apparently for Professor Grudzinskas, on 28 February, while I was on leave. Before finalising his reports, Mr Bourne saw the original of the mothers' notes in at least four cases. His final report, dated 9 April, produced after nearly six months, consisted of eleven short pages, distilled from some 550 pages of medical notes.

On the basis of this document Francis Cumberlege decided to suspend me, bringing to an abrupt halt the work to which I had devoted my entire adult life.

Friday, 19 April 1985. Dr Richards to Gordon Bourne:

> The Chairman joins me in offering you our sincere thanks for the enormous amount of work you have put into the reports recently submitted.
>
> The Chairman has decided that these provide a *prima facie* case for suspension under Section 112 of the 1961 Act, and Mrs Savage is being suspended from her Honorary

> Clinical Contract. The College will then decide whether to suspend her from College activities for which she is totally paid by them. Following submission of the evidence to her, and her replies, the necessity for a full enquiry will be decided upon.
>
> I would be grateful if you could submit a fee which would be appropriate for us to reimburse your time and expenses.
>
> Please may I thank you again for all the work you have put into this problem.

Mr Bourne waived his fee.

Chapter 5

The Muted Response of the Medical Establishment

> ***I will maintain the honour and noble tradition of the medical profession. A clinician shall behave towards his colleagues as he would have them behave towards him. A clinician shall deal honestly with patients and colleagues and strive to expose those physicians who engage in fraud and deception.***
>
> Geneva code of ethics for the medical profession

I was not simply a doctor: I also taught medical students at the London Hospital Medical College, part of London University. When I was suspended I assumed my academic colleagues would support me. On the day following the suspension of my honorary clinical contract, I received the following letter

25 April 1985. Professor Grudzinskas to Wendy Savage:

> Dear Wendy,
>
> I regret that following a discussion with Dr Jean Richards this morning concerning suspension of your Honorary Consultant Contract, I think it is in your interest and the interest of the Medical College that you should be withdrawn from all teaching and research activities in Obstetrics and Gynaecology in relation to under- and postgraduate student teaching until resolution of the present situation.
>
> I wish this to take effect forthwith.
>
> Yours sincerely,
>
> JG Grudzinskas

Mr Leigh dictated a letter in reply that I took in to the college that night. He advised against writing to the Academic Board but sent a copy to the dean.

26 April 1985. Hempsons to Professor Grudzinskas:

> We have been instructed by the Medical Defence Union and their member, Mrs W. D. Savage, with regard to your letter of the 25th April. In that letter you assert your view that it is in our client's interest that she should be 'withdrawn' from teaching and research activities in relation to under- and postgraduate student teaching until resolution of the present situation. Our client does not agree.
>
> You also said that it is your opinion that it is in the interest of the Medical College that this should be so. You do not say why this may be. You will be aware that for a doctor of our client's standing to be suspended from an academic post without notice and for no more precise reason than that it is 'in the interest of the Medical College' is gravely damaging. All our client's rights with regard to this step are reserved. In the hope that the damage

> which follows from this can be limited, we request you to withdraw the suspension forthwith.
>
> In the event that you decline to withdraw our client's suspension we should be grateful if you would explain precisely why it is in the interest of the Medical College so that we can advise our client further as to the remedies available to her...
>
> We are sending a copy of this letter to the dean.
>
> Yours sincerely,
>
> Hempsons

As Mr Leigh finished dictating this he told me that this letter virtually told the professor that he might be sued for libel and I felt cheered that at least I would be able to teach whilst I endured the suspension from my clinical work.

The Threat to Academic Freedom

At the Academic Board meeting on 29 April the 'suspension from clinical duties' of an un-named senior lecturer was announced 'sadly' by Professor Blandy as an addition to the routine report of the Academic Division of Surgery, of which I was a member. Professor Grudzinskas then said he 'deeply regretted this matter' and the dean clinched the identification when he said that the college would continue to pay *her* salary.

The dean added that the matter was *sub judice* and could not therefore be discussed. (Francis Cumberlege later prevented discussion at a DHA meeting by asserting that my case was *sub judice*. This effectively closed off other avenues of approach and ensured a major public confrontation. In fact, *sub judice* was used incorrectly in the context of my suspension, and there was no legal reason why my case could not be discussed openly.)

That night several people phoned wanting to know what on earth I could have done that was so dreadful as to require my suspension. Seducing the patients? Embezzling NHS funds? I replied that I had been suspended for alleged incompetence, but that no, I hadn't killed dozens of patients. Following Hempsons' advice, I said nothing more. It was a strange feeling being under suspicion like this and I felt sad that people would doubt my competence after all those years of working in the same hospital. Some of them had recommended me to their wives. Did they regret that now? Did they think they had had a lucky escape?

In the hospital the next day I noticed how some people did not look at me as we passed in the corridor. Some even crossed the street rather than have to speak to me. Part of me felt hurt; another part saw that it was very useful to see who was and who was not going to support me in the coming battle.

At the Academic Division of Surgery meeting on 1 May I read out a statement in which I denied the allegations of incompetence and said I would fight to restore my good name and professional reputation. I insisted that this be minuted and included in the report to the Academic Board and this was agreed by the chairman.

Many people expressed concern about the way I had been banned from teaching. It established a precedent, as although professors have overall responsibility for the direction of teaching, in practice the individual academic is free to present the subject matter as she or he sees fit and the concept of freedom of thought and speech is jealously guarded in universities in Great Britain. They were also disturbed by the fact that this had been announced to the Academic Board without consultation with the division or myself. Professor Blandy defended himself by saying it was the dean's decision but, 'if one of my chaps was operating badly it would be ludicrous to let him teach Academic Urology'. He gathered his papers and left.

It seemed I was to be assumed guilty until proven innocent. I continued to go into work and eat in the Medical College Blizard Club lunch room; I was not going to allow people to think that I was ashamed of my actions, or act as if I was guilty of these charges.

I received more than twenty letters of support from GPs and midwives in the first four days after my suspension. Yet after the Academic Board meeting, only a handful of hospital doctors and Medical College staff wrote to me. The contrast was striking.

The medical students were very upset by my suspension. Several of them joined the Support Group and helped with the march even though finals were approaching. They had a noticeboard in the common room where they put press cuttings about my campaign. Later they asked me to give them some lectures before finals. They found a school hall near the college and I was encouraged by the large number who attended. The dean told them, after a routine lecture, that it was to 'save Mrs Savage from emotional trauma' that I had been asked not to teach. His words were greeted with incredulous laughter.

Between June 1985 and February 1986 I wrote six letters to the Academic Board, appealing to my professional colleagues to support my request to be allowed to continue to teach students. In October the Board voted not to support my request by seventeen votes to twelve.

The Royal College of Obstetricians and Gynaecologists

The irony of receiving the highest award to a member of my profession, the Fellowship of the Royal College of Obstetricians and Gynaecologists, came home to me when, suspended from my post, I attended the award ceremony in June.

Each year the fellows are circulated with papers inviting them to name people whom they consider deserving of fellowship status. Acceptance is not automatically granted but is awarded by a Fellowship Committee for 'advancing the science and practice of obstetrics and gynaecology'. Of the 764 consultant obstetricians and gynaecologists in England and Wales, there are eighty-eight women (11.5 per cent). This is reflected within the committee structure of the RCOG where 10 per cent of the members are women. However, in 1986 only one woman was elected to the council, and all but one of the twenty-six committees are chaired by men. Male members and fellows are invited to join two clubs, the Travellers and the Gynaecological Club, and membership is limited. Excluded from the cosy male get-togethers where, it is rumoured, all the consultant posts are 'fixed', women have formed their own club but it does not seem to be an effective pressure group for women, either as obstetricians or as patients. The incongruity of a specialty devoted to women being almost totally controlled by men has always struck me forcefully.

The official position of the RCOG is that it represents the interest of all members and fellows and must remain neutral in disputes. Its position of not taking sides meant that the 'Savage' case has never been mentioned officially in its newsletters. On a personal level, senior council officers have been supportive towards me, and I was told informally at the highest level that they would have been happy to sit down with the obstetricians at Tower Hamlets to try to find some way forward. Nevertheless the college declined to comment on what it termed 'the difficulties' until a conclusion had been reached.

The General Medical Council

Through the General Medical Council, which has almost one hundred members, both appointed and elected, the medical profession sets its own standards and disciplines its own members.

One of the most important principles of the practice of medicine is that of clinical autonomy, which allows a fully trained doctor the responsibility for deciding which mode of treatment is best for his or her patients. In practice, clinical autonomy means that consultants and GPs are of equal status, are responsible for their own clinical decisions and should not be criticised by their colleagues as long as these decisions are 'within the broad limits of acceptable medical practice'. The GMC's handbook also states that the deprecation by a doctor of the professional skill, knowledge, qualifications or services of another doctor could amount to serious professional misconduct.

Throughout the time that Professor Grudzinskas was asking me for case reports I had maintained to the MDU and Hempsons that he had no right to ask me for these reports as he was not my clinical superior.

I decided to raise the matter with the president of the GMC.

17 November 1985. Wendy Savage to Sir John Walton:

> At the moment I am not seeking to lay a complaint against my colleagues at the London Hospital, but am seeking your advice about matters of interprofessional relationships which do not seem to be covered by the 'Blue Book', but which I had thought were part of the code of practice between doctors.
>
> Firstly, I believe that doctors holding either honorary or normal NHS consultant contracts are independent consultants in their own right and that; whilst a professor is academically superior to a senior lecturer, as far as clinical matters are concerned, he has no more right to criticise or direct a senior lecturer than one of his NHS colleagues.
>
> Secondly, is it ethical to ask for case reports from a colleague in order 'to defend you against gossip' and then use these cases to boost a complaint via the HM 61/112 procedure?
>
> Thirdly, is it usual for another consultant to order notes belonging to one of his colleagues in order to prepare case reports about clinical care, without the knowledge and consent of that person and in the absence of a complaint by a patient or formal enquiry of which the department is aware?
>
> Fourthly, I enclose a letter which, as you can see, was widely circulated within the hospital, was not marked private and confidential, and which I was advised was not libellous, despite the fact that parts of it are untrue, because it was 'privileged'. Does the GMC concern itself with matters of this nature?

Weeks passed and there was no reply, so on 21 December I wrote again, having by now seen the statements made by my colleagues in preparation for the forthcoming enquiry. On 6 January 1986, I received a reply and an apology for the delay from Sir John Walton. In essence, he confirmed that academics did have clinical autonomy, and referring to the pamphlet ‘Professional Conduct and Discipline: Fitness to Practise’ that doctors would normally only disclose confidential information about patients to other doctors who are looking after or taking over responsibility for that patient, he continued:

> I would not normally think it proper for a doctor to take an initiative in disclosing confidential information about one of his or her patients to another doctor for any other purpose, unless that was a purpose covered by other aspects of the Council’s guidance, such as disclosure at the order of a judge or other presiding officers of a court. Similarly, I would not regard it as usual practice for a doctor to request access to the clinical notes of another doctor’s patient for any other purpose other than one of those mentioned in the Council’s guidance; any doctor who does so and who discloses the information so obtained should therefore be prepared to justify his action, in accordance with paragraph (3) of the Council’s guidance.

The Official Hospital Response

In February 1985 Sam Cohen, Professor of Psychiatry, became Chairman of the Final Medical Committee and Medical Council. He is a quietly spoken man who has always been pleasant to me. I made an appointment to see him the week after I was suspended and told him briefly about the five cases. I said that even if I were incompetent it seemed to me that my suspension raised questions that needed to be discussed, not just for me, but for all doctors at the London. These were the use of suspension before I had been given a chance to defend myself and the secretive way the case had been built up. Sam was shocked by my suspension and expressed his support for me.

I wrote to Professor Cohen after the DHA on 9 May 1985 had not agreed to my request for the suspension to be lifted and Mr Cumberlege had said publicly that an enquiry was going ahead:

> I enclose the letter [see Ch. 4, p. 41] which started off the enquiry process under the HM(61)112 procedure, which could lead to my dismissal. Unless I accept the charges of mismanagement, which I do not, the next stage, after I have replied formally to the DMO within twenty-eight days from 24.4.85, is a formal enquiry with two obstetricians and a legally qualified chairman.

I then went into details of the U case, the ‘worst’ of the five which I allegedly mismanaged. I ended the letter:

> It was then alleged, in retrospect, that my registrar who had delivered the baby, had done so badly, and that a tentorial tear had resulted. This is an extremely rare occurrence in a term baby delivered by Caesarean section. What I am being condemned for is allowing the woman to have a trial of labour with a scar in the uterus and a breech presentation. Both the woman and her husband wanted her to try and deliver vaginally, and declined the offer of a Caesarean section twice during the labour.
>
> *At neither time did I consider that the baby’s condition was such that I should force the*

> *couple to agree to an operation* and this is a matter of clinical judgement. There was no post-mortem at the couple's request.
>
> I do not think that this is the way one expects one's colleagues to behave and I also think that the Chairman of the Health Authority has been poorly advised.
>
> The result will be bad publicity for the hospital and the college which I regret.

I had copied this letter to two people whom I knew would speak in my defence at the FMC meeting on 16 May 1985. (The FMC is made up of the chairmen of the hospital divisions and meets monthly. In addition all consultants are members of the Medical Council which meets three times a year. The same person chairs both bodies.) There was considerable discussion and concern about how I could have been suspended without the chair of the FMC knowing about it, and the damage being done to the hospital by the publicity which had already occurred. The committee asked Professor Cohen to speak to Mr Cumberlege.

What passed between them I do not know, but Mr Cumberlege was not swayed by the opinions of the hospital consultants expressed through the chair of the FMC.

Between June and August I asked members of the Medical Council to raise the manner in which I had been suspended. I was disappointed not to be invited to the June meeting; nor did they discuss the matter because the debate 'might have got out of hand' and 'people might say things they regret later'. Most people apparently thought that nothing could be discussed until I was reinstated. At the July meeting of the FMC the committee asked its chair to see again if there was any way of resolving the matter; Professor Cohen wrote to me, the Chairman of the Division of Obstetrics and Gynaecology and the Chairman of the Health Authority to offer the services of senior medical staff. I replied as follows on 31 July 1985:

> Dear Sam,
>
> Thank you for your letter and offer to help in any way possible.
>
> I certainly would welcome anything that could be done to make it possible for us to work effectively and harmoniously in the Department of Obstetrics and Gynaecology.
>
> At present affidavits have been prepared and my solicitor tells me that the case should be lodged with the High Court on Monday, 5.8.85.
>
> Two professors and one reader have said that the five cases were not sufficient material to suspend me and two of them said that any enquiry into the two they thought did show errors of management should include the whole department. We are suing for reinstatement on the grounds that my suspension was unlawful and a breach of my contract.
>
> Any steps that could be taken to make reinstatement as painless as possible for everybody concerned I would welcome. The latest offer from Professor Grudzinskas through an intermediary is 'if WDS will resign we will drop all the charges', so I find it difficult to see a way forward in the present climate and with court proceedings almost inevitable.
>
> I deeply regret the divisions in our department that taking evidence from the junior staff will almost certainly bring. I wonder if your good offices could be used to assist them to

> make the difficult decisions that will be forced on them? I understand that the DMO has now written to say that as the notes could not be released they should be perused in her office and the doctors' report on their personal involvement be prepared there. I have advised the junior staff to discuss this with their defence societies, but perhaps they would like to talk to someone from outside of the department as well...
>
> Thank you again for your offer of help.

In August no FMC meeting is held and by September it was known that the High Court case for immediate reinstatement had been lost and that an enquiry would take place in November.

In October, I was refused permission to attend the Medical Council meeting the next day. That night was one of the 'low spots' in the time since my suspension. It seemed that the – as I saw it – male professional view was that having been unjustly accused I had to accept this injustice and await the slow creaking HM(61)112 enquiry procedure, however much it cost the NHS or me personally. If I gave up and threw in the sponge it would show that I wasn't tough enough to stand the pace of a teaching hospital consultant life. In a way I felt that many people hoped that I would give up and then the whole affair could be smoothed over and forgotten and people would not have to face the fact that those they worked with, referred patients to, or drank tea with in the consultants' room, had behaved in such an unusual way.

At that point I thought that I would stop trying to get my hospital colleagues to act.

Chapter 6

The Public Protests

> ***Off stage there have been unedifying antics. Some doctors who complain about 'trial by the media' seem to find nothing repugnant in 'trial by gossip'.***
>
> Michael O'Donnell, *British Medical Journal*, 14 September 1985

In the months following my suspension the position of the medical establishment became clear to me. Meanwhile, however, my case had aroused enormous national interest and concern.

Word of my suspension had travelled quickly. The news certainly reached some organisations before I was formally suspended. It seems that a health visitor, pregnant and booked under my care, had overheard a conversation between a midwife and a GP after a lunchtime meeting. She was so shocked that she immediately rang Sue Hadley, the Tower Hamlets National Childbirth Trust (NCT) teacher, whom I knew slightly. They agreed that this outrageous action should be fought and even before my meeting with Jean Richards they had rung the NCT national office. The NCT then informed the press.

At the time, I was still in a state of shock. I had not thought about publicity. I still hoped that the MDU and Hempsons would somehow get an injunction to stop what was so obviously unjust and wrong. In retrospect, although I would have preferred to inform the press on my own terms, it was probably just as well that it was done for me. In less than twenty-four hours, doctors, midwives, a neighbouring Health Authority member, the Community Health Council and medical correspondents from the national newspapers had all left messages on my answerphone.

The Local GPs Respond

On Thursday, the professor told the GP representatives on the Maternity Services Liaison Committee (MSLC) that I had been suspended. Unknown to me, on Friday evening, forty-eight hours after my suspension, local GPs and midwives gathered at South Poplar Health Centre, one of the four practices I visited as part of the community obstetric scheme. Fifteen GPs came, including several of the older ones, like Dr Bernard Taylor who had been in practice for thirty-five years in the East End and Dr Nebhrajani, speaking on behalf of Asian women. They decided to form a committee, later to become the Appeal Fund. Mary Edmondson, Tony Jewell and David Widgery were elected as members.

Mary Edmondson had had both of her two young children at Mile End. I had worked with Tony Jewell at the Mile End when he was Peter Huntingford's Senior House Officer and I had looked after his wife during both her pregnancies. She was then due to have her second baby in three weeks' time. Several of the younger GPs had done their vocational training at the London, as had Tony Jewell, and had either worked for Peter Huntingford or myself.

I am told that it was their contact with me at a clinical level as GPs, and their respect for the support I had tried to give them as professionals (both in providing the kind of care that they wanted for their patients, and in encouraging them to take on more antenatal and intrapartum maternity care) which made them act. Many had small children and as young GPs were still building up their practices. Writing and circulating petitions, and later writing and talking to the newspaper, TV and radio journalists was a heavy and time-consuming burden for them all, and I am grateful to them for that invaluable support.

The many doctors who say to me, ‘But how could you go back and work in Tower Hamlets after your colleagues have attacked you like this?’ perhaps do not realise that sixty-eight of the eighty-three GPs in Tower Hamlets signed that first rushed petition which the GP Committee presented to the Chairman of the District Health Authority. They continued to support me throughout this long struggle – even though, initially, they knew nothing about the details of the cases. They knew, however, that I was not incompetent. In many ways GPs are in a better position to judge competence, as they are responsible for the long-term care of patients and have more contact with consultants than consultants often have with each other.

On 6 May, Bank Holiday Monday, the GP Committee, now with the addition of Dr Jo Shawcross from the third practice I visited, met and planned a small press conference to be held on the 9th (the day of the monthly District Health Authority’s next meeting) at Steele’s Lane Health Centre.

The DHA meeting was packed. Around sixty people turned up, in small groups or on their own initiative, to demand my reinstatement. Beverley Beech of AIMS (the Association for Improvements in the Maternity Services) collected their names.

Mary Edmondson presented the GPs’ letter calling for my reinstatement and also presented a petition from the medical students describing me as ‘an inspired and conscientious teacher’ – despite the 7.45 a.m. ward rounds! A further petition from the Mile End Hospital had been signed by 150 people from all grades of staff.

The Wendy Savage Support Group

The Wendy Savage Support Group was formally launched on 16 May 1985, in the basement of a local community centre in Bethnal Green. More than fifty people were crammed into the room – GPs, midwives, nurses, medical students, local mothers, and a few fathers, and representatives of the national consumer movements like AIMS which, through Beverley Beech, had been active from the day of my suspension. Sue Hadley and Heather Reid attended for the NCT and Christine Smith and Ron Brewer represented the Community Health Council, the NHS watchdog group for patients. There were women from the Maternity Services Liaison Committee which is a link group between women from ethnic minorities and the antenatal service. Many of the women were former patients of mine. They decided to hold a march on 13 June, the day of the next Health Authority meeting, and to write individually and collectively to Mr Cumberlege and other people in positions of authority.

Posters were printed and badges produced with the slogan ‘Wendy’s Best – Investigate the Rest’ and ‘The Savage Cut – Who Asked Us?’ Car stickers showing a baby with the slogan ‘Reinstate Wendy Savage Now’ were provided free of charge by Malcolm Crowe, whose wife had chosen to have her first baby at home with my blessing, and had been looked after by Mary Edmondson.

The public response was overwhelming. Women stood in street markets, toddlers at their feet, collecting signatures for petitions. Petitions went around nursery schools, GPs' surgeries and Labour Party meetings. Vast numbers of posters advertising the march appeared all over the borough virtually overnight – on hoardings, bus-stops, in clinics and libraries, and in the windows of people's homes.

Both Beverley Beech and Sheila Kitzinger of the NCT were veteran campaigners for women's rights in childbirth, and using their connections the Support Group added to the national media coverage of the issue. Sheila's article, 'Battle of the Birth Rights', in the *Sunday Times* on 19 May and pieces in *New Society* and the *New Statesman* carried news of the march. The *East London Advertiser*, the *Guardian*, *Hospital Doctor* (distributed free to all doctors working in NHS hospitals) and the *Nursing Times* all carried features about different aspects of the case and the campaign for my reinstatement.

Taking the advice of Hempsons, I was refusing to speak to the press, concentrating my efforts on the hospital and Medical College in the hope of an internal solution. I spent my time conferring with Mr Leigh, my solicitor, drafting letters, gathering statistics and dictating notes on the five cases.

At the time, I was not aware of the immense efforts of my supporters behind the scenes and it was only later that I realised, with gratitude, their work on my behalf.

As the press coverage widened, letters of support flooded in daily and I began to question the lawyers' advice to avoid publicity. On 28 May, five weeks after my suspension, I decided to change my solicitors. Although I had no reason to doubt their integrity, I had been feeling, increasingly, that Hempsons were part of the same medical establishment which I felt was attacking me. Mr Leigh was on first name terms with Mr Dibley, the Health Authority's solicitor, and I realised that they were usually on the same side, defending doctors against patients. I, on the other hand, was supported by my patients against some of my fellow doctors.

Helena Kennedy, a barrister, had recommended Brian Raymond, of Bindman and Partners, to me. He had just successfully defended Clive Ponting in the 'Belgrano Secrets' trial. He had time to take the case, and I went to meet him the next day.

I drove to Bindman's offices in Finsbury Park. The contrast could not have been more marked. Bindman and Partners are known for their interest in civil liberties and their staff reflected their principles. I went up a narrow staircase to the top floor; the office was small and functional, crammed with papers. Brian Raymond, shorter and less angular than Mr Leigh, was in his shirtsleeves in the sunny, uncurtained room. The atmosphere was relaxed and informal. I immediately felt at ease and although it was painful having to go through the details of the suspension and its aftermath again, I knew I had made the right decision. Brian's view was that rather than shunning the publicity, I should use it to my best advantage.

I was still hesitant about using publicity, and although I had known since February that I was to be elected to the Fellowship of the Royal College of Obstetricians and Gynaecologists, I had kept quiet about it. It was therefore a surprise to me when I opened my *Guardian* on 1 June to read, 'Top Award for Suspended Doctor'. The article went on to describe how Professor Chamberlain, the junior vice-president of the RCOG, had publicly supported me. The solicitors, Hempsons, had asked him for a report on the five cases to be submitted to the District Health Authority. I knew he had seen the criticisms and the case notes, and felt doubly cheered by his stand.

On Sunday 2 June, Katherine Whitehorn's regular *Observer* column was headlined, 'Who's Hysterical Now?', referring to the medical establishment. Apparently an attempt to oust me, using 'mental instability' as an excuse, had been considered but rejected.

On Wednesday 5 June, I went to the Royal College to receive the award. I evaded the press photographers outside, leaving the taxi by another door. All the old photos in the press files were from the days when my hair had been long and straight so they didn't recognise me with my comparatively new hairstyle. Instead they beseiged my stepmother, under the mistaken impression that she was me.

On 7 June Brian Raymond and I had met with the Support Group for the first time. Although I wanted to go on the march we thought it best that I did not because its focus was the feeling of the *community* about the effect of my suspension on the women of Tower Hamlets. If I were there, the press and the District Health Authority could dismiss it as simply being a personal protest and this it was not. Three of my four children went. I dropped them outside the Mile End Hospital at 1.30 p.m. There was a handful of people there and I felt that anxiety I always feel when giving a party, when everything is prepared and the time for starting approaches, and I think no one will come. But more than a thousand people turned up, pushing prams and push chairs. MPs Jo Richardson and Ian Mikardo, who had sponsored an Early Day motion in Parliament calling for my reinstatement, marched along with the Maternity Service Liaison workers, women from Bangladesh and Somalia and women's health organisations. Led by a small band, they marched from Mile End Hospital, along Whitechapel Road to the London Hospital, Whitechapel, where the DHA meeting was to be held. There the Assistant District Administrator was sent out to face the well-behaved crowd and its police escort, whilst Mr Cumberlege and Sotiris Argyrou kept a low profile. The Support Group had done a magnificent job. In four weeks they had organised a very big event, on a shoestring, and with no previous experience of doing anything quite like this. I learned afterwards that a senior professor, who had watched the march arriving from an upstairs window, remarked, 'Who would have thought to see the day a rabble marched on the London Hospital?' That's no rabble, I thought; those are your patients.

The next day's press coverage lifted my hopes even further. Several papers carried pieces about the march and over the weekend the *Observer* carried a feature on my suspension, following up a series of *New Statesman* articles which had investigated the medical-political background to the events and the extent of my colleagues' involvement in private practice. Francis Cumberlege's response to the protest was quoted by the *Observer* as, 'I was in the tea business: I was out in Bengal from 1946–1953. I don't want lectures from women on what Bengalis want.'

Because I had decided to leave Hempsons, it was estimated that I could face legal costs of around £50,000. Brian Raymond told me not to worry. When he had defended Clive Ponting people spontaneously sent money in without any public appeal from him.

Sam Smith, a seventy-six-year-old ex-Tower Hamlets GP, staunch socialist and a fighter for justice throughout his life, rang me on 8 June to say that he had been sent a cheque for £100 and suggested that an appeal fund should be set up. He embarked on an enthusiastic one-man telephone campaign to local GPs, which raised several hundred pounds. Then a group of GPs took on the extra work involved by forming the Appeal Fund Committee. The press coverage of the High Court hearings in August and September mentioned that I had to pay my own legal fees. The public response was astounding. By mid-September the fund had reached £2,000; by mid-October £5,000, and by the time the official circular asking for donations was printed, it stood at £9,000. Eventually the Appeal Fund was to reach £60,000.

The gulf between what women were seeking in obstetric care and what the medical profession wanted to provide became clear from the different responses of the community and the medical establishment. The doctors and health workers who worked in the Tower Hamlets Health District were willing to become publicly involved in my case because they knew, and liked, the kind of care I provided – and that I was competent. Their public declaration of support gave me strength. They and the women's health organisations who were involved from the beginning of my suspension ensured that my case caught the attention of the media: my case was no longer the fight of the individual for her livelihood but a focus for a countrywide debate on the future delivery of maternity services.

The strength of feeling about the case and the whole issue of maternity services must have surprised my colleagues and taken the medical establishment by surprise. Many doctors were horrified at the prospect of the profession washing its dirty linen in public. From the beginning, when the chairman of the Health Authority declared the matter *sub judice* and the professional bodies refused to become involved, it was clear that their overriding concern in my case was for a discreet and private conclusion to the affair. The public silence of my consultant colleagues contrasted strongly with the willingness of many of them to talk behind the scenes. One journalist said to me after some days of talking to doctors: 'I've come to the conclusion that if I said to a doctor, "Do you put on a gown and gloves to operate?" he would say, "Off-record, yes."'

Gossip thrived in the corridors not only of the London Hospital but also amongst examiners for the Royal College of Obstetricians and Gynaecologists and members of the General Medical Council. Michael O'Donnell, the well-known medical journalist, writing in the *British Medical Journal* in May 1986, said:

> Some doctors who complain vociferously about trial by the media are themselves active proponents of that traditional medical pastime, trial by gossip. During the Savage case I decided to document this practice by noting items of gossip that were offered to me or passed on in my presence, and then investigating them as best I could to see if there was any substance to them.
>
> I found it a depressing assignment. The gossip, for instance, included allegations about Mrs Savage's sexual inclinations and marital history which if those who uttered them had bothered to make but the simplest of inquiries they would have learnt to be untrue. Yet these personal smears were passed on in conversation by some of the most senior people in medicine and accepted unquestioned by others as evidence for the prosecution in the court of gossip. There were also professional smears.
>
> I intend to publish the full dossier one day but now offer one example to advance my argument. Here is an excerpt from a letter I wrote last November to a professor of

> obstetrics and gynaecology, a man that I had enjoyed meeting and whose work I much admire: 'You may remember that, in conversation, I was interested in your views on the "Wendy Savage case", and you said that "we have to do something about someone who has cut six ureters".
>
> 'The conversation was private so I would never attribute the remark to you but I've recently been examining the extent to which our profession indulges in "trial by gossip" and have been trying to find out just how true are some "received truths".
>
> 'It's taken a long time to track down the details – for reasons you can easily guess – and, though I can't be certain, it seems likely that, during Wendy Savage's time at the London, only two of her patients have had "ureteric complications". One, operated on by her registrar, had a ligature put round one branch of a congenital double ureter; the other suffered ureteritis after a ligature had been placed close to it but not around it.
>
> 'I don't expect you to tell me who told you about the six ureters though I hope that you will have a chance to pass back this bit of "counter information" and would be interested to know what his or her reaction is.'
>
> He eventually replied: 'It was very good of you to write. I have asked around since you were in touch and, although the rumour seems to be widespread, as you suggest, there is no real substance. I think we all have learnt a lesson from this but unfortunately, whatever the outcome, medicine, the practice of obstetrics, and the individuals concerned in the London debacle cannot benefit.' And so say all of us.

In the month following my suspension there were more than twenty articles about it in the national and medical press. They struck a chord with women all over the country who wrote in their hundreds to explain that their own experience of birth had made them want a different kind of care. Regular press reports – particularly in the *Guardian* – throughout the fifteen months I was suspended, ensured that the issues were kept alive. Television and radio coverage, once I had decided to 'go public', helped me to reach millions of people. I made two rules for the media – I would not discuss my colleagues or the cases. I was only prepared to talk about the issues involved as I saw them: the provision of obstetric care, who makes the decisions and disciplinary procedures for doctors. The public campaign was, I believe, essential if justice was also to be a factor in the resolution to my suspension. But there was another, more important, aspect of the publicity. Women throughout the country have realised that they have the right and the power to see that the health services they get are the ones they want.

Chapter 7

The Legal Battle

Your power in the court is directly proportional to your power outside the court.

Brian Raymond's advice to Wendy Savage when they first met

At the DHA meeting on 9 May 1985, Mr Cumberlege had said publicly that an enquiry would go ahead, although I had, in accordance with the circular HM(61)112, four weeks to reply to the written criticisms of the five cases that Jean Richards had handed me on 24 April. It took three of those weeks before the case notes were sent to Hempsons. Whilst we were waiting for them, Mr Leigh had told me that if 'safety' were mentioned in connection with a 112, an enquiry was virtually certain to take place. In view of this I decided not to reveal my defence. Hempsons wrote on 22 May to this effect, but no reply had been received when I decided to change my solicitor a week later.

Brian Raymond and I decided that our first task was to see if the DHA could be persuaded to change its mind about holding an enquiry in view of the community support for me and mounting public pressure.

Then, on Monday 3 June, Jean Richards phoned me to see if an HM(61)112 enquiry could be avoided. I replied in writing that while I must take every possible step to preserve my reputation and career, which had already suffered as a result of the action taken by the chairman of the DHA, I was prepared to forgo a public enquiry providing certain conditions were met. On the assumption that a final decision had not yet been made by the chairman as to whether a *prima facie* case existed, I would assist him in making this decision by putting forward my own account of these cases to an independent senior obstetrician of standing, from another district. He would then advise as to the existence of a *prima facie* case of professional incompetence on my part in relation to the five cases taken in the context of my overall practice as a consultant since 1977.

Jean's reply was surprisingly swift, and the ground had changed somewhat. There had been 'a little bit of a misunderstanding', she wrote:

> My proposal was that you should sit down with one or two outside assessors from the Royal College and then *meet with our obstetricians to see if a* modus vivendi *was possible* (my emphasis). On that front I understand from the Royal College that they now feel that a reconciliation is not possible... In addition we now have the formal letter from Hempsons instructing us to proceed to... a 112 enquiry... I must point out that the enquiry is in private, not in public as you state in your letter...

What Jean had in fact suggested to me on the phone was that if I were to sit down with someone from the RCOG, herself and the chairman, maybe we could go through the case notes together and avoid a 112. The other obstetricians had never been mentioned.

On 5 June 1985, while I was having lunch after receiving my FRCOG, a senior official of the Royal College had told me that the district had in fact approached him with this idea on Monday but had withdrawn the suggestion on the Wednesday morning.

Brian wrote to all members of the District Health Authority on 11 June, just before the DHA meeting on the thirteenth. It was a long, four-page letter, and made several points:

I. We appreciated the responsibility the DHA had to provide services, and heed the advice of their medical advisers. However, they would also wish to be fair to any individual doctor whose competence had been challenged.
2. The evidence that came from patients, GPs, the RCOG and the perinatal figures we enclosed did not suggest that my competence was in doubt but rather that there were differences in opinion about the way that obstetrics was practised.
3. It was well known that there were differences of opinion between the obstetricians in the district.
4. Although the DMO had given me twenty-eight days, until 23 May, to respond to the criticisms, the chairman had announced publicly on 9 May that an enquiry was to take place in any event, and the dean confirmed this in a conversation with me on the eleventh. I had therefore reserved my defence, but if it was not the case that an enquiry was already scheduled, we were prepared to take part in a review of the cases to establish whether or not there was a *prima facie* case. We suggested someone of the standing of one of the vice-presidents of the RCOG acting in a private capacity.

Brian's letter concluded:

> It will not be necessary to emphasise that this issue has aroused strong feelings in many quarters over the past few weeks, not least in Mrs Savage, who feels herself the subject of wholly unfounded allegations. At this stage, however, our purpose is to find a satisfactory resolution to the present situation, rather than to criticise those responsible for bringing it about. It is unfortunate that the Authority has become involved in what is clearly a dispute between practitioners over clinical practice and judgement, but having done so, we respectfully suggest that the matter can be dealt with most sensibly in the manner proposed above. At the same time we feel that it is only fair to point out that in the absence of a satisfactory resolution, at an early stage, Mrs Savage will be forced to protect her rights in this matter by means of action in the High Court, although this step would be taken with the greatest reluctance.

I had been pleased to find, when I had worked out the perinatal mortality figures for the London Hospital, that my rate was numerically the lowest, although with such small numbers the differences were not statistically significant. (A perinatal death occurs when a baby is stillborn or dies in the first week of life. The perinatal mortality rate, or PMR, is the number of deaths per 1,000 total births.) We had included a table giving these figures with the letter. The morning of 13 June, Jean Richards rang Brian and thanked him for the approach but said my perinatal figures were meaningless, comparing 'apples and pears'. Her argument was that I didn't get referrals or difficult cases at Mile End. In fact, I had checked on as many variables as possible which affected perinatal mortality, and told her so. 'But, anyway Wendy,' she said, 'it's not that your practice is dangerous... it's just that it is different from the others.' For a minute, I was completely speechless.

It was at this point that I made the biggest mistake of the whole campaign. Earlier that week, when talking to Eva Alberman, Professor of Clinical Epidemiology, she had asked me if Professor Dennis from Southampton would be a suitable person to review the cases. I respected his work in the Wessex region on abortion services, and knew he was one of the Regional Assessors in Maternal Mortality. Eva said he had been suggested by the RCOG.

When Jean Richards rang me she put forward his name, and still thinking that we were going to sit down with the lawyers and the chairman to work out the exact way to do this review, using my considered responses to the allegation, I said I had no objection in principle to him. I did not know that Jean Richards had already sent the note, *with Gordon Bourne's adverse comments*, but without my considered responses on which I was still working, to John Dennis the previous evening.

I was taken aback to find a message from Professor Dennis on my answerphone that Saturday. On Wednesday 19 June I travelled to Southampton with the first draft of my comments about the five cases. John Dennis hardly looked at these but we had a long conversation. He was very sympathetic, and said he didn't agree with Gordon Bourne about most of the cases but he thought that with Mrs D, I had had a brainstorm. I tried to explain my policy of allowing a woman to experience labour even if I think the chance of success is small, but I could see that this was a foreign concept to him. I also told him a little bit about the problems in the department and gave him the perinatal figures by consultant, including the variables of social class, age, parity, gestation at delivery, birthweight and serious medical illness. On the way back in the train, I felt relieved and reassured.

The next two weeks were hectic as Brian and I went through the case notes and translated my comments into legal language. By this time Brian had moved back to the head office of Bindmans, opposite King's Cross. We sat in his room over an amusement arcade. It was hot, and the tinny strains of *Für Elise* interrupted our thoughts every now and then.

We worked till the small hours gathering the facts together. These formal comments to the chairman were finished on 28 June. The report which Hempsons had commissioned from Professor Chamberlain some six weeks ago reached us on the 27th. It contained nothing new; if anything, he was less critical of my management of the five cases than I was myself.

Friday, 28 June 1985

We checked our document early on Friday morning and sent it by special messenger to the Regional Legal Adviser at his offices, along with the report from Professor Chamberlain. We both felt pleased. We had finished a mammoth task, it read well, and Brian had given them a deadline of 5 July – or we would go to court. Brian had spoken to John Dennis on the phone and had heard reassuring noises.

This euphoria was wiped out when I returned in the late afternoon. I took one look at Brian's face and knew something was wrong. He handed me Professor Dennis's report – it was terrible. The words 'bizarre and incompetent management', 'consistent aberration of clinical judgement', 'confusing to junior staff and midwives' sprang out of the blurred, old-fashioned type. I turned to the individual case reports. Apart from AU, they were less damning. How had he reached such a devastating conclusion? Had he not done a second report after he had spoken to me and received my draft comments, which filled in the gaps in the case notes?

I felt I had let Brian down by misinterpreting Dennis's friendly behaviour and the, as I thought, frank discussion we had had. Brian had fought so hard for me and he had trusted my judgement. Would he now be wondering if I *was* incompetent? It was one of the worst moments since my suspension. Was I deluding myself? Was Brian's faith in me shattered?

I pulled myself together and apologised to Brian for my misreading of John Dennis. We decided to write a letter to confirm that I did dispute three facts – Trevor Beedham's letter of 21 May 1984, the cause of baby U's death, and the professor's statement that I had failed to make adequate arrangements for my study leave. This was important: if there was no dispute about the facts there need not be an independent enquiry.

It was nearly seven when I left, a hot sticky evening and I had neglected to find myself a partner for the Students' Summer Ball. I rushed home, rang a friend – yes, but no dinner jacket – borrowed one from a neighbour, and we arrived. I had been suspended for nine weeks and two days.

That weekend I showed all the notes, the criticisms and my comments to Professor Ron Taylor and he wrote the following note for Brian:

> I have looked carefully at the five cases which are the subject of dispute between Mrs W. Savage and the Tower Hamlets District Health Authority. I think that there are matters here where my clinical judgement may have differed from Mrs Savage but in these issues I accept that there is no certain correct management. The issues must be 'was reasonable care exercised' – not 'did the consultant play safe'. We can all play safe to our own advantage and the detriment of the patient. I think very good care was exercised in all these cases – although in two specific incidents, an incorrect decision was made in the absence of the consultant. To my mind there was no question of negligence in any instance...

Ron Taylor and I could not be further apart on the issue of abortion, yet his tolerance of my pro-choice stand was in such contrast to the attitudes of some of the other people I knew. It was a relief to hear his judgement. I felt ready to continue the battle.

Tuesday, 2 July 1985

Brian was asked to meet the Deputy Regional Legal Adviser at Addison House, the headquarters of the Regional Legal Office in Chart Street, Islington. After the meeting he called in to my house to tell me the news. The Deputy Legal Adviser had said that there were difficulties with cross-cover between consultants because of our difference in approach. Basically the offer was that if I would go away for six months or so to Oxford or Edinburgh (why not Siberia? I thought), my colleagues, who had been upset by the one-sided publicity, might be able to work with me again. Brian had pointed out that logically that meant that these five cases were not evidence of incompetence or I could hardly come back without having had an enquiry, but the DLA did not want to accept this. He said that if I didn't accept this offer, and suggestions about changing my role to do 'community obstetrics' (i.e. no labour ward work), they would go ahead and have an enquiry. Right at the end, he said this was a 'without prejudice' meeting, that is 'off the record'. I was beginning to understand how the administrative establishment works. This seemed to me to be yet another attempt to get me out of the way now that it was likely that the charge of incompetence would not stick. I told Brian that I was not going to go back as a second-class consultant. If there had to be an enquiry, so be it.

The High Court Action

Our deadline for my reinstatement, 22 July, passed. We had not yet taken counsel's opinion, hoping that it would not be necessary, but Brian rapidly prepared a brief and the following day we met in Old Square, Lincoln's Inn. Upstairs, we each sat at a huge desk, surrounded by bundles of papers tied up in dark pink tape, the bookshelves full of leather-bound tomes. John Hendy, in his late thirties, had been recommended by Brian as an expert in employment law. He said there were three possibilities: defamation, judicial review or breach of contract, and he outlined the pros and cons of each. He thought the third was our best bet, but warned that courts were reluctant to enforce contracts. I felt that he was sizing me up, deciding whether to take the case or not. Suddenly I knew he was going to do it. Rapidly he gave Brian a list of people from whom he would want supporting affidavits, and outlined the way he saw the case being presented.

Our long days and eighty-hour weeks of preparation began again. We began to collect our affidavits. I asked the two vice-presidents of the RCOG and the immediate past-president whether they would swear affidavits. Brian told me titles always went down well with judges but the college was keeping its strictly neutral stance and they all said no.

Monday, 5 August 1985

I went to LBC radio to talk about the issues involved in the case and why we were going to court, and then met Brian and John in Old Square. The Court began at 10 a.m. Outside the Law Courts I greeted the Tower Hamlets women and their babies who had come to support me. We walked in through the back door and found Court 16. The court was crowded. It seemed a pity to be inside this dark, cramped, old-fashioned place, with the barristers in their sombre gear, on such a nice summer day. John Hendy's wig, I noticed, looked a bit untidy, a curl or two loose. I warmed to him for striking a blow for informality. John stood up and explained why we thought an injunction was necessary to force my immediate reinstatement: the loss of service to patients, the damage to me personally, the fact that there were not adequate reasons for my suspension, the long delays common before enquiries under HM(61)112. It sounded convincing to me, but then I was biased. James Badenoch, representing the DHA, rose next and read the most damaging words from John Dennis and Gordon Bourne. My heart sank. I had thought that once inside a court the full evidence would come out, and the tactic of using selected quotes could no longer be used.

Then John stood up and quoted from Professor Taylor's draft affidavit: 'What is happening to Mrs Savage is not a dispassionate enquiry into her competence but rather a deliberate attempt to manufacture a case against her for the purpose of dismissing her from the staff of the London Hospital Medical College.'

The judge gave the Health Authority two weeks to prepare the case in response to ours, then ten days for us to see their affidavits and prepare our response. We had cleared the first hurdle. I kept calm and tried not to think about the headlines the next day. In fact the press were kind – they picked up the conspiracy theory in the headlines, and quoted Professor Dennis in the body of the text. It could have been much worse.

By 22 August the district had definitely decided to go ahead with a 112 enquiry – and they said it would be held in October. Was it worth going back to court to get my suspension lifted while preparing for the enquiry? We were sceptical about the DHA's date for the enquiry and decided we had nothing to lose.

On 24 August, we received from Mr Dibley the terms of reference for the 112 enquiry which were as follows:

> 1. In accordance with paragraphs 8 to 15 of circular HM(61)112 to enquire into and report upon the professional competence exhibited by Wendy Diane Savage in her treatment and clinical management of the following cases: Denise Lewis; Susan Payne; Ms X (1986 substitution); Linda Ganderson; AU (1986 substitution).
>
> 2. Arising out of the findings and conclusions reached in the enquiry to make such recommendations to the District Health Authority as to any disciplinary action in relation to Wendy Diane Savage as may be deemed appropriate.

What these terms told us was that the enquiry would not concern itself with how the case came into being or my overall practice.

So, four and a half months after my suspension, we had a decision about the enquiry. Preparing for the court case had been like working again, even though all those words weren't quite the same as the joy of a delivery, the satisfaction of a well-performed operation, or working out how to help a woman with a sexual problem.

2 September 1985. Return to the High Court

Both my daughters came this time, and the Support Group were there in force. Several women filed into the court, the saris of the Bangladeshi women and the colourful African cloth of the Somali women bringing some colour and life into the place. Once again, the press were overflowing their benches.

This time we made two gains. Firstly, if I was not found to be incompetent I must be reinstated or we could come back to the High Court; and secondly, the judge ruled that the enquiry must take place in a reasonable time.

It soon became clear, however, that even November, the date proposed in the High Court which had influenced the judge's decision not to allow our case to be heard, was not going to be possible, as the members of the panel had not yet been selected.

Going to the High Court had not been a waste of time. Although the affidavits hadn't been read by the judges, they were now available for other people to read. And preparing them had given Brian some idea of the strength of our case.

Chapter 8

The Five Cases

Alas, doctors are judged by their peers not by their patients.

Francis Cumberlege, Chairman of the Tower Hamlets Health Authority

Through all the frustrating months leading up to and during the enquiry, I held on to my conviction that my suspension was *not* about my competence, but was based on an intolerance to a different approach to obstetric care.

Of the five cases, three concerned breech presentation – when the baby is lying bottom, not head, downwards – and one of these women also had twins. Four women were delivered by Caesarean section after labour had been tried, and the fifth had delivered normally, but sadly the baby had died before labour began. Approximately 3 per cent of women will have a breech presentation at term, one in a hundred has twins, and only one woman in a thousand has twin breeches.

In the Mile End branch of the London Hospital the Caesarean section rate, like that in the country as a whole, was about 10 per cent in 1983–4, although in 1984 my personal rate was just over 8 per cent. So clearly these cases had been carefully chosen – 80 per cent of this small group of women had been delivered surgically and 60 per cent had breech presentations!

The Rising Rate of Caesarean Section

In the 1958 national survey done in one week in March, 2.6 per cent of women were delivered by Caesarean section, twice the proportion of those who had this operation in the previous survey at the end of the war in 1946. By the time of the third survey in 1970 the proportion had risen to 4.8 per cent.

Official statistics based on a 10 per cent sample of inpatient records for England and Wales (HIPE), show that the rate continued to rise, to 6 per cent by 1975 and 8.7 per cent by 1980. The 1983 figure for England was 10.1 per cent, and a detailed study in Scotland showed an overall rate of 13 per cent with rates varying from 4.9 per cent to 19.2 per cent in different hospitals in 1982.

Some younger obstetricians speak as if there is no longer any risk to a Caesarean section. It is certainly much lower than ever before, but all surgical operations carry a risk, comparable to those we take willingly every day when we travel by car, cross the road or take part in various sports; Caesarean is no exception. What is clear is that it is safer for the woman to have a vaginal delivery – and moreover she has less 'morbidity', that is infection and haemorrhage and other rarer complications, and she recovers more quickly from a normal birth. After any operation people feel pain in the wound and they feel tired. Looking after a newborn baby, establishing breastfeeding, getting up at night, does not seem the ideal way to recover from surgery.

Although most women cope well with the new baby, more of those delivered by Caesarean section become depressed after they return home, and some studies have shown subtle differences in the ways in which they relate to their babies. In addition, the uterus is scarred, which means a higher chance of an operative delivery next time round, and some work suggests a slightly lower chance of getting pregnant when the woman wants to.

Also, most people think that a Caesarean guarantees a normal healthy baby, but statistically about one and a half to twice as many babies die following a Caesarean operation than if they are delivered head first vaginally. Some of this risk is because the woman may have a complication such as bleeding (ante-partum haemorrhage) or high blood pressure, and it is probably in this area that the balance of risk in suggesting one type of delivery over another is most difficult for the obstetrician, with his or her duty to two patients in one body.

The rate of surgical delivery in the USA has risen even faster than on this side of the Atlantic. In 1970 our rates were similar, 4.9 per cent for England and Wales and 5.5 per cent for the USA. By 1983 it was twice as high here, 10.1 per cent, and four times as high, 20.3 per cent, in the States. In 1980 a National Institutes of Health Consensus group – the Task Force – met to discuss the use of Caesarean section in the States, as women and obstetricians were concerned about this rise. They found that breech presentation, repeat Caesarean and 'dystocia' (literally, difficult labour, in practice used loosely to cover 'prolonged' labour, failure to progress, suspected cephalo-pelvic disproportion, etc.) were the most important reasons for the rising rate. The Task Force made several recommendations, including encouraging vaginal birth after previous Caesarean delivery, and allowing vaginal birth for breech babies under 8lbs in weight.

Their recommendations with regard to legal action were:

> 1. The courts should recognise that if a vaginal birth resulted in a 'less than perfect baby', this does not necessarily mean that the physician was negligent for not performing a Caesarean birth.
>
> 2. Physicians should make a determination as to the need for Caesarean section delivery based solely on sound medical judgement.
>
> 3. Physicians should support the patient's right to participate in the decision-making process concerning whether to have a Caesarean by proper application of the doctrine of informed consent.

In this country, the legal concept of informed consent is not so strictly drawn, but I have always tried to obtain truly informed consent from a woman by explaining how things are done and why they are necessary.

The Task Force failed in its attempt to halt the steady rise in Caesareans and the provisional figures for 1985 in America are over 24 per cent, almost one woman in four. This is madness. One can only hope that women, midwives and obstetricians will prevent it happening here.

In 1978 the rising rate of Caesarean section at Mile End had caused Peter Huntingford and I to look critically at our practice. When booking a woman for her second or third pregnancy, looking at case notes at the height of the induction era (1974, before Peter had returned to the London) one often saw this sequence of events: induction of labour, often for not very clear reasons, poorly established labour with contractions produced by syntocinon, 'failure to progress', mild fetal distress, 'emergency' Caesarean section – and a healthy non-distressed baby born. Often the conclusion was drawn from this pattern of events that the baby was too big to go through the pelvis (i.e., 'borderline cephalo-pelvic disproportion'), but in the next pregnancy, if allowed to go into labour naturally, four out of five of these women delivered normally – and often the babies were bigger, showing that the suspicion of disproportion was wrong. (Disproportion means that the leading part of the baby is bigger than the bony pelvis and cannot safely be delivered vaginally: if the head is first, then it is called cephalo-pelvic disproportion; when the baby is breech first then it is usually referred to as feto-pelvic disproportion.) I also tried to spend more time in the labour ward with the new registrars, and we arranged some lectures on the interpretation of fetal heart traces (CTGs).

The Caesarean section rate at Mile End, which had risen from 6 to 9.5 per cent between 1975 and 1977, stayed at 9.5 per cent to 10 per cent up to 1984, the last full year I worked before my suspension, but at Whitechapel, where the neonatal intensive care unit is situated, it continued to rise, from 8 per cent in 1976 to 17 per cent in 1985. This may be because more women who are 'at risk' are being referred there, but further analysis needs to be done to establish the reasons for this rise.

Breech Presentation

The question of whether or not women with a breech presentation should be allowed to labour and deliver vaginally or should have a planned Caesarean section – especially if it is a first pregnancy – is one of the most hotly debated topics in obstetrics today.

The evidence about the best way to deliver a baby by the breech is vast, and confusing, and that is why two obstetricians reading the same papers can hold opposing views.

My view is that if the labour goes well in both the first and second stages, and the breech descends on to the perineum naturally, there is no significant risk of the 'obstetrician's nightmare' – that the body of the baby will be delivered and the head becomes stuck above the brim (the top opening) of the pelvis. It was calculated fifty years ago that if the buttocks of the baby would go through the brim of the pelvis then so would a normal-sized head. But it is possible for the head to be held up by an incompletely dilated cervix or if the head is abnormally large, and I think this is where the anxiety stems from.

My own view is that in circumstances where the choices are evenly balanced, the woman's own feelings about the birth should be the deciding factor.

Trial of Labour

If the obstetrician is unsure whether or not the head will pass through the pelvis, a trial of labour is recommended. This means that labour is allowed to progress normally but that preparations are made for a Caesarean section, should this become necessary. In my practice I try to get the same person to do all of the vaginal examinations which tell the doctor how well the labour is progressing.

Sometimes it is necessary to augment labour (strengthen the contractions with syntocinon) to ensure that the woman has had a real 'trial'. Obstetricians also differ about whether or not one can use syntocinon with a scar in the uterus, but my view is that if this is used carefully it is no different from the contractions of normal labour, and one must produce good contractions or the woman will not deliver vaginally. There is no set time for a trial of labour: it depends on the size of the baby and the pelvis, the position of the baby's head and the way that the mother and the baby respond to the labour. As long as there is no maternal or fetal distress I believe that labour can continue although in practice few women are undelivered within twenty-four hours.

Length of Labour

In 1981 I looked at the figures from the hospital computer obstetric databank and found some very interesting differences. My own Caesarean section rate was considerably lower than that of the other consultants: 6.5 per cent compared to a range of 10.9 to 11.9 per cent. This was in part due to the fact that I had more women having their first babies (because I was the newest consultant then) so there were fewer women needing a repeat operation, but in part it seemed to be related to the length of labour. The higher rate at Whitechapel was almost entirely due to the much smaller number of elective Caesarean sections at Mile End (that is, operations planned to be done before labour, compared with emergency sections, which are done once labour has begun or a complication develops).

Of women under my care 12.3 per cent had a labour lasting over twelve hours, compared with between 1.7 per cent and 3.9 per cent under the care of other consultants. It was not that my rate was particularly high – in the 1958 survey a third of women have labours lasting over twelve hours and by 1970 about 20 per cent did so: it was that the others had very low proportions. There was no difference in the percentage of babies needing extra resuscitation at birth or who had low Apgar scores (a measure of the baby's wellbeing at birth).

I looked up the literature about length of labour. I was convinced that one of the reasons for the rising Caesarean section rate was that we were pushing labour on too fast. I went back to the 1958 perinatal mortality survey and here I found some evidence that for women having their first babies, twelve to twenty-four hours labour was associated with the lowest 'mortality ratio'. Why, I wondered, had the survey in 1970 used eighteen hours as the definition of a long labour?

My Obstetric Philosophy

1. Women are different, and each woman and each labour should be managed individually.
2. Midwives and doctors must have clear reasons for procedures and birth management options.
3. Communication between the woman, with or without her partner, and members of the clinical team should be frank and complete.
4. Choice for the woman is important, and midwives and doctors have to overcome their authoritarianism (reinforced by their training) whilst accepting responsibility for life-saving decisions.

In essence these are my ideas on how to approach labour – without rigid rules or routines.

The five cases which Professor Grudzinskas had selected from about 800 women who had had babies under my care during a fourteen-month period in 1983–4 were, as Mr Leigh from Hempsons pointed out to me, 'not my five best cases'. Even so, my policy of having individual plans of management to suit each women had been followed, even if those plans hadn't always been carried out as well as I would have liked. Four of the five cases were very unusual and the fifth, Linda Ganderson, was the only one to have a normal delivery.

When I presented my twenty-two pages of comments on the cases to the Chairman of the Health Authority on 28 June 1985, Brian and I prepared the responses about each case in three parts, the plan of action, where there were departures from ideal management, and my answer to Mr Bourne's specific criticisms.

In July I circulated all members of the Health Authority with the first part of the document and short summaries of each of the cases, which did not reveal the women's identity and which I have used in this chapter.

The criticisms of the professor and Mr Bourne which led the chairman to suspend me have been put separately from those of Professor Dennis, a couple of sentences from his covering letter having been used by the chairman at the July DHA meeting to reinforce the case for the continuation of my suspension.

Professor Chamberlain, affectionately known as 'Bodger' after a rugby player, had been asked by Hempsons to comment on the cases. These reports on the cases were to help the Medical Defence Union advise me to fight or to accept the *prima facie* case of the DHA, and Professor Chamberlain was *not*, as Mr Cumberlege stated, 'the champion selected by Mrs Savage herself'.

The Five Cases

The brief summaries of each case are versions of those I prepared for the Health Authority members in July 1985.

X (initials withheld 1986)

Single. Age 15. 4ft 10in tall. Delivered 26.9.84.
Trial of labour planned and carried out by my new registrar. Difficulty with the delivery of the baby's head when Caesarean section carried out. Lecturer (honorary senior registrar) called. Next day baby thought by paediatricians to have suffered a fractured skull (extremely rare). Mother and baby well at post-natal examination, done by myself at six weeks.

What were the problems? The baby was lying with its head facing towards the mother's abdomen rather than her back. This happens in 6 per cent of babies coming head first at term, and these labours tend to be longer and more painful.

A trial of labour – one where you are not sure if the baby will be able to pass through the pelvis or not – went well, but at the Caesarean section, it was difficult to deliver the head. This does sometimes happen if the head has been pushed firmly into the pelvis. It requires a knack to release the pressure but this was not an anticipated problem, so I was not there to assist my registrar.

The baby was irritable at birth, which is not uncommon after an eighteen-hour labour and a difficult delivery, and after a skull X-ray, which I did not see at the time, a fracture was diagnosed by the paediatricians caring for the baby.

What went wrong: I should have been there to assist my registrar, so that the anxieties about a possible skull fracture would never have arisen. My registrar had never felt the 'eggshell' sensation of the moulded head where the bones are overlapping one another. Although X and the baby were well at six weeks and the baby has developed normally it was not the best start for a young mother.

Criticisms made before my suspension: Both the professor and Mr Bourne said that the labour lasted too long and said respectively that labour should have ended after twelve or six hours. Mr Bourne thought that the pelvis had not been properly assessed, whereas the professor did not mention this but said that 'it is unfortunate that a more senior person was not present at delivery'.

Comments after my suspension: Professor Dennis said, 'The decision to manage this patient with a trial of labour was justified. The problems occurred at delivery...' Professor Chamberlain was sympathetic: 'One can well understand the reluctance of the consultant to do a Caesarean section on a fifteen-year-old girl...'

Statements before the enquiry: None of the expert witnesses thought that the management of this young woman's labour could be criticised.

What I think about the case now: Although my registrar did not ask me to assist her, I regret not getting up at 2.45 a.m. as it would probably have made things easier for her and for Ms X but I think it was the right decision to allow her to try and deliver normally. Many of the expert witnesses before the enquiry found great difficulty in understanding why this case had been brought as an example of any shortcomings on my part.

The criticisms were based on a rigid approach to labour, measured in terms of arbitrary timescales rather than observing individual women, and it is this approach that I believe leads to unnecessary Caesarean sections.

AU

Bengali. Age 23. Married. One previous child delivered by Caesarean section. Delivered 26.4.84.

This couple wanted her to try to deliver vaginally and I agreed to a short trial of labour. This commenced on 26.4.84 and AU was delivered that day.

The trial was not conducted as I had outlined. Despite this the baby was delivered in good condition and was noted to be ill forty-eight hours after birth. There was no post-mortem at the parents' request, and I believe the paediatrician's diagnosis can be disputed.

What were the problems? This woman had had a previous operative delivery because of fetal distress after a dysfunctional labour during which the contractions had been augmented with syntocinon. She had not wanted to have a Caesarean but agreed to an operation when advised that the baby was showing signs of distress. However, when the baby was born, he was very active and healthy and her husband who was in the theatre had the opportunity to see that he was not distressed.

When she became pregnant this second time she wanted to deliver vaginally if at all possible. She had a scar in the uterus, and a smaller than average pelvis. It was agreed that she could have a trial of labour and then the baby turned to be a breech. (Breech babies have less time for the head to mould as it goes through the pelvis and so a baby, who could be delivered head first, may not go through in the breech position, even though it is the same size.) Then her labour was dysfunctional again, which might have been because the baby was too big (although that is not as likely a cause in a second pregnancy as in a first), but it needed augmentation if we were going to let her have a proper trial of labour.

What went wrong: I was not aware of the opposition of the lecturer to allowing this woman to experience a trial of labour, which led to some difficulties in communication. This meant that the labour lasted longer than I had planned.

The critics' response: Mr Bourne had a list of nine criticisms which can be summarised as:

- Trial of labour is contra-indicated if the pelvic inlet is less than 10cm (the normal range is 10–14cm with an average of about 11.5 in British women).
- If the baby is presenting by the breech, syntocinon should not be given.

Mr Bourne and the professor would have done an elective Caesarean section, as I would have if the woman had not wanted to do otherwise. Mr Bourne said, 'This patient was not managed by normal standard practice and a disastrous outcome was almost certainly inevitable.' But he did not commit himself to saying why the baby died.

Professor Dennis said that the woman would 'almost certainly have agreed' to an elective section – but of course he had not spoken to her! He considered that my management was 'bizarre and incompetent' (a phrase that Mr Cumberlege read out in the July DHA meeting).

Professor Grudzinskas stated that the cause of death was thought to be a tentorial tear leading to intracerebral bleeding, but Professor Dennis considered that the baby died 'from anoxia caused by strong uterine contractions affecting the placental circulation in the presence of disproportion'. Professor Chamberlain, who did not have the criticisms of this case sent to him, speculated that 'the ultimate bad outcome may have been related to hypoxia in labour'.

Anoxia means no oxygen and hypoxia means a shortage of oxygen, but in my experience, if a baby has been starved of oxygen for a damaging period during labour or delivery it has fits soon after birth because of the damage to the most sensitive tissues in the body, the brain cells. This new theory of the cause of the baby's death was to be a major focus for Mr Kennedy's cross-examination during the enquiry, but had not been a criticism in the original *prima facie* case against me.

What I feel about the U case now: I regret that I did not understand how opposed the lecturer was to allowing the woman to experience labour, even though I knew that the chance of her delivering vaginally was remote. Had I done so, I would have taken over the case completely in the morning.

The principle that a woman should be able to have a trial of labour, even if I do not think she will succeed, as long as she and the baby are all right, is one that I stand by, but I wish I had spent longer explaining the situation myself to the couple.

I also feel deeply saddened by the way the enquiry into my competence has affected the Us and their ability to mourn for their baby in privacy, and with the understanding of their own doctor.

One of the worst moments of the last fifteen months has been the sight of Mrs U on television saying that she had trusted me, and my awareness that she thought I had let her down.

Denise Lewis

English. Married. Age 26. Twins 1976, 8lb 10oz baby 1980. Delivered 5.7.84.
Breech presentation of both twins, raised blood pressure and anaemia. The major criticism was of the management of labour which was conducted by the lecturer and my registrar when I was on study leave. The professor was asked for his advice about this woman at 3 p.m., ordered no specific treatment, and did not see her until 7.50 p.m. Caesarean section was performed at 9.20 p.m. and resulted in the delivery of two live, healthy children. The mother also did well. I had made adequate arrangements for my cover whilst on leave.

What were the problems? Denise developed anaemia, which did not respond to the usual treatment with pills and then injections. She later received a blood transfusion for this. She also developed high blood pressure at the end of her pregnancy, and as soon as this happened I arranged for her labour to be started off, in case of any risk of eclampsia (fits). The syntocinon drip which was used to do this did not work. I was on study leave but in order to minimise the burden on David Oram, the consultant who was 'covering' my cases, I came into the hospital at the beginning and end of each day.

What went wrong: Medically speaking, nothing went wrong but communication was not good. The message that I gave to my SHO to give to the lecturer was apparently not clear enough for him to understand. When my registrar took over at lunchtime he and the lecturer did not speak directly to each other, so the registrar was unclear about the plan of management. He then rang the professor who was the duty consultant but was not standing in for me during my study leave.

Criticisms made before my suspension: The anaemia had not been investigated adequately, or treated properly. They said she had had severe pre-eclampsia in June (which was not correct), and that she should have been delivered by elective rather than emergency (done after a trial of labour) Caesarean section. My plan of management was 'insufficiently defined' and my arrangements for study leave were criticised.

Comments after my suspension: Professor Dennis thought that her 'problems were not treated with adequate urgency and I must judge the patient fortunate not to have suffered more severe complications'.

Professor Chamberlain said he would need more information before commenting on the administrative matters and as far as elective Caesarean section was concerned, 'It might be expected that labour would proceed apace and Mrs Savage's view could probably be defended.'

Comments made at the enquiry by expert witnesses: Gordon Stirrat's reply to the question of any incompetence on my part in this case was: 'In no way, shape or form can Mrs Savage's management be described as incompetent in this regard. If it were I would suggest that the majority of obstetricians in this country are similarly incompetent.'

What Denise thought: Denise, who has been one of my most stalwart supporters, appeared with her two sets of twins and her daughter at meetings and demonstrations, and offered to give evidence at the enquiry. She did not want to have a Caesarean, and was glad to have had an opportunity to try to deliver normally. She had nothing but praise for her care.

What I think now: I should have spoken directly to the lecturer so that no confusion could have arisen.

Susan Payne

English. Married. Age 24. First baby. 6ft 1in tall. Delivered 5.8.83. Breech presentation: for planned vaginal delivery. The second stage lasted longer than usual, and although it is not my usual practice, I used syntocinon to see if vaginal delivery could be achieved, as the baby was not large (6lbs 13oz). There were problems with communication, but I assisted my new registrar with the Caesarean section and mother and baby were well. She has since delivered a 7lbs 11oz baby vaginally after a 2½ hour labour, under my care.

What was the problem? After normal first stage of labour lasting about twelve hours, the cervix was fully dilated but the labour virtually stopped. Because this was so unusual, I thought it might be because she had had an epidural (a pain-relieving injection of anaesthetic round the spinal cord) which had then been repeated twice, so I thought we should wait for this to wear off as both mother and baby were well.

I expected the contractions to return, but they did not, and having checked personally the size of the baby and the bony pelvis, I thought we would augment labour with syntocinon. The baby had still, inexplicably, failed to descend into the pelvis, so she had a Caesarean section, with which I helped my registrar.

What went wrong: I should have gone to assess things as soon as my registrar telephoned me, which would have saved some time. However, the mother and baby were well and this did not affect the outcome.

Criticisms before my suspension: Professor Grudzinskas and Mr Bourne said I should have done a Caesarean section as soon as the second stage – defined as the time when the cervix becomes fully dilated – was prolonged, and that I should not have used syntocinon to strengthen the contractions with a breech presentation. Interestingly, in his draft reports Mr Bourne said: the use of syntocinon is 'totally and completely' contra-indicated and there was a third paragraph which read: 'It is possible and highly probable that this patient survived only because this was her first child. Had this been anything other than her first child then it would seem reasonable to suggest that because of this delay her uterus would have ruptured and a disastrous situation would have followed.'

Uterine rupture in a woman having her first baby is exceedingly rare – and as the reason that Susan's labour was not progressing was because her contractions had virtually stopped, this risk was a non-starter.

Criticisms after my suspension: Professor Chamberlain found this 'the most difficult case to defend, for eight hours in the second stage in a breech presentation is well outside the normal range of behaviour', whereas Professor Dennis described my management as 'eccentric'. At the enquiry these criticisms were changed halfway through my cross-examination after John Hendy had exposed the weakness of the case.

Comments before the enquiry: John McGarry had this to say: 'This, however, is a highly unusual case and I do not believe that Mrs Savage's management can be faulted. It seems extremely curious to me that this case is used as an example of poor management on Mrs Savage's part', and he suggested that it should have been written up 'for a scientific journal as an example of a wholly inexplicable occurrence, namely the failure of the breech to descend and pass normally through what must be regarded as a gigantic pelvis.'

What Susan thought about her care: Susan was very satisfied with her care, otherwise, as she pointed out, she wouldn't have chosen me again as her consultant. On TV later she said, 'When I heard that she had been accused and my baby's birth was being used against her, I just left the children and went into the kitchen and had a good swear – even my husband said, "It can't be possible."'

Linda Ganderson

English. Married. Age 27. First baby. Delivered 22.4.84.
The baby did not grow well, this was recognised by the GP when I was on holiday. The woman was admitted to hospital for investigation, allowed home for Easter, and came back with a small amount of bleeding. Immediate action was not taken and the baby died undelivered the next day. Since then she became pregnant again and has safely delivered. Despite careful monitoring, growth retardation again occurred late, her GP alerted the hospital and Trevor Beedham induced her labour and all was well.

What were the problems? At thirty-two weeks the uterus was noted to be small. Was this because the baby was not growing well or because she conceived after her monthly egg had been produced late? When it was decided that the baby was not growing well some weeks later, she then had a small amount of bleeding. The question was, should her labour have been induced then?

What went wrong: Due to an administrative error I did not see Linda at thirty-six weeks when I had planned and this meant that I was on holiday when a week later her GP correctly made the diagnosis of intrauterine growth retardation (IUGR).
When admitted to hospital no consultant opinion was obtained, and with hindsight one could see that the significance of the baby's growth retardation was not appreciated.

Criticisms before my suspension: Mr Bourne had seven paragraphs on this case and said that, 'Obviously this patient was mismanaged, but the apportionment of blame is difficult because everybody began to assume that the intrauterine growth retardation was caused by "wrong dates".' He, like the other commentators, John Dennis and Bodger Chamberlain, did not know that I was on holiday when Linda was admitted.

I had had considerable correspondence with Gedis about this case and had sent him a case report so he could answer the 'gossip' he said had occurred after the May 1984 perinatal mortality meeting. He agreed with Mr Bourne that shared care should have ended as soon as growth retardation was even suspected, and said she should have been classified to 'full consultant care' and that her delivery should have been earlier. He did know that I was on holiday.

Criticisms after my suspension: John Dennis said, 'The diagnosis of intrauterine growth retardation was made in good time. The action taken as a result seems to be sluggish. The infant died in utero as a result of an error of judgement. Such an error can occur in the experience of any obstetrician on an occasional basis.'

Comments made by experts before the enquiry: Professor Taylor said that, 'I cannot accept that admitting this woman at thirty or thirty-two weeks would have been a sensible way to proceed.' Edmund Hey said, 'I find it difficult to see what objective grounds we have for faulting management until thirty-four weeks after the last menstrual period and Mrs Savage has already conceded that an error of management occurred at that time.' John McGarry: 'I cannot see any reason why this woman should not have received shared care.'

What I think about Linda Ganderson now: One of the most difficult situations for any doctor is explaining to a patient that something was not done perfectly – especially if the end result is bad. Nobody is perfect and mistakes do occur, so all mature doctors will have had to face the fact that their good intentions have sometimes resulted in harm – sometimes even death. In obstetrics, maternal deaths are now rare, and the average obstetrician qualified in the last ten years will not have more than two or three women under his or her care die in a lifetime. However, one baby in every hundred dies inside the uterus or in the first week of life so most obstetricians will have between five and ten women a year who leave hospital without a live baby. In about a quarter or a third of these women, a different course of action would probably have saved the baby's life. As an obstetrician one's own feelings of guilt in this situation can be overwhelming, and the doctors must be honest, with themselves primarily, before they can discuss things honestly with the parents.

One of the most difficult tasks is to ensure that one deals with the parents' feelings of grief, whilst admitting to one's own errors in such a way that the trust between the parents and the doctor is not destroyed. One must not unload guilt to make oneself feel better but the parents worse. The most difficult situation for me is trying to be honest with the parents whilst not criticising actions of the junior staff who, because of their inexperience, may have missed something which I probably would have seen. As a consultant, the responsibility for the work carried out by junior staff is yours – though one cannot be in the hospital twenty-four hours a day, fifty-two weeks a year. I try to do ward rounds or visit the antenatal wards every day, to be at the end of a bleep or a telephone, and to create a climate in which they feel free to discuss potential problems as well as situations which need an immediate decision.

When I returned from my holiday and was told of Linda Ganderson's stillbirth I felt responsible – not because I had delegated care to the G P for which I was so heavily criticised by the professor, Gordon Bourne and John Dennis – but because I had not been there when the GP picked up the IUGR, and not there for my registrar or the senior registrar to consult when she was admitted. I explained to Linda that probably there had been a further amount of bleeding on the morning the baby had died which had been the last straw as the baby had not been growing well for some time.

I have Linda's permission to use her case, and she has seen successive drafts as I have written them. For her the publicity of the enquiry was painful and opened old wounds, but I hope that by sharing her experience with other women – and doctors – we will all learn to the benefit of women in the future.

Chapter 9

The Run-Up to the Enquiry

The law is not about justice; and justice is expensive.

Brian Raymond

Preparing the Defence

We had agreed with Mr Dibley that Brian and I would prepare the typewritten transcript of the case notes to be used in the enquiry. The first task was to get the various missing parts of the case notes, the CTG's, the X-rays of the mothers and babies, and the ultrasound scan for Baby U from the hospital records department. We also needed to track down the notes of Baby X which had never been sent to us; I had done my comments for the chairman of the Health Authority from the mother's notes. We wrote off for these and then began to go through the material with a fine tooth comb.

I knew that a baby of 2.9 kg with a normal sized head could be safely delivered through a pelvis with an inlet of 9.5 cm because of my experience in Africa. I spent some time in the library checking these references.

We had still not received all the notes, and as we were going through them I noticed other omissions: the treatment sheet and some of the nursing notes in the U case, the first EEG report on baby U, the pre-eclampsic toxaemia (PET) charts on Denise Lewis, the labour CTG on Ms X, one of Susan Payne's X-rays, some laboratory forms. By mid October we still had not received the ultrasound scans of Baby U, and I learnt that they had been sent to Mr Dibley without copies having been made for us. I rang him myself – and he told me that to do so was quite improper, I had to communicate via my solicitor. Such strict protocol seemed very strange to me. I needed them urgently because I had asked Sid Watkins to look at the notes and scan with his neurosurgical eye, and he was going away. So, finally I went to Addison House where Mr Dibley worked, and demanded to see him. When he came down to the lobby with a photocopy, which was not adequate for our purposes, I said I had to have the copy film by nine the next morning. I offered to take it and have it copied myself. He was horrified at the very thought. But if he was adamant, so was I, and I got the film the next morning in time to give to Sid.

On 3 December Mr Dibley sent us the full list of charges (see Appendix I). Now we were able to start the detailed rebuttal of these fifty-nine items. As we finished each case, these responses and the annotations were sent to brief our counsel. By the second week in December we still did not have Baby X's notes along with the other details we had requested, so I asked Brian to ask Mr Dibley if I could go to his office and search for the missing items from the original notes. This time he agreed, and twice that week I spent five hours going through the notes and listing what was needed, including copies of the CTG traces.

I collected Baby X's films from the hospital a fortnight later. I had never seen these X-rays before. Two radiologists were in the room. I took them out of the packet and looked at them carefully. I could not see any skull fracture. I passed them to one of the two radiologists. He looked at them in silence and passed them to the second who scanned them both. 'Who reported on these?' he said. I read out the registrar's name. They looked at each other and said nothing. I knew I was right – there was no fracture. This was confirmed by the expert paediatricians when I sent the copies to them.

Brian's secretary, Hilary, was snowed under with annotations and my lengthy comments. Over Christmas and the New Year, with all the information together at last, both Brian and I and a temporary secretary worked for hours on the transcripts, checking them against notes. It seemed endless.

The starting date of the enquiry was Monday 3 February 1986. It struck me that if a woman had her last menstrual period on the 24 April 1985, the day I was suspended, her estimated date of delivery would be the first of February. The third was the first working day after this. It seemed fitting somehow that a case centred on obstetrics should have this kind of time scale. By the time the enquiry was over the pregnancy was well beyond term!

The Selection of the Expert Witnesses

Although an enquiry panel is set up to look into the accused doctor's competence, there was no doubt that this one was going to be, in effect, a trial, and its adversarial nature was made very clear on 1 December when we received the list of the prosecution's witnesses (and their statements): my four consultant colleagues, the lecturer and one of the senior registrars involved in Linda Ganderson's case, one registrar and two senior house officers. The junior staff had written statements about their personal involvement in the cases, but my colleagues had also put in their own opinions, criticising my management in strong terms. We wondered who their expert witnesses were going to be. Even at this point I thought John Dennis might refuse. After all, he had done his report very quickly, in one day, and at the time he lacked all the documentation. I had been told that he had not given his permission for his reports to be read out in the High Court.

I also wondered if Gordon Bourne would appear. Professor Taylor had given evidence in his affidavit that Bourne's report did not constitute 'any form of external scrutiny in that he was closely associated with Professor Grudzinskas when the latter worked under him at St Bartholomew's Hospital'. Peter Huntingford's affidavit had recounted how Gordon Bourne had opposed my appointment at the London and he, in turn, denied this in his own affidavit. However, just before Christmas we had heard that Bourne and Dennis were to be the Health Authority's expert witnesses.

I found the whole question of involving junior staff as witnesses for my defence difficult, fearing that their support for me could damage their careers. I deliberately chose to ask those of my staff who were not planning to continue a career in obstetrics, except for one who particularly wanted to give evidence in my defence because of her commitment to women and to feminism. She was in a good training scheme so I did not think her support of me would damage her. When I was preparing my case for the High Court I had asked two of my registrars for affidavits. One was doing venereology and one was a principal in general practice. Katie Simmons had done a locum registrar post for me, had worked for Peter Huntingford and had also finally decided to do general practice. The SHOs I asked were now all doing general practice.

What we needed were expert witnesses to discuss the disputed points of management. We decided not to use all the people we had asked to give affidavits, partly to keep the opposition guessing and partly because we were now looking at the details of the five cases, whereas in the summer when we went to the High Court we had been arguing that my suspension was unjustified. For the first time we had an advantage; instead of responding to other people's initiatives, we did not have to reveal our witnesses until the case started.

Ron Taylor's understanding of my approach, combined with his own wide clinical experience and knowledge of community antenatal care, made him an essential expert witness. He was also a man of principle: I thought that this attribute was the most important. People might have different ideas about the best clinical management, but those with principles would accept that in most cases in medicine there are different approaches to the same problem and would understand my viewpoint – even if they themselves would do things differently.

Rather than calling only London obstetricians, whose day-to-day contacts with my colleagues might become an embarrassment, I thought it would be better to call medical witnesses from different parts of the country. I also thought this would broaden the debate. As far as the paediatricians were concerned, I asked Peter Dunn, Reader at Bristol, whom I had heard speak a couple of times; he was also President of the British Perinatal Paediatric Group. On the advice of a colleague of Sid Watkins, I got in touch with Edmund Hey, whom I had never met. And through Carole Desateux, a paediatric senior registrar at Great Ormond Street who had her baby under my care and whose partner works as a GP in the South Poplar Health Centre, I approached Professor Campbell in Aberdeen. I had never met him either.

John McGarry from Barnstaple, whom I knew through Doctors for a Woman's Choice on Abortion, was one of the obstetricians I asked. Another, James McGarry, I had heard speak thoughtfully about Caesarean section at a conference. From Glasgow, he had worked in Nairobi before I was there. Glasgow University had a link in Nairobi, and I always felt that my most important formal obstetrics training had been Glaswegian even though it had occurred in Africa. I wanted a woman, and Marion Hall from Aberdeen, whom I knew slightly, had done a lot of work on antenatal care.

Again I knew nothing of her practice, except that, on the whole, Scottish obstetricians spent more time in the labour ward than their London counterparts. Iain Chalmers, who runs the National Perinatal Epidemiology Unit, I had met through work; we were both members of the Forum of Obstetrics and the Newborn. I chose him because I wanted an obstetric epidemiologist to put the range of opinions into a scientific framework – and to comment on the validity of the selection of five cases as a way of assessing competence. Gordon Stirrat, Professor at Bristol, I did not know personally and I knew nothing about his research interests or obstetric practice, but I knew he was a Christian and opposed to abortion. When we met in Brian's office soon before Christmas I found him impressive and intelligent.

Along with the letters going to and from the witnesses, I sent them case notes, affidavits, and copy X-rays. Hilary and I worked till 5 p.m. on Monday 23 December making sure that the last of these parcels, containing the photocopied CTGs, and the missing bits of notes received from Mr Dibley, got there in time for our experts to use the Christmas break to study them.

In the new year Brian Raymond embarked upon a tour of the country, going to Glasgow, Aberdeen, Bristol and Barnstaple to collect the statements from our experts in relation to the specific charges – a massive task, but he returned from these expeditions more and more cheerful as he realised what a strong case we had.

I spent many hours going through the transcribed notes, line by line, with John Hendy. Every day I drove down to Lincoln's Inn with large files, references, books and papers. I had borrowed one of the bony pelvises and dolls we used for teaching, and I showed John the mechanics of breech delivery and the difference between a footling and a complete breech and a frank breech. One day we went to Queen Charlotte's and the radiologist explained to him all the features of the pelvimetry and the ultrasound films that we had. I was amazed at the way all this information was absorbed and how he could find his way through the mass of papers.

We finished our preparation by Friday, 31 January. There was nothing more that we could do. The transcripts had been checked by the Health Authority, amended, interleaved with photocopied notes and put into different coloured folders. Large cardboard boxes were used to transport them to Addison House where the enquiry was to take place.

A friend of mine had bought me a respectable suit in a Jaeger sale, and on the Saturday I went out to buy a blouse. I returned some hours later with several blouses, shoes, matching handbags, a leather jacket, a bookcase and an Amstrad computer. As my youngest son unloaded the car, he looked in disbelief, 'I thought you went out to buy a blouse, not the whole of London.' The day before the enquiry we unpacked the Amstrad, attempted to understand the manual and assembled the bookcase so that I had somewhere other than the floor of my study to put all the reference material overflowing from my bookshelves. I had only just taken down my Christmas cards and needed the string in the hall to put up all the cards that had been arriving to wish me good luck.

That night I slept well: a medical training prepares you as well as most for this kind of situation. We had done the work, now the exam was ahead and we would either pass or fail.

Chapter 10

The Enquiry Begins

Who shall decide when doctors disagree.

Alexander Pope, Moral Essays

The Prosecution Case

On Monday 3 February I woke at 6 a.m. and left the house in the dark. Brian had arranged for me to do BBC Breakfast Time as well as TV AM, which had been booked for weeks, followed by LBC in Gough Square before getting to Addison House. He arrived to collect me in the taxi, and we drove to Lime Grove. Denise Lewis and her incredibly placid eighteen-month-old twins were also on the programme, quite relaxed in front of the lights, and the short interview went well.

The next interview was more difficult – I was asked if I thought all this would have happened to a man, and I really had not thought about that for ages; I answered as best I could but I didn't feel that I had done it well. LBC, on the other hand, was much more relaxed. I decided again that I much prefer doing radio to TV and it doesn't take half as much time. As we left another radio reporter was there with his machine, and then we were arriving at Addison House.

It was a cold grey morning, but already at 9.30 there were dozens of women and their babies outside, plus press photographers and TV cameras. Heather Reid's son, Matthew, gave me a bunch of flowers from the Support Group, I posed for photographs with Carol Lefevre and her twins, seeing all the familiar faces of women I had cared for and those who had fought for me over the last ten months – Sue, Myra, Beverley, the MSLS workers. A clergyman carried a banner saying 'Justice for Wendy Savage'; I hoped he would be proved right. Clutching two large ring-binders, a large bouquet of flowers, a bunch of freesias and cards from well-wishers, I went through the door into the foyer where we were greeted by the woman in charge of the arrangements and shown to our room – about ten feet square, windowless, cream paint stripped off where sellotaped notices had been removed, a cardboard-wrapped filing cabinet and two desks, and the boxes from Bindmans with all the case notes in folders, the affidavits, the pelvis and doll. This was to be our base for the next five weeks. I met our clerk, Phil, a medical student having a year off. John arrived and we moved the furniture around, got permission to use the new filing cabinet, and checked out the phone. Then it was time to start, so down the corridor past the security guards. I didn't wear my badge – I assumed they would know who I was!

The room where we were to sit was the Council Chamber where the Area Health Authority had held their meetings. Today as we entered, I saw that the opposition were on the left; the middle tier of three rows was packed with the press, and we were to sit at the front on the right. Phil sat behind with the tape-recorder and our supporters, almost all women, sat in the top third row. As we sat down, I studied the other side: Mr Ian Kennedy QC, glasses, slightly receding dark hair, mid-fifties, a little overweight, setting up a folding lectern for himself. Next to him in the front row, James Badenoch, who had represented the THHA in the High Court, fairer, younger, a more open face, turning to talk to Gedis Grudzinskas, sitting in the second row. On his left a very heavy-set, middle-aged man and next to him another slighter, more dapper lawyer with a watch chain across his waistcoat. On the professor's left sat Mr Dibley, his bushy eyebrows twitching as he rustled the papers anxiously, and then a smaller man with a goatee. And in the back row, a very neat, young, dark-haired man, their law clerk. The contrast between this phalanx of sober-suited men with their often loud middle-class voices and the less formally dressed women on our side, with John Hendy, tall 'as a beanpole' as Jeremy Laurance from *New Society* put it, and Brian and myself in the front row, reflected the battle of a group of establishment men versus a somewhat non-conformist woman.

The door on the opposite side of the room opened and in came the panel – we all stood up just as we had in the High Court. The panel, set up by the Joint Consultants Committee of the BMA, comprised Leonard Harvey, the BMA nominee, Consultant in Obstetrics and Gynaecology from Rugby; Christopher Beaumont, the chairman, a barrister chosen from the panel maintained by the DHSS, and Peter Howie, the RCOG nominee, Professor of Obstetrics and Gynaecology in Dundee. Len Harvey I'd met once – he came and sat nearest to us; the chairman was obviously the tall, white-haired man who took the middle chair, and Peter Howie, the Scottish professor, sat farthest away from us on Beaumont's left. Cameras flashed as the panel, ourselves and the other side were photographed. Then everything settled down and at about 11.15 Mr Beaumont opened the proceedings: the timing of the meetings, the request for tape-recording the proceedings so that Clare Dyer of the *BMJ* could do weekly reports and Mr Kennedy's grudging acceptance. Then lunch and tea arrangements – it seemed we would never get down to the case itself. Sitting at a little table between the lawyers in front of Mr Beaumont and facing us was the shorthand writer, writing rapidly. In the space between the seats was a larger table on which were piled the five ring-binders containing the case notes. Brian, referred to formally by John as 'my instructing solicitor', handed duplicate sets of these to the panel members. They did not have enough room on their curved table for everything so some went on the floor.

The chairman referred to 'Mrs Savage being the only one on trial' when the lawyer with the watch chain identified himself as Mr Conlin from the Medical Protection Society, there to represent the interests of all the London Hospital doctors. The chairman then mentioned that this was somewhere between an enquiry and an adversarial system. When he ruled that the women would be referred to by their initials, Mr Kennedy pointed out that that would not be sufficient 'cloak' because of the publicity, and John Hendy told the chairman that we had permission from Mrs P., Mrs G., and Mrs L. to use their names publicly, but not the others. Mr Kennedy introduced the 'compendium' of all the criticisms and my comments in a sixty-nine-page 'bundle', and the documents relating to my appointment, including the 1977 curriculum vitae (CV). John Hendy said he thought my up-to-date CV was more relevant, and casually mentioned that we were proposing to put that in with the affidavits which had made up our case to the High Court. I waited for the chairman to say that they were irrelevant, but he said nothing, and neither did the other side. Finally Mr Kennedy got to his feet.

I could hardly believe my ears as he started off with a long speech about what this case was *not* about – *not a contest between the old and new, or between technology and the woman's freedom to choose how, when and where to have their babies.* He must have been reading the press cuttings: *my colleagues in no way criticise or do not subscribe to many of the philosophies that Mrs Savage supports*. Good news – so when they are reassured about my competence we'll all be able to work together again seemed the logical extension of that line of argument. *The question is not about the principle. The question is about the way that it was put into practice in these five individual cases, and it is an enquiry not into theories, but about dangers in obstetrics*.

Here we go again, I thought: the same argument put forward by the professor to convince the DHA that obstetrics should be centralised at Whitechapel. The barrister will put forward the views of his client, transformed into legal language, but that is in essence his job, to make the best case, however poor the material. *Of the five cases, one resulted in neonatal death and another in a stillbirth. One does not like to have to advance these matters in a public debate, but since it has to be in public it has to be in public, but one must say that the evidence we would call will suggest that both these sadnesses could and should have been avoided. In the remaining cases the management was outside all normally accepted principles and exposed the mothers and their babies to risks which were both real and not necessary.* I looked at the press scribbling away furiously – it sounded very convincing. To me it was not new. Would Andy Veitch, who had covered the case so well in the *Guardian* since the beginning, wonder if he had made a mistake? *The answer has been made in a number of instances that no harm was done and this has been relied upon as justification of the judgement at the time, but we must remind ourselves that this is also the answer of the driver who rounds a blind corner on the wrong side of the road...* He went on in the same vein – one hour to get a Caesarean at Mile End so must tailor practice... confusing junior staff... plans inadequate... I should have been there... I was critical of junior staff... perinatal death led to a complaint... other cases came to light because of the concern of my colleagues and junior staff... end of preliminary remarks. Now I thought he would list the charges, maybe not all fifty-nine, but suitably shortened. However, he did not.

Instead he began to go slowly through the case notes, almost as if he was reading them for the first time. He began with Susan Payne. Suddenly Professor Howie leant forward and in his quiet, accented voice he said, *There is a technical confusion. At one point it says that there is a footling presentation and at another point it says it's a complete breech. These two are mutually, exclusive and that is a matter of considerable obstetric importance*. Kennedy turned to Professor Grudzinskas and after a whispered discussion said that it was not clear what the presentation was. My spirits rose; obviously Peter Howie was not going to allow sloppiness. Gedis had incorrectly described the presentation in his summary and Gordon Bourne and John Dennis had accepted this. Peter Howie asked for the X-rays. They were not forthcoming. Kennedy looked irritated: *your point will be attended to*. He continued his slow progress through the notes. I began to see how they had thought we needed four weeks. He came to a *notation in the left hand margin*. John Hendy rose to his feet: *it was the professor's telephone number at Whitechapel where Mrs Savage was going*. Suddenly the scene sprang to life – it was not all paper and words – a ripple of laughter ran round the room.

Mr Kennedy continued on through the notes and then summarised the criticisms.

Professor Dennis said I should have been there all the time; Gordon Bourne said there was *no reason why the section should have been delayed for so long*. I'd explained in June 1985 how it happened. Then Kennedy read out the whole of Professor Chamberlain's comments on this case – naturally – as Bodger had found it the most difficult to defend and had thought that I had not come in to do the operation, which I had. Mr Kennedy could have seen that in the typewritten transcript, even if he couldn't read my registrar's handwriting in the notes. Gedis could have told him, had they sat down and gone through the notes as John and I had. John Hendy corrected the error, *Thank you. I do not know how he came to make the mistake, but there it is*, said Kennedy.

He turned to Linda Ganderson, and Professor Howie showed that he had read the notes as he directed Mr Kennedy to the redrawn antenatal page which we were all to have indelibly imprinted on our memories by the time the case was finished. Several times John Hendy drew his 'learned friend's' attention to errors as he went through the notes. I had not been prepared for the pauses: the turning over of pages of the notes to find the evidence, the picking up and slowly finding the place in the compendium. I realised that my idea of court procedure was heavily influenced by films and plays in which the drama, not the tedium, comes over. Kennedy criticised me for not intervening earlier. John asked him to read the part of my comments where I explained I was on holiday, thus destroying his argument. But Kennedy raised the question of the 'uncertainties of the junior staff'. It was lunchtime.

I realised that my period had started – I hadn't had one for three months and thought I'd reached the menopause, glad that it seemed I was to be part of that 20 per cent of women who don't have symptoms like hot flushes. I looked in my new handbag, I had not put in any tampons. Somehow it seemed symbolic – men never had to think about such things interrupting their lives. There was no handy chemist and the tight skirt and high heels I was wearing made it impractical to nip out to Old Street and look for one. I spoke to the woman in charge and she found some for me. We smiled at each other as I disappeared into the toilet.

We took the lift to the top floor, queued behind the opposition in the canteen and then watched them enter the 'directors' dining room', a little closed-off, glassed-in room up two steps, opening on to a roof garden. We had a screened-off area at the other end of the canteen – the food was plentiful, rather like school and provided free; the women serving were very cheerful and everybody was very nice to us. We reviewed the morning – no worse than expected – I understood the meaning of the phrase 'he hadn't read his brief'.

Then back to the chamber where the windows are covered by long, thick curtains kept drawn, and the ceiling curves up into a strange inverse turret of wood and dark glass. With the soft carpet, the subdued lighting and the closed curtains, it was like going into a space capsule, and as the day went on the feeling of unreality became stronger. That afternoon Kennedy made several errors as he went through AU's notes – as well as making his position clear when reading out my explanation as to why I had allowed a trial of labour: *if a repeat Caesarean was deemed necessary she would feel that she had had a chance to deliver normally. Again, with respect* – I understood that whenever a particularly telling point is being made the lawyers drew attention to it by saying 'with respect', as

Kennedy did now – *a slightly remarkable statement because most women would be prepared to accept the advice of their consultant.* I felt that was his own view of the world. He stressed that my management was likely to result in severe damage or death, but only when he came to the fourth case, that of Denise Lewis, did he actually list the criticisms. They were in essence that, 1: it was a 'case for section'; 2: labour went on too long and, 3: I had not delegated things properly.

The last case of the 4ft 10in teenager was not so alarming, *but there are serious features to it.*

In conclusion, two threads ran through the case against me; there were direct criticisms of my actions and decisions and, secondly, of their effect on the junior staff.

Apart from his opening remarks, it was a lacklustre performance. I had been told that Kennedy was a tough criminal barrister, but if he continued like this we ought to beat him hands down.

It was a strange experience to hear oneself criticised in public, but I knew that the first week would be the worst and I had to endure this before we could put the record straight.

We reviewed the day. The word incompetence had not been mentioned; the charges had not been listed. John thought Kennedy must find them an embarrassment. It could have been much worse. With some friends I went home to watch a TV programme, Panorama, about the case.

John had to read through his handwritten notes of Kennedy's opening speech and Brian went to sort out the affidavits that Hilary had been photocopying. Lawyers have a bad press, but I now understand that the court day is relatively short because of all the other work that has to be done.

Day 2. Tuesday, 4 February

The *Guardian* headline stretched right across page 2: 'Savage's "deficient care caused avoidable deaths"'; *The Times*: 'Obstetrician exposed mother and babies to danger, inquiry told'; the *Telegraph*: 'Babies' deaths "could have been avoided"'. But other papers changed the emphasis: 'Mothers' anger as Wendy faces "trial"' said the *Express* and 'Dr Wendy's big fight to win back her job', said the *Daily Mail*. I opened my encouraging post, took some blutack and thought I'd stick some of the postcards on the wall to cheer us up.

The morning started slowly; Mr Kennedy introduced Denise Lewis's letter complaining first about her notes being used without her permission and sent to all sorts of people, which she saw as a breach of the law of confidentiality, and secondly about the use of her case, as she had no complaints about her care, to prosecute me. Thirdly, she said that initials would not protect her confidentiality. She ended by saying how angry she was that they had tried to use her to damage me. Mr Kennedy treated her complaint dismissively: *her notes are the property of the department, and we as the Health Authority have the custody and use of these... there is no question of this patient or that saying that they are not prepared to have their case examined because, after all, they do not have the knowledge that the profession have about whether this is right or wrong... desire for publicity has come from the other side... no wish to discuss in public.*

John Hendy made it clear that his instructing solicitor had spoken to her. She accepted that the publicity was now unavoidable but was still angry that her case was being used without her consent.

My up-to-date CV and an abbreviated one for Professor Grudzinskas were handed out. Kennedy took Grudzinskas through his 'evidence-in-chief' as it is called. He ran quickly through his CV and then the professor was asked to describe his philosophy about intervention: *Mr Kennedy, before I start, I would like to say at this point that only with extreme difficulty can I speak to this enquiry in public because, as a doctor, we are trained to consider matters concerning patients, and administrative matters relating to patients, as an aspect of serious confidentiality, and for that reason I prefer not to discuss any aspect of clinical matters, or the administrative related clinical matters, in public at all.*

I knew that unless the debate was public, even if I was exonerated, the destruction of my reputation would continue. Kennedy gave the chairman time to think about this request as he took Professor Grudzinskas through the 'philosophical' part of his evidence. Again he started off with an apologia, stressing that the London was not a high-tech unit, listing the area's social problems. Kennedy tried to put him at his ease and asked him about the 'old names' for Tower Hamlets. He didn't know them and I was allowed to tell the panel that Tower Hamlets included Stepney, Bow, Bethnal Green, Poplar and Spitalfields. Professor Grudzinskas stressed how counselling was used and parents' wishes always taken into account and how he had been associated with the equivalent to the National Childbirth Trust in Australia. I thought back to Mr Beaumont's words the previous day that 'only Mrs Savage is on trial' but the first hour of Gedis's testimony was devoted entirely to an attempt to defend and justify himself – eloquent evidence of the success of the press campaign. He then introduced the 1985 obstetric figures for intervention rates and perinatal mortality. The enquiry was supposed to be about my competence: would the chairman not intervene?

The outlining of the staffing, beds, duties and so on of the department took over an hour. Finally Kennedy moved on to the cases: *I suspect this is where you would like to discuss the sort of patients other than publicly?* It was a tense moment as the chairman turned to John Hendy: *The decision has been made that it should be conducted in public... My learned friend did open these matters in public.*

The members of the panel put their heads together as we watched anxiously. Finally the chairman straightened up: *We feel this evidence should be in public... I understand the professor's feelings, but he has done his duty.* As Mr Kennedy took Gedis through how the cases *came to his attention*, I made notes for John Hendy of where there were discrepancies between my recollection of the letters we had. We reached Susan Payne. Professor Howie brought up the question of whether or not it was a footling or a complete breech. I saw the chairman look puzzled. I whispered to John, 'Shall I get the pelvis?' He nodded. When I gave it and the doll to him, he offered it to Mr Kennedy via the chairman. Mr Kennedy looked at it without enthusiasm; Mr Dibley carried it across to the professor who pushed it away. Mr Beaumont said he thought a visual impression might be useful. Mr Kennedy: *Right. Can you put the baby into a complete breech?* The professor looked miserably at the pelvis. *Well, chairman, I have failed to put a baby into a complete breech using a doll on many occasions when I have tried before, and I have no reason to think that I can succeed now...* I watched him in amazement for it is something that most obstetricians teaching students do frequently; it really is quite easy to bend the soft doll's legs into any position you want to. Finally he put the doll into the position which fitted my drawing in the notes. Professor Howie: *That is what I would have said that a complete breech was*. Gedis: *Well, I regret, chairman, to disagree with Professor Howie... this doll may not accurately be representing what Professor Howie is trying to convey to us*. Then as he talks on he realises that he is describing a complete breech: *I would be guided by his view here.*

On and on it went. I could feel the women behind me watching these two professors having such difficulties in understanding each other. Mr Harvey could stand it no longer; he turned to the chairman and explained the differences between different kinds of breeches, concluding *...I would accept this as a complete breech.* Peter Howie was not to be deflected: *Is it possible that the X-rays may give us some help?* Mr Kennedy produced copies, the originals having been lost. Mr Harvey commented on the poor quality of the film: *It looks like a snowstorm.* Mr Beaumont: *So you both accept that it is a complete breech?* They did. Then Gedis said, *I shall be guided by the opinion of the enquiry. That is not a useful X-ray.* I wondered what had happened to the original after our copies had been made.

So the panel were doing our work for us, showing that the criticisms were not completely accurate. Laboriously, Gedis explained his criticisms of my care: the second stage was too long and I should not have used syntocinon. Then Mr Harvey asked if he would absolutely rule out the use of syntocinon in this woman. Gedis responded: *It is possible to consider a place for syntocinon usage in women in circumstances similar to this, but I do not think that in this instance, this instance was such an occasion when I would consider the use of syntocinon*. Kennedy tried again and Gedis launched into a lengthy explanation of how he would have used syntocinon in this woman only if she had been transferred to the theatre. I looked at him in amazement – the theatre, that cold clinical environment totally unsuitable for birth. Mr Harvey was looking at Professor Howie over Mr Beaumont's head.

Mr Kennedy did his best to repair the damage and after a few more questions about the timing of syntocinon which, after all, did not seem to be completely ruled out, he turned almost with relief to question Gedis about Linda Ganderson. Slowly and painfully we went through the notes. In short the staff didn't act when I was on holiday because they were confused.

On to AU, better photocopies of some pages were provided and handed around. The word counselling was used a lot when what Gedis meant was advice. At one point the chairman asked what was the difference between a trial of labour and a trial of scar. Mr Kennedy helped him out: *Your concern is whether it is going to get unzipped along the old scar line.* Again I felt conscious of the women behind me – so mechanical it sounded, not like one's uterus, the place where a child is nourished and grows. Gedis committed himself firmly about the cause of death: *It is extremely difficult to entertain any other possible cause here than some degree of trauma associated with the birth process.*

Denise Lewis came next, and after about an hour Professor Howie pointed out that one of the charges was 'factually incorrect': the length of labour was given as fifteen hours. Mr Kennedy tried to work out how the mistake had occurred, that it should read eleven hours – as the criticism was about the length of labour. Professor Howie asked if it should still stand. Kennedy said he would have to consult his experts. It was never changed.

On to Ms X; again Professor Howie intervened to confirm that Gedis thought the trial of labour should have ended at 22.30 hours. *In my view yes.* Peter Howie, his fingertips together, leaned forward: *Could I put it to you that at that point the membranes were still intact, there was no caput succedaneum reported, and the registrar… thought that only two-fifths of the head was palpable. Now do you think on the basis of that you would be absolutely able to predict inability to deliver vaginally in safety?*

Gedis replied to the effect that he would not have got into that position in the first place. Mr Harvey then asked about X-ray pelvimetry and Gedis answered that, *In this respect, like many of the other views I share with Dr Savage, I would not have done an X-ray pelvimetry*. This differed from one of Gordon Bourne's criticisms.

I noted the way Gedis referred to me as *Doctor*, for in England as a whole obstetricians are considered as surgeons and called Mister rather than Doctor. Somehow there is a subtle downgrading of women obstetricians by referring to them like this rather than as Mrs, Miss or Ms. He had always called me Mrs Savage or Wendy before – why the Doctor all of a sudden? Mr Kennedy sat down. John Hendy rose, *Thank you*, he said, looking at Kennedy.

A short break was taken and we resumed at about 4 p.m. John Hendy stood up again. Mildly he asked whether these cases could be considered *unique, or is the sort of criticism raised in these cases, the sort of criticisms that might be raised on other obstetricians, in other circumstances, on other cases?* Gedis replied: *Chairman, is Mr Hendy actually referring to the collection of the cases – that is, the circumstances enclosed in the five particular cases?* John tried again: *The sort of criticisms which are raised in these five cases, are they criticisms which you think could be found on other cases dealt with by other obstetricians?* Gedis answered, *It is possible*.

John Hendy again: *Are they similar to criticisms which you feel that you could level at yourself looking back over your years as an obstetrician?* Gedis frowned, *If I can just consider that for a moment or two, chairman?* John replied, *Of course*. There was a long pause – everyone held their breath – *In specific detail, in specific clinical detail, it is possible in relation to at least one of the patient's cases that we are discussing here.* John paused to let this admission sink in and changed tack: *The way that these cases grew into the enquiry... is that you referred – yes, I think it was you – the case of AU to the District Medical Officer. Is that right?* Gedis reached for his glass: *I don't recall that to be the case.* John then asked, *That case, the case of AU, was referred to the DMO, and you were asked to express a view on it? Is that right?* Gedis pulled a file towards himself and began to leaf through the letters: *I was asked to express a view – I am referring to my notes here in order to be absolutely precise in my answers*. He turned the pages over, back and forth. I reflected that I had not seen him at close quarters since the previous summer. He looked uneasy; his hair had receded quite a bit. After what seemed an age he said he didn't have the correspondence in the file; he gave the impression that the District Medical Officer had asked him for reports but John made it clear that Gedis had volunteered some of them. Gedis said, *I believe that the DMO passed the reports... to the*

Regional Obstetric Assessor who I learned later was Gordon Bourne. My sympathy evaporated: Gedis had been lecturer at Bart's, worked for Gordon Bourne, presumably read the Confidential Enquiries into Maternal Mortality which lists the Regional Assessors – Gordon Bourne had been one since 1974.

Soon after John asked, in the same even tone *When did you form the view that Mrs Savage was dangerous and incompetent?* A hush fell on the room. *I do not think, chairman, that I have ever expressed that view.* I heard an intake of breath behind me. *Does it follow it is not your view?* Gedis said how difficult he found it to speak publicly about *clinical matters, and the behaviour of my colleagues*. The chairman ruled firmly that the enquiry was a public enquiry and that I wanted it so and that John was putting questions on my behalf. Gedis replied: *Thank you. That is very helpful. It is difficult for me to answer the question directly in that it is so difficult to comment on who is dangerous and who is... I am not sure of the other word, Mr Hendy?* A gasp of incredulity ran round the upper benches, echoed by Mr Beaumont's *'incompetent' is the other word.* Gedis continued: *On who is dangerous and who is incompetent and when it occurs and how often it occurs and for how long it occurs at any particular time. It was my view that Dr Savage was an extremely hardworking individual with many, many, many commitments, and in the course of our discussions I urged her to consider a review of her many commitments so that she could give her important duties – in particular her heavy clinical duties – the attention they deserved. I sought the support of my other colleagues of the Medical College in the hospital in this respect.* I felt a sudden wave of anger, but it soon subsided; it was as if it was Gedis who was on trial today. And his reputation was not being enhanced.

Another long pause, then John said, *I'm sorry. That was your answer to the question, was it?*

Mr Kennedy produced the Particulars of Case which had been sent away for photocopying. *You were consulted over the formulation of those charges?* John asked. In a firmer voice Gedis replied, *That is correct*. Quietly and reasonably John asked him, *Does it follow that you are in general agreement with those charges?* Gedis agreed. The afternoon was over.

John Hendy had put the case clearly: it was about incompetence. We had a set of charges and the professor had been responsible for setting the case into motion. He handed the panel members the bundle of affidavits; they would have time to read them before the professor took his place on the witness stand the next day.

Day 3. Wednesday, 5 February

The *Guardian* headline read, 'Breach of confidence claim rejected' and a smaller 'Savage inquiry considers disputed evidence about "too long" labour'; *The Times*: 'Professor shared dilemma' and an editorial entitled 'Educating Patients' considered that an 'all-important cause had been served. It is the cause of professional demystification... doctors disagree even about fundamentals... at Mrs Savage's expense, their assent might in future be better informed.' I was glad that *The Times* thought it was important – but not quite sure how I felt at being the person on whom all this hinged.

John Hendy started this third day by going through the professor's CV, bringing out his relative lack of clinical work and his twelve years' experience against my twenty-five. I had realised that John would cross-examine their witnesses, but it was not until he began to ask Gedis about Professor Taylor's evidence that I understood that it was not all going to be their case against me in the first ten days. When I thought about it, it was obvious that the witness would have to be given a chance to reply to allegations that were going to be made – another part of the rules of evidence that I learnt as we went along.

John read from the affidavit '*...I can remember that on one occasion at the time of his appointment, he told me his first task was to change his senior lecturer. I know that he has expressed similar sentiments to other people.' That must be a matter of hearsay, but is it right you have expressed that view to other people?* Gedis described discussions about the Academic Unit and my role and the Medical College. John asked politely, *What is the short answer to the question, Professor Grudzinskas? Were you at the time of your appointment expressing the view that you wanted to get rid of Mrs Savage?* Gedis looked down at the floor: *Absolutely not* – but his voice dropped and the chairman had to ask him to repeat what he had said. This allegation was not new – it was in Professor Taylor's affidavit that we had used for the High Court proceedings some six months earlier. I was surprised that Gedis has not gone to greater lengths to refute it. If true, it would mean that all his evidence on the medical side would be open to attack as being influenced by personal bias, yet we had not received a sworn affidavit actually denying this on oath.

John then turned to the evidence of Peter Dunn, and read out part of his statement, made after he had read my colleagues' statements but before he had read the affidavits which made up the High Court case: '*...In a busy hospital misjudgements, failures in communication and frank mistakes are bound to occur to the best of doctors. It is usual to show understanding and sympathy when such events occur to a colleague, yet I find no trace of such support in any of the statements of Dr Savage's colleagues, which are not only highly critical, but tend to over-emphasise the adverse aspects, with at times the aid of hindsight. In no case is Dr Savage given the benefit of the doubt. In no case is the possibility that on occasion she might have been poorly served by her junior staff ever mentioned.' You can appreciate I do not want to ask you about this word for word but would you generally agree with the tone of that?*

Gedis replied, *No, I would not, but I would actually like to consider the precise wording of that letter, but the general theme I think is incorrect. I wouldn't agree.* A firm answer and John continued reading: *'I can say without hesitation that if the worst five of my own cases over the period of a year were put under a microscope, it would be possible to create a dossier similar to that of Mrs Savage. I believe the same could be done of every consultant obstetrician that I have ever worked with.'* Neonatal paediatricians probably know much more about obstetricians' practice than do fellow obstetricians, as they get the results of their work. I had been very encouraged when I had first seen this. The professor asked to have the paragraph read more slowly, then replied, *I think it is possible, chairman, to select the five worst cases of anybody, of any consultant in any discipline, and discuss the matter in some detail as can occur... could Mr Hendy read to me the latter part of the statement, because it is here some confusion arises in my mind.* John read the passage through again and Gedis responded, *I would not agree with this particular statement when we come to the word 'similar', because it is the dissimilarity in the clinical events that we are considering here, and which caused so much concern for these matters to come to the attention of the District Health Authority.*

Yet in June 1985 John Dennis, who was to be one of their expert witnesses, had expressed the view that it was the 'congruence' of these cases which led him to support my continued suspension – whereas here was Gedis saying it was their differences! John went on to deal with shared antenatal care, focusing on the 'agreed guidelines' which Gedis had mentioned the day before. This had been news to me as I thought we all had our own individual plans. Gedis produced a document; there was a pause while we looked at it. A murmur of astonishment ran around the room. He had produced a paper which dealt with home deliveries, a completely different subject! The chairman intervened, unusually revealing some impatience, and Gedis admitted that there were no written guidelines. Before going on to the issue of clinical autonomy, Gedis asked to be excused. I was quite glad of these breaks because of my period.

Professor, can I ask you whether you would agree with the proposition that Mrs Savage, like any other consultant, is not accountable either to you or to the Health Authority for the quality of her clinical judgement so long as she acts within the broad limits of acceptable medical practice? This was the cornerstone of our legal case and a fundamental principle of the NHS. Gedis, however, did not agree. *You disagree with that? In what respect do you disagree?*

In respect that her clinical practice may have implications on the academic responsibilities that the unit must discharge. Gedis expanded on this point that clinical autonomy is different in a teaching hospital. This will hardly go down well with those consultants, I thought. He continued, *In a teaching hospital it is necessary, I believe for clinical autonomy to be considered in a different way from a non-teaching hospital.*

What does that mean? John Hendy asked. And Gedis replied, *Excuse me, Mr Chairman, what was the question?*

John rephrased Gedis's words and Gedis then agreed that, *if one holds an academic unit position, then the clinical autonomy may have to be modified.* I thought that this was an issue that senior lecturers throughout the country might unite on, and certainly explained his behaviour towards me. But after several more lengthy replies Gedis conceded that he meant I should explain my actions fully, and in answer to the question. John then asked, *What you are not suggesting is that any of the decisions that she makes should be modified because it is a teaching hospital?* Gedis replied, *No, I am not.* But maybe he was confused by the negatives!

Before he started on the cases John passed around my annual and study leave dates in 1984, and about 11.15 a.m. he began with Denise Lewis. We had gone through her case first because of the different clinical points and the 16 charges, although chronologically she was fourth on the list. It was a very shrewd legal move because it exposed the weakness of the case against me very clearly. John asked how my management of her anaemia demonstrated incompetence. Gedis said it didn't, then it did. The chairman tried to get him to give a straight answer. Inadequacies; then overseeing the management; I was responsible for what went on in the district; I should not have shared care with the GP. Mr Kennedy tried to help him out. Professor Howie intervened. With ruthless logic,

John Hendy showed that the Charges 1 to 3 referring to shared antenatal care with the GP and investigation and treatment of the anaemia were nonsense: *...the first charge we can really strike out as far as you are concerned. That is not a demonstration of incompetence on her part.* John had already got Gedis to accept that shared care with the GP was a reasonable decision. I thought at last we would have the answer, yes. But instead: *In certain circumstances, no.*

Mr Beaumont: *Well, we are asking about these circumstances.* Gedis would not have chosen to share care. *I understand that but happily for you, your competence is not on trial – it is Mrs Savage's*, replied John. *You concede that she is not incompetent in prescribing this patient for shared care. It must follow... that Charge 1 against her can be struck out as far as your evidence is concerned from this charge sheet. No, I'm afraid not, sir,* Gedis responded. The initial decision to share care was not wrong, it should have been revised when seen by the registrar. Was I incompetent for leaving the decision to him? *No. So... where is the incompetence in relation to Mrs Savage in relation to shared care?*

Sir, may I come back to the question of consultant responsibility here, in that in my mind the deficiency here is that there does not seem to have been an adequate consideration of the suitability of this lady continuing her care in a shared care system which would provide for her medical needs satisfactorily.

John decided to move on to pre-eclampsia. He demolished the fourth charge, alleging that Denise had severe pre-eclampsia in June. Then to the 5 July note: again Gedis's criticisms were difficult to pin down. It was a relief to us all when 4.30 came.

We discussed the day. We had only gone through four of the fifty-nine charges with one of their witnesses. John said that it would be quicker after today but I was worried about the slowness of Gedis's evidence.

I drove to the hospital, collected my mail and, seeing Sid Watkins's car in the consultant's car park, went to see him to ask if there was any way that the district's case could be speeded up. As I walked through the door into the Alexandra Wing, Gedis passed me, walking hurriedly and looking anxious. Sid's door was open; I told him my fears about the slow progress and he said they were shared by the professor. That was a relief to me. When I had been in Mr Dibley's office in December he had told me that they had set aside four weeks because if we weren't finished in two it might take months to reconvene the panel and lawyers. I could not face the thought of another six months' suspension from my work.

Day 4. Thursday, 6 February

'Hospital chief "wanted Savage out as lecturer" – replacing accused consultant was seen as first task' was the *Guardian* headline with a picture of Professor Grudzinskas who 'helped to draw up charges'. *The Times*, 'Savage plot is denied'.

As I drove into the car park at Addison House, it was still grey and cold. I saw Gedis arriving in a taxi with the thick-set man who, although he looked like a heavyweight boxer, I had discovered was the MPS solicitor. Gedis looked less worried than the night before.

I decided to show how intervention in birth at the London Hospital was rising, and the number of deliveries by consultant, just to get the record straight. And now that the obstetric figures for 1985 had been introduced, it seemed likely that we could also introduce figures. I took the London Hospital annual obstetric reports and piled them up on our desk and drew up some graphs whilst listening to the cross-examination.

We started at 9.30 a.m. and John Hendy took Gedis rapidly through the rest of Denise Lewis's notes – the birth plan interpreted as a set of inflexible instructions, but not well enough defined, according to Gedis, who would not accept that I could have expected the senior registrar to use his discretion. John asked, *You are suggesting, are you, that she should have explicitly set out all the options, and the factors to be taken into account in deciding for and against each or something?* The professor replied, *That would have been one way of dealing with the situation, yes.* But he did not accept that this was – a counsel of perfection in a busy hospital? The professor did not.

Susan Payne was discussed next. John took him methodically through the charges. Gedis said that the reason that syntocinon should not be given with a breech was the risk of feto-pelvic disproportion. But he was reluctant to accept that this risk was negligible although, finally, he agreed that in a woman with a large pelvis like this, syntocinon was not ruled out – thus getting Charge 2 out of the way.

We moved on to Linda Ganderson. Gedis betrayed his unfamiliarity with the Dundee chart (an ultra-sound chart to show fetal growth) which has been in use in our district since 1982. He questioned its validity. The point of this chart was that it showed that the GP's note on 12 March 'Wrong dates likely' was a perfectly reasonable conclusion and that there was no need in the circumstances to admit Linda to hospital, *at thirty weeks... or at the very latest 12.3.84,* as had been one of the charges against me.

Gedis admitted that the chances of the baby surviving would have been high if delivered on 18 April and that he knew that I was on holiday then.

In the case of AU, John attempted to summarise the eight charges running to over two A4 pages: *the essence of what is said against Mrs Savage here is that there should have been no trial of labour?...* Gedis agreed: *I think that tends to summarise what is in the particulars of the case.* It was mid-afternoon; the close air in the dimly lit chamber made us all feel tired. I noticed Mr Kennedy looking at Gedis with a detached, almost quizzical air. We turned to the compendium and John returned to his original question about trial of labour. Again, by a series of logical questions, John showed that Gedis did not support all the charges. We went through the notes line by line, decision by decision. Professor Howie intervened to clarify whether Charge 2(i) should stand after Gedis had said that AU need not have had an elective Caesarean.

At about 3.45 p.m. we reached Ms X. Over and over again John tried to get the professor to define in what way the trial of labour carried out was not a trial of labour, as stated in Charge 1. The chairman tried to help. As to the delivery, Mr Beaumont asked: *Was it wrong for Mrs Savage to leave it to Dr Robinson?* Without hesitation Gedis replied, *I believe so, yes.* But four questions later he agreed that it would depend on what information I had had from the registrar.

The afternoon was finally over.

Day 5. Friday, 7 February

Nothing in the *Guardian*. 'Experts clash on birth', said *The Times*.

That morning John introduced the graphs which I had drawn, the deliveries by consultant and the perinatal figures I had submitted to the DHA the previous June. Gedis looked puzzled and said he'd never seen the latter before, although on questioning he agreed that he'd seen the report in *The Times*. (Nicholas Timmins had quoted the figures I'd given to the DHA, saying that 'her perinatal death rate in the 16 months to April 1985 was 11.3 against an average of 13.7 for the other four consultants at the same hospital'.

John tied up a few ends; on sessions, Gedis was uncertain; Was the community antenatal care scheme at risk? Mr Kennedy attempted to repair the damage – but Gedis stated that there was no time for consultants to go into the community. We would need another consultant. Mr Beaumont asked if there was anyone doing my work. Gedis replied that there was a locum but she was not doing all the work. He left the witness table after three days and half a morning.

Next came Mr and Mrs U. I was saddened to see them – I felt and still feel both anger and regret that I have been unable to help them with their understandable grief. After lunch the two senior house officers involved with Denise Lewis, one also with Mrs U, gave evidence. I expected the professor or Mr Conlin to ask if they could give their evidence in camera – and I would not have objected at all – but they did not. It was a relief, they answered 'yes', 'no' and 'I don't know'. If they couldn't remember they said so and their evidence confirmed mine on several points. And neither of them said they were confused by my management.

We finished at 4 p.m. The first week was over and now things ought to move faster. We weighed it up: the chairman had not drawn the terms of reference narrowly; we had introduced the affidavits; John had shown up the paucity of their case. The professor had been unimpressive; we had introduced the perinatal figures. And the press coverage, apart from the first day, had been better than expected. So far so good. There was some anxiety about time; Kennedy had said they needed ten working days for their witnesses, but he had been so slow – and so had the professor. Would we have time for all of ours?

The following day the *Guardian* headline was: 'Consultants end pioneering scheme for community care of pregnant women'. *The Times* and the *Telegraph* had picked up the perinatal mortality figures: '"Fewer babies" were lost by obstetrician' and 'Obstetrician had the best success rate', the former I accepted, the latter was not scientifically accurate without more data analysis! It was not until I really knew the details of what was being reported that I understood the power of the subtitle writers and how infuriating it must be for the responsible journalist to have his carefully worded report appearing under a 'sensational' headline.

I started to reply to the letters and cards that had come during the week. Many people had sent cheques as well. It was good to feel supported.

Chapter 11

Expert Witnesses for the Prosecution

It is the customary fate of new truths to begin as heresies and to end as superstitions.

T. H. Huxley, *Collected Essays*

Mr Nysenbaum, the lecturer, was a very confident witness, but there was considerable discrepancy between his recollections of when we met with the Us at 8.30 in the morning in the labour ward and mine. Fortunately for me the evidence of the SHO and Dr Fay differed from his memories. At the end of his evidence on the Monday afternoon, Mr Kennedy asked him about another woman – nothing to do with the five named in the terms of reference. John Hendy objected; the public were sent out and although John argued strongly against this, Mr Kennedy said that this was evidence to back up the general charges that my management was confusing to the junior staff. His plea was accepted, and everyone trooped back in. There had been some mention of this case before lunch and over the meal I had told John and Brian all about her: I recalled her name, her considerable social problems, her severe pre-eclampsia, a violent partner, possible drug addiction, threats to 'thump' the staff, and how angry I had been when Tony Nysenbaum had refused to carry out my instructions. I had spoken to him late the following evening and kept a record of the conversation in August 1984. He had described my management as 'dangerous', but had withdrawn the remark after I had said I found it offensive. After this conversation I had had no further difficulties with Tony.

Kennedy took him through this case and all Tony could remember about the woman was that he had refused to give her intravenous prostaglandin when I had asked for this to be done. In cross-examination he said that he had done this *eyeball to eyeball* whereas I remembered him ringing me in the antenatal clinic.

To me this exemplified the difference in approach which I felt divided me from some of my colleagues: Tony had no memory of the woman or the obstetric problems in her case – just the use of the drug prostaglandin. I remembered him saying that she ought to have a Caesarean, not that the dispute was about the drug. I remembered vividly the labour, the social problems and how I had delivered her. At the end of the day, I drove to Mile End, went to the records department and got the case notes. I then rang Jean Richards, and said they had raised a sixth case and I wanted to take the notes in to the enquiry the next day. She sounded shocked but agreed. Then I went and sat down in the labour ward and went through the delivery book, counting the number of patients of mine that Tony Nysenbaum had looked after before and after this episode. This confirmed my recollection that there were no other 'problem cases'. I got home at 10.30 p.m. It had been nice to see the midwives, and one of my patients had delivered whilst I was there, though I didn't go into her room.

The other junior staff did not give any evidence to support Mr Kennedy's case that I had confused them, and some of their evidence was very helpful for my defence. For example, Toby Fay, the registrar who had spoken with the Us at 4 and 5.30 in the morning of 26 April 1984, confirmed that he had put the options of Caesarean section or trial of labour to them – the pros and the cons – that Mrs U was not in labour at that time, that I liked to be kept informed, and that I usually knew about my patients, although he thought I had unconventional views.

John Dennis, Professor of Obstetrics and Gynaecology, University of Southampton: The first of their expert witnesses was John Dennis, who like so many distinguished obstetricians had trained in Aberdeen in the days of Sir Dugald Baird. He is a short man, and was very relaxed in the witness chair, a complete contrast to Gedis. He gave his evidence in a conversational tone, talking to the panel members as if in a hospital rather than a courtroom. But under cross-examination he was not impressive. His emphasis on protocols; no problems in his unit once the oldest consultant had retired; his labelling of women at booking on the basis of risk factors betrayed a rigidity of approach which at times I found oppressive. Professor Howie asked him: *Do you think that enforced uniformity could be a barrier to progress?* His answer: *If it is never analysed or reviewed,* of course, suggested to me that innovation would be unlikely to happen in his unit.

Taking up a point from his second letter to Dr Richards on my workload John asked him, *Would it be right to take from your evidence that she is a lady who is, as an obstetrician, incompetent?* He replied, *It is impossible to answer that, because for that I would really have to know much more about the rest of her work. So I cannot – I'm not saying yes and I'm not saying no. I do not know.* I looked at him with new eyes. This was the man who wrote those damning words 'bizarre and incompetent', 'consistent aberration of clinical judgement', but when asked a direct question he wouldn't commit himself.

That is a very cautious answer, professor. He smiled at John. *It has to be*. He admitted that unless you worked closely with someone it was hard to judge, he had a lot of sympathy with many of the things I stood for, he wondered how incompetence was defined. Everybody laughed.

John tried a different tack: *Mrs Savage was suspended, or part of the basis for the suspension was that she was dangerous. It would have been dangerous if she had continued in office as it were. Are you able to express a view? Would you agree that she was dangerous on the basis of the notes that you have seen?* There was a pause. *Dangerous is a strong word.* He circled round the point. *I am avoiding the word dangerous.*

Throughout the cross-examination, I passed John notes covering various points under discussion. John glanced down at one of the notes and remarked: *We know that dysfunctional labour is often a manifestation of disproportion, is that right, professor? Is dysfunctional labour a manifestation of disproportion in a multiparous woman?* Dennis frowned: *Not usually, unless, of course – he paused – I cannot remember now how far she progressed in her first labour...* John asked astutely, *It got to 4½ cm ... how would that affect it?* Dennis replied, *The uterus is then more likely to function like a primigravid uterus than a multiparous one.* He leaned back in his chair. John pressed him further, *Is that a view based on research?* Dennis twisted a little in the chair: *No, it's not. Just experience.*

There was quite a lot of laughter during the two days of his evidence, but there was one point where every woman in the room shuddered with distaste. Ian Kennedy was asking him about Susan Payne's long second stage. He responded, *I myself have extended the second stage in a breech delivery on a few occasions, but I was sitting beside the patient.* Kennedy smiled down at him: *Literally?* Dennis turned towards him and said, *Well, at the bottom end.* They both sniggered. Again it emphasised the gulf between the two sides of the room.

He thought the majority of British obstetricians would not allow a trial of labour with a scar in the uterus if the inlet of the pelvis was under 10 cm but conceded that at thirty-four weeks he might if the head was well down in the pelvis. He thought that a baby of 2.6 kg was the largest that would safely go through an inlet of 9.75. (There is published evidence that a breech baby of this weight can pass safely and if it is head first, it can weigh as much as 2.9 kg.) He retracted his earlier allegation about 'imminent eclampsia' by redefining it: *It does not mean to say that eclampsia is going to happen in a minute or two.* (Doesn't it? I teach the students that it requires urgent action because fits may occur at any time.)

He accepted that the pre-eclampsia was not severe in June, that the criticism of the management of the anaemia not being treated energetically was not a severe censure. But despite this, when asked by John Hendy if his agreement to Charges 6, 7 and 9 in Denise Lewis *does do justice to your position?* he changed ground again. *The problem about this investigation is that things have to be put in black and white, and given the limits of this process I agree with 6, 7 and 9.* I looked at him in amazement. Didn't he realise that this 'process' had prevented me from working for forty-one weeks and could destroy my professional reputation and career for ever?

Lastly John reached the case of AU: *Your criticism there is that in spite of adverse signs, Mrs Savage decided to continue with a trial of labour. Dennis refined his criticism: The possibility of vaginal delivery, yes.* John: *That is really the only clinical decision that you challenge on Mrs Savage's part.* Dennis: *Well, as I said in my original summary, all the other cases apart from AU could have occurred. I could have seen those in the practice of many other consultants.*

So it seemed to me that unless the other consultants were incompetent or all practising 'outside the limits of acceptable medical practice' he had destroyed the Health Authority's case, as earlier he had said that one case could not be used to prove incompetence. John: *Of the other cases you say it is the congruence of these cases which troubles you, but now having examined each one of them, the panel may find it difficult to understand how the congruence of these cases reveals anything about the competence of Mrs Savage at all.* Professor Dennis shifted his position in his chair. He looked uneasy for the first time. *We are all human and we can all make mistakes. It is the frequency with which we make errors which reveals our overall competence.*

Professor, that goes without saying. That is understandable, but where the errors, so-called, amount merely to what is demonstrated in those four other cases, and where the errors, so-called, are so different in nature, they really do not reveal anything about Mrs Savage's competence at all, do they? Professor Dennis turned towards the dais: *Well, that is for the panel to decide.* Very quietly John said to him, *It is also for you to express an opinion about.* Professor Dennis looked at him: *Well, I think if I put it another way, had there only been the four cases, I think the conclusions I would have reached would have been different. Would that satisfy your question?*

I am a hard man to satisfy, professor. Your emphasis on the congruence might be understood if all the so-called errors in these cases were of the same nature, if they were all failures to intervene with a Caesarean section, or if they were a consistent pattern of lack of instruction to general practitioners for antenatal care. But those four cases other than AU all demonstrate different things, do they not? John Dennis looked down again: *Well, yes. I think that two of them have a hint of reluctance to do a Caesarean section apart from AU as well. Three altogether have that.* He leaned back again, crossing his legs. *But apart from that there is not a lot of similarity between them? No that is right.*

John read out the passage in Professor Dennis's second letter about reducing my workload, having established that perhaps the whole workload of the district might be looked at to see if some people were doing too little rather than it being me at fault for doing too much. And then he said, *Can we take it from what you say that the very last thing you would recommend is that this lady should be dismissed on grounds of incompetence?*

If all the evidence of incompetence is encompassed by what has been discussed here, I would be sad to see that. John pressed him a bit harder:

More than sad, it would not be right, would it? Dennis shifted in the chair again: *I think I will leave the panel to judge that.* I wondered if he had ever been responsible for assessing a consultant's competence before – he looked glad that he was not the one to make a decision – but it was his report in June that had enabled the Chairman of the DHA to maintain my suspension.

Gordon Bourne, Regional Assessor for Maternal Mortality: Gordon arrived on day 11, Monday 17 February. I had not seen him since just before I was suspended – we used to meet once a month at Bart's as part of the Joint Academic Unit along with Gedis and Tim Chard and the Bart's consultants. In my affidavit Brian had translated what I had said about his attitude to me into 'had displayed personal animosity towards me' and in the rush I had not corrected this. I felt I owed him an apology: I greeted him and said I was sorry – the statement was not quite accurate. He had always been perfectly polite. We chatted together amicably until Trevor Beedham sat down as the panel filed in.

Gordon Bourne took the stand just before lunch. In his well-cut suit, with the carnation in the button hole, and greying hair, although looking younger than his sixty-five years, he is a typical Harley Street obstetrician. Retired Senior Consultant at Bart's, he had also worked at the Royal Masonic Hospital. He answered the questions in a very soft voice, almost inaudible at times, with an occasional intonation of the vowels which reflected his North Country origins.

We stopped for lunch. By chance I was behind him in the queue: 'Not much fun.' 'No,' I replied, 'it's rather like a viva, isn't it?' 'Rather a long one,' he looked uneasy. I replied deliberately, 'Yes, Gedis looked pretty sick after three and a half days in the witness box.' Ahead of us, Gedis was collecting his plate, talking to one of the lawyers. He looked completely relaxed. I wondered what was going on inside his head. That afternoon Kennedy took Gordon Bourne through his evidence. He talked rapidly, fluently, his speech peppered with words like disaster, dangerous, dire consequences, life of baby at stake. His position at one end of the spectrum of obstetric opinion emerged more and more clearly: *No woman should ever be allowed to go into labour with a haemoglobin under 10 Gms'.* He dismissed the risks of antenatal X-rays even when pressed by Professor Howie, although he retracted his criticism that there had not been satisfactory antenatal assessment of the pelvis when Howie pushed him harder. *I accept absolutely that a clinical pelvimetry done by a consultant on this patient is perfectly acceptable.* The charge about fetal distress he also retracted after Professor Howie had intervened. With AU he would have strongly warned the husband of the dangers: *rupturing her uterus... the life of his child is indeed at very, very grave risk.* He ended by saying in that characteristically mild voice (it sounds so reasonable that one almost doesn't hear the strong words, the dire threats, the ominous fears, the undercurrent of anxiety about normal pregnancy): *the messages tend to be different, don't they* – he is discussing my style of management, so he doesn't agree with John Dennis. *There is somewhere a lack of responding to warning signals and lack of reaction to situations that may become dangerous and in some instances do... if there is a theme here it is a lack of reaction to conditions which might have been – or in some circumstances should have been, responded to.*

Brian had decided, with John Hendy's agreement, to cross-examine Mr Bourne the next day, a move that Mr Kennedy obviously regarded with suspicion. John Hendy was not a QC and now a mere solicitor conducting a cross-examination – it was like asking the SHO to take a consultant to task!

Brian, assisted by Peter Howie, who intervened more than he had done before, exposed the rigid, authoritarian view of obstetric practice that Mr Bourne represented: the treatment of Denise Lewis's anaemia was outside accepted limits; women with pre-eclampsia should stay in hospital; it was difficult to draw the line between severe pre-eclampsia and eclampsia. For a woman to go past thirty-eight weeks with a haemoglobin less than 9 Gms was dangerous. Acceptable practice was what was in student textbooks and standard practice in teaching hospitals – although he did modify this after Mr Beaumont pressed him near the end of the day. No wonder the professor and the lecturer who had both worked for him were so 'anxious' and saw as 'dangerous' plans of management which deviated from the narrow pathway they had been taken along by Mr Bourne.

Brian put it to him that he was wrong about his view about the spectrum of practice in the profession at large. *No, I'm not*, he said more firmly than anything else that day. But he could not accept that in Ms X Professor Dennis had said there was no case to answer. *Would it be impertinent of me to say that Professor Dennis is at fault?* There was a burst of laughter from behind me. Mr Kennedy looked annoyed. The professor, sitting staring into space, did not react.

At one point Bourne showed emotion, delivering a lecture about Linda's baby: *These are the babies that die*, he said in a choked voice (and without any good scientific evidence). *I'm sorry... I didn't mean to bang the table.* It was an impressive performance, but it left me cold. I remembered those who had told me about Gordon Bourne's skill at politics, his charming manner towards me whenever we had met, in contrast to his role in my suspension, to which Brian now turned. He denied that he had anything to do with it despite Jean Richards' letter of 26 September 1984 asking him to look at the case reports to see 'whether there was a *prima facie* case for suspension', and the tone of his own affidavit in August 1985 (both Mr Kennedy and Mr Conlin objected to this line of questioning by Brian). Brian then tried to establish exactly how Mr Bourne had approached the task of assessing the cases – obviously a sensitive area. Mr Kennedy kept leaping to his feet like a jack-in-the-box and Mr Conlin, in contrast, quietly glided up when he intervened. Clearly here was a difference in the way the panel reacted: Peter Howie did not look convinced by many of Gordon Bourne's answers to his questions and could see that there was an important point here and wanted to pursue it. The chairman backed the lawyers on the other side. And Len Harvey leaned back, fingering his unlit pipe.

The day finished with Mr Bourne saying he had used the word 'mismanagement' advisedly, but, *putting life at risk or in jeopardy was one definition of incompetence*. He agreed with Mr Harvey that there had to be persistence of error and here the underlying philosophy was important. He accepted Professor Howie's point about acknowledgement of error needing to be taken into account. Mr Beaumont then asked, *So you can envisage circumstances in which competent practice could be something other than that which is set out in the standard textbooks and teaching practice?*

Yes, sir. Because that is really the only way we move. Had he realised that the answer he had given so firmly to Brian six hours before put him out on a limb? Mr Beaumont looked at him benignly: *That is the way medicine advances*. Mr Bourne smiled at him in return: *That is the only way we move forward.*

That completed their expert witnesses' evidence and we did not think that they had produced a very convincing case. But this is where Mr Kennedy would come into his own in trying to break me and then discredit our expert witnesses. He was not familiar with the notes and from his line of questioning it looked as if he had almost abandoned many of the original fifty-nine Charges and was busy constructing a new case.

On Friday evening the lawyers had decided to look into the possibility of extending the hours we worked and the next week it was agreed to do this; then, as the time still seemed insufficient, to sit for another week. Five weeks for five cases – it seemed incredible. But the legal process was extremely slow and tortuous – and Mr Kennedy's stubborn attempts to win his case extended this. At the end of the prosecution case I felt how ridiculous it was to continue. But part of me wanted to show clearly what the defence was and another part of me knew that once the system was set, it had to go through all the motions, however nonsensical they seemed.

Chapter 12

I Defend My Practice

It is not ultimately a matter of High Tech versus natural childbirth. The doctor does not necessarily always know best. A woman having a baby is doing what she was designed for and that equips her with a kind of knowing. Surely humility and respect on both sides is what is needed... The awareness of the paper-thin divide between life and death can be life-enhancing or can shake your confidence completely.

Mary Ellis, *British Medical Journal*, 25 January 1986

The case for the prosecution ended just after lunch on Wednesday 19 February – the last lunch I was to have with Brian and John until I had finished giving my evidence. It seemed to be an extraordinary rule that, during this time, when I needed them most, I discovered that I was not allowed to speak about the case to my legal advisers – but that is how the system works!

The Defence Case Opens

After lunch on day 13 of the enquiry, John Hendy rose to present our side of the case. I looked across to Mr Kennedy; he looked almost bored, leaning with his back towards the professor sitting in the second row, expressionless, almost as if he were detached from the proceedings. Kennedy now looked at the panel, and I supposed he was watching them for signs of reaction to John's opening speech. I thought about the differences between their two voices: Kennedy had that plummy, public-school, accented voice and used phrases like 'jolly good'. When his line of questioning had not produced the desired results he would say, 'Very well' in a curt tone. John Hendy, on the other hand, had a neutral accent with occasional words that reminded one of his West London background. He began his speech by presenting extracts from my comments to the chairman which had been drafted very lucidly by Brian the summer before. This set the scene. John defined incompetence very clearly, and then pointed out that imperfection was not uncommon in medical practice, however hard doctors tried. He then outlined what was left of the prosecution case: he dismissed Ms X – there was no case to answer, according to one of the two Health Authority experts, but what of the others? In the case of Susan Payne, was I incompetent because I decided to wait and see how the labour progressed in a woman with a large pelvis? As for Linda Ganderson, was I incompetent because I had not ordered a first-trimester scan and had delegated care to the GP? And regarding Denise Lewis, was I incompetent because I had not ordered prophylactic iron and folic acid, had I ignored the pre-eclampsia, and was it incompetent to induce with syntocinon? He said I would admit that I had not written this note perfectly, but was it incompetent to ask the senior registrar to 'sort it out', i.e. use his discretion?

In the case of AU they had to decide whether I was incompetent to ask Toby Fay to speak to the woman at 4.30 in the morning, to decide on a trial of labour at 8.30 and to continue it at 12.15 p.m. As for the allegation that *my conduct of the cases confused junior staff, there was not a shred of evidence to support that.* It was said that I failed to appreciate or understand the risks involved, but in fact I was an obstetrician who weighed up every risk; it was also said that I lacked insight because I referred to the good outcome in three of the cases, but this was absurd.

I Speak for Myself

Finally, it was my turn to speak. I was to give my account of the management of these cases after exactly forty-three weeks of suspension, and after two weeks of hearing other people's criticisms of the way the cases had been handled. I walked to the table and sat in the chair where I was to sit for the next week, facing the panel, with John Hendy and Brian Raymond on my left and Mr Kennedy and James Badenoch on my right. I couldn't see my supporters very well because of the subdued lighting, but I could feel their presence behind me. The press benches were almost as full as they had been on the first day.

John took me through my curriculum vitae, my philosophy and attitude to childbirth, my timetable at work, what I knew about the setting-up of the HM(61)112 and the collection of the cases. I felt quite relaxed because of the work that we had done and the way that John had such a clear and thorough grasp of the case. As he asked the questions (which we had not rehearsed), I was very glad that I had changed to Brian Raymond; I felt that not only had I got good lawyers but that we understood each other. It was a bit like being interviewed on radio or television: when you feel on the same wavelength as the interviewer, the programme goes well.

The next morning the headlines differed. The *Guardian* had 'Savage spells out her case'; *The Times* 'Savage a victim of colleagues', the *Telegraph* 'Men frightened of birth pains' and the *Daily Mail* 'Natural birth doctor answers critics'. My age, which had been reported as lower and lower since I had been suspended and had reached forty-two, was now correctly given as fifty. All four of the papers had also quoted part of my answer to John's questions about my approach to obstetrics: *...I think that obstetrics spans the whole spectrum of attitudes from what I call the 'pessimistic approach', that no labour is normal except in retrospect – and I believe that Mr Bourne and Professor Dennis tend to that end of the spectrum – to the other end which I call the 'optimistic approach', which I think reflects my own personality, that everything is normal until something goes wrong. Pregnancy is not an illness. It is a very important part of a woman's life, a couple's life together, and it is of enormous psychosocial significance. I think that it is very important that the people who are assisting a woman during pregnancy allow her to feel in control of the situation and not feel taken over by the hospital, by the doctor, by the system, because if she does feel that way, she is far less able to be this autonomous new person who is a parent.*

John asked me how the two views differed in practice. I referred to John Dennis labelling women as high-risk, preventing them from feeling that they were healthy pregnant women (although obviously some women did need extra special care, but you had to be careful not to label almost all women as being 'high risk'). *What about the male/female approach you referred to just now?*

I think that men, who are not going to actually physically give birth, but are onlookers and bystanders, have the feeling that they have got to do something about the pain, about the way labour is progressing, whereas women, who know that they will probably go through this experience, even if they have not already been through it, understand that it is a very important part of how a woman functions in life, and that there are worse things in life than pain, and that to go through the process of pregnancy and labour and be in control of it is a very important part of a woman's self-esteem. Now, I did not learn that from my own experience of giving birth, I must say. I learned it from women that I looked after. And most notably from Peter Huntingford when I came to work for him in 1976.

Day 14. Thursday, 20 February. I Transgress the Rules of Evidence

We started at 10.15 a.m. Both Mr Kennedy and Mr Beaumont had travelled in by train from the country and had been held up by the wintry weather. It was when John had asked me about the Trevor Beedham letter of 21 May 1984 that Mr Harvey asked me a question which I found really upsetting. We had been discussing the phone calls which had gone on behind the scenes, when he suddenly said to me, in his quiet unemotional voice, *Did you find that a little sad, that Dr Fay had not communicated with you?* I *had* found it very sad, and I had been even more saddened as I had listened to his evidence because I felt so terrible that the junior staff should have been mixed up in all this struggle among their seniors. I answered noncommittally, and then he asked me if I had had it out with Mr Fay. I suddenly remembered, vividly, speaking to Toby on 22 May after I had received Mr Beedham's letter.

I forgot I was sitting in this room, surrounded by lawyers, the press, my judges and women, I just remembered the feelings and the conversation, and I recounted it as I recalled it: *I said to him, 'I do not think that this baby died because of her labour or because of her delivery and I think this baby died because of a rare blood disorder.' He was obviously upset about it, and feeling responsible about it, and I said to him, 'Look, I knew I could trust you to put across the case of having a Caesar or having a vaginal delivery because I knew that you wanted – you thought it was the correct thing to do a Caesarean section so you were not going to be pushing the vaginal delivery aspect.' And he said to me, 'But you know, I didn't want to do any Caesar because I was tired.'* When I had finished there was a moment's silence and then Mr Kennedy was on his feet. His objection – which was only later explained to me – was that the normal court rules of evidence require the defendant's case to be put to the witnesses on the other side so that they can 'put their case', and because I had never discussed this conversation with my lawyers, and it was not part of our defence, I had transgressed the rules. But I was unaware of this, so was completely confused by all the fuss.

With all this talk of points and Mr Conlin also rising to his feet, I saw that they were all taking this remark as being a criticism. But that was not how it was meant. I wished I had never spoken, all my feelings about the disruption of the relationships with the junior staff and midwives, the way pressure had been put on them not to talk to me or go on marches, the suspicion in the department, the division of loyalties, the split between the GPs and the obstetricians in the district, the gynae ward shut – that terrific team of nurses disbanded. These thoughts flashed through my mind as I heard the lawyers discussing whether to recall Mr Fay. As they finished, I said to the chairman, *I'm sorry that Mr Harvey asked that question. I do not think that I have ever discussed that conversation with Brian Raymond or John Hendy. It was just...* I could not go on. I thought that I was going to cry – I fought the tears back; I couldn't cry here, it wasn't the right time or the right place. Mr Beaumont helped me out: *Sometimes things do come out that have not been anticipated.* I asked the press not to put that remark in, as I hadn't discussed it with Toby and Mr Beaumont reinforced my plea.

The rest of that day was taken up by my evidence about Susan Payne, Linda Ganderson and Denise Lewis. John Hendy took me through each case, but the obstetricians on the panel also asked me questions, so that it was much less like a trial and more like a viva or at times even a discussion between professionals.

That evening I went to collect my mail at Whitechapel, and met Toby Fay in the lift. I said I was sorry that he had had to come back, but I supposed that it would be wrong of me to explain the reasons, as we were in the middle of this legal battle. I wish now that I had explained things, because it might have limited the damage.

Day 15. Friday, 21 February. Emotions, Fatigue and Training

Guardian: 'Savage felt isolated from decisions'; *The Times*: '"I was isolated", Savage tells inquiry'. I read the *Guardian* article while waiting for the kettle to boil. It wasn't by Andy Veitch but by someone I had never met, and right at the end he had put in the quote, as had Nick Timmins in *The Times*, which I had hoped they would not.

Reading those articles was bad enough, but the atmosphere in the chamber was even worse. John Hendy asked Toby Fay about my statement: *Do you remember saying words to the effect that in your heart of hearts one of the reasons connected with you not doing a Caesar during the early hours of the morning was that you were tired?* Toby Fay replied: *That's not it* and John Hendy continued: *The only question that arises from that: was it, in fact, the case that, on the night before the delivery of the AU baby, you were tired?* Toby Fay: *I am always tired!* There was a burst of sympathetic laughter from those in the audience who included that morning some GPs who had done SHO jobs in our department, but Toby did not pick up the fellow feeling and said somewhat defensively, *Most of the junior registrars are.*

John Hendy: *Was that a reason for doing or not doing anything in particular in relation to that?* Toby Fay: *Absolutely not, and I think the implication is* – he paused and he sounded angry – *the implication of saying that I would not do something because I was tired is not right.* John Hendy: *And something you would resist?* Toby Fay: *And resent, I might add.*

Mr Conlin rose to his feet: *With your leave, with the greatest respect to my learned friend, Mr Hendy, I submit it is not putting properly what Mrs Savage said in the witness box yesterday.* Mr Kennedy stood up and said, *It is not, but the ground, I observe, is moving. What she said in the witness box yesterday was: 'He said, "I did not want to do another Caesar because I was tired."' There was no question of shilly-shallying yesterday.*

At that moment I could have shaken Mr Kennedy. The words were the same but the mood, the emotion behind them was quite different. My attempt to convey the emotional nuances of a conversation two years ago was twisted and thrown back at me. His tone said it all: I was lying, prevaricating, shifting my ground in order to hide the truth. We were not taking part in a dispassionate scientific enquiry – this was the Old Bailey style at its worst.

Although John tried hard to state clearly on my behalf that no criticism of Mr Fay was intended, I could see he felt criticised; he would not look at me. Later I tried to repair the damage when I came back to give my evidence-in-chief. John gave me the opportunity: *I think you had better tell us your best recollection of that conversation*. I started by speaking about the emotion experienced in a department when a baby dies. I then repeated the conversation I'd had with Toby when I remembered him saying that he did not really want to do a Caesarean because he was tired. I continued: *We both knew that often when you are woken up in the middle of the night, in your heart of hearts all you want to do is to turn over and go to sleep. But your professional training overcomes that, and you get up and you do go in and you do the Caesarean section or whatever. In no way did I think that Toby was reluctant to do the Caesarean section. When you have conversations like this, they are not really for public discussion. They are sensitive and about emotions, and they do not take well to being dealt with in this kind of forum and being reported in newspapers, which, after all, summarise things and do not tend to get at these kinds of subtleties. But in no way did I feel what Toby said meant he would not have done a Caesar if a Caesar was necessary. At that time he did not think the woman was in labour, and I did not think that the woman was in labour. Had that been the case, I certainly would have come in and assessed the size of the baby myself, and all that kind of thing.*

When I had finished there was a moment of silence. I could feel the women had understood me, and my lawyers too, but had I made the men in the room, those on the panel, understand what I meant? Then John asked me the 'legal' question: *Knowing Dr Fay as you do, do you think it conceivable that he is the sort of doctor who would let fatigue interfere with his medical judgement?* I answered, *No, I do not.* Mr Beaumont asked that: *any corrective reporting should be given the same prominence*. I thought of how genuine and heartfelt Toby's reply that morning had been: *We're always tired*. Surely we should not have a training scheme which left people feeling like that? We as a profession should be able to organise it better. Part of the problem at the London was that there was never enough time to deal with all the interpersonal relationships properly. Maybe, though, that was a result of our training that men on the whole did not think that emotions were important. I was glad I had put these ideas into the enquiry – I hoped that they would be understood. After all, it was Mr Harvey's use of the word 'sad' which had started off the whole train of events. The *Guardian* did print my support of Toby and discussion of the emotions, but *The Times* reported Toby's understandably angry reaction. On Sunday, Annabel Ferriman wrote a very sensitive piece in the *Observer*. At the lunch break two women came up to me and said that they had found my explanation very moving. I hoped the panel had.

The Forgotten Charge

In essence, my defence was much the same as that given in June 1985 to the Chairman. However, when the AU case had been discussed (before the baby died) at the Wednesday paediatric meeting, and in Professor Grudzinskas' and Mr Bourne's original criticisms, fetal distress had not been an issue. It *was* a point that I had addressed in my comments to Mr Cumberlege because of Professor Dennis' theory of fetal anoxia when I spoke to him in June and I had obtained evidence from an expert that the CTG did not show evidence of fetal distress.

When I had come back to the labour ward about midday to see Mrs U, I had been angry with the lecturer for not carrying out my clear instructions which included re-examining the woman in two hours and letting me know the result in the theatre. I then quickly examined Mrs U myself, put a catheter into the bladder because I anticipated that we would take her to the theatre then and there, and I did not go all through the partogram or read the notes – as I usually do – but spoke to the midwives about the progress of labour. Then the husband said she had not had the two hours of labour that I had promised them. I felt so badly about not delivering the care that I had promised them that I agreed to let the woman have another two hours of syntocinon-induced contractions as the CTG was reactive – a sign that the baby was in good condition. However, I also got his agreement that if there were decelerations – a hard sign of fetal distress – that he would agree to a Caesarean. I had noted meconium when I examined her, but this I put down to the pressure on the baby, which had entered the pelvis by this stage. (Meconium is a substance in the bowel of a baby which, in a breech presentation, may be forced out by pressure on the baby's abdomen. Sometimes the baby will open its bowels and pass meconium because it becomes distressed in the uterus. This often follows a shortage of oxygen.)

As I was talking to the couple I heard Mr Nysenbaum come in behind me, but when I left the labour ward he was no longer there. Then, as I began to read his note, I saw the words 'ARM – unable to reach buttocks'. ARM means 'artificially rupture the membranes', and in my opinion it should not be done until the presenting part is engaged in the pelvis, otherwise the cord may prolapse and an emergency Caesarean Section has to be done to save the baby, as its blood supply is cut off. I was so furious that I stopped reading, turned the page over and wrote my own note. I did not see that Mr Nysenbaum had found meconium at his 8.50 a.m. examination. After the baby became ill and I was going through the notes to see if there was any reason why this should have happened, I finished reading his note and realised that I had missed this alleged sign of fetal distress. However, there were some puzzling inconsistencies. Firstly, if the baby was so distressed as to be passing meconium at 8.50, it seems unlikely that it would have been in such good condition at birth five and a half hours later. Secondly, the liquor round the baby was clear at the time the baby was born, so if the baby was as high as Mr Nysenbaum thought, it should have meant that the baby must have started to pass meconium at the moment he ruptured the membranes – which is possible but not very likely. Thirdly, the CTG, though not of good technical quality in parts, showed accelerations right up to the time the operation was done. Although my registrar thought that the CTG showed type 2 dips (a sign of distress) I thought that what he was seeing were in fact accelerations from the base line (a sign of a non-stressed baby). Lastly, although Mrs U was not thought to be having effective contractions, and although the cervix had not changed much over twelve hours (which would support this), the breech seemed to have descended quite a lot between the 8.50 examination and my examination three and a half hours later.

When John Hendy and I were going through the brief that Brian had prepared so carefully and comprehensively, I asked John how I was going to deal with this issue. He suggested that I might bring it in myself at an appropriate moment. I decided to do this in my examination-in-chief when we reached the decision I took at 12.15 about the AU case: *There is another charge here which nobody has thought of.*

The Times headline on 22 February was 'Savage defends view on labour'; the *Guardian* had 'Savage's feelings clouded judgement', but that referred to my admission that I felt I had let the parents down and had not been firm enough in my advice. Both reports mentioned that I had been angry with the lecturer and had failed to notice the entry, but it seemed understandable. As an obstetrician said to me, 'When I read that in *The Times* I thought, that's terrible, and then I thought back over the years and I know there have been times when I have felt like that.'

After this evidence I had quite long discussions with Mr Harvey and Professor Howie about the management of AU's labour. Then I asked if we could go into camera to talk about the Us' evidence, which we did. We spent over three hours talking about the U case, and by mid-afternoon we reached Ms X.

I felt the day had gone better than expected, but I was worried. Three weeks had gone by and I hadn't even finished my evidence. How would we finish in time?

Day 16. Monday, 26 February

The fourth week opened with John just tying up a few loose ends. Then I asked if I could say something because over the weekend I had been thinking about an interchange I had had with Mr Harvey on the question of *fire brigade obstetrics* when I had pointed out to him that women did not die immediately if they had a post-partum haemorrhage (bleeding after the baby is delivered). At one point he had said, *Think of the obstetricians' coronaries*, and without thinking I had replied, I don't think we should be planning our obstetric services on the basis of obstetricians' coronaries, and there had been a burst of spontaneous laughter from the benches. So I thought I needed to emphasise that I was not casual in my approach. Mr Harvey had seemed very attuned to Gordon Bourne when he was giving his evidence, and might tend towards the pessimistic end of the spectrum. I was worried that Mr Harvey might go away with the impression, because of my Third World experience, that I was a bit too relaxed about warning signs. *I am not casual, but I believe in looking at the whole person and not just one thing in isolation.*

The Cross-examination

I turned slightly in my chair away from my lawyers and towards Mr Kennedy as he rose to his feet, his round glasses catching the light. He opened with, *Mrs Savage, when Professor Grudzinskas was appointed, that was the first of January 1983, that he took up his appointment, was it not?* I said, *He came on the fourteenth of January because he went skiing for a fortnight first.* This reply clearly irritated him and set the scene for his cross-examination of me, which was to last for over two days. He asked me sharply, *Why did you think it was important for the committee to know he went skiing? To show he was an idler? Why did it matter that he went skiing?* I said, *That is the way my memory works...*

Looking back on it, I think that Mr Kennedy made an error in the way he approached his cross-examination of me. I had always thought of the law as a very dry and unemotional process, but sitting in the waiting room sometimes at Bindmans and observing the other clients – noting how Brian, as well as having this objective assessment of people and their motives which was quite detached and unemotional, was also very sensitive to my need to talk about all aspects of the case, not just the legal ones, and seeing at close quarters how he and John had approached the whole enquiry once it started, I realised that there was a lot of psychology involved. I saw too that the whole planning of the case and how to introduce the evidence and how to cross-examine people was just like the best medicine – approaching the topic as a whole, seeing the person in context. Mr Kennedy had had the opportunity of seeing me questioned by the panel and led through my evidence by John Hendy for three days – and only once had I nearly broken down, when Mr Harvey had asked me if I felt sad.

On another occasion I had responded sharply to Mr Harvey, and that was to do with my feelings about obstetrics being organised for the provider, not for the woman. Having taken note, as he clearly had from his line of questioning, of the events since my suspension, Kennedy could have seen that I was a fighter. If he had been sympathetic and been sensitive to my feelings, I think he might have reduced me to tears, and made a case out for me being emotionally unstable or not up to the stress of the job, or something of that nature.

As it was, his treatment of me was unpleasant. He attacked not only my clinical judgement and decision-making but also me as a person, and his approach converted the atmosphere into that of a criminal court. As the March Bulletin of the Institute of Medical Ethics put it, 'Daily reports of the enquiry proceedings did not always reflect the intense distaste that many who attended felt for the event. That distaste centred on leading counsel for Tower Hamlets who seemed to think that an enquiry into a professional's competence required the same style of advocacy as prosecution for a mass murderer.'

Another aspect of this forceful approach was that it seemed to me that the chairman usually deferred to him if he rose to object to John Hendy's questioning, and for example the fuss made about my inadvertent transgression of the rules of evidence on Day 14 was minor compared with the way that the chairman allowed Mr Kennedy to present evidence outside the terms of reference, for example the first two hours of the professor's evidence on Day 2, and another example is given on Day 18.

The way the case was pursued also perpetuated the personal differences in attitude and approach that underlay the whole affair. It has damaged the relationships between the Tower Hamlets Health Authority and the women in the community of Tower Hamlets who it is meant to serve, and between myself and the GPs and the Division of Obstetrics and Gynaecology. In addition, it added to the unfavourable impression of the profession which this affair has given to many people.

The next two and a half days are not so clear in my mind: the endless slow progress through the case notes, the new allegations, the battle of wits as Mr Kennedy kept on trying to trap me, his manner varying between condescension and irritation with my thoughtful answers. There was a moment of laughter when he produced the copy of my circular letter to the Academic Board of Monday 24 February and asked me if I planned a warlock hunt, which made the *Guardian* headline the next day. There was another moment in the afternoon when he, in response to my comment that Susan Payne had told me that she had gone to sleep during her labour, expressed scepticism that she would remember. I told him that even the grandmothers in the room would remember every detail of their labours, and a murmur of agreement ran through the room.

Day 17. Tuesday, 25 February

Mr Kennedy started with some letters from Professor Ritchie who had been dean, pursuing his point of the previous day about how Gedis had tried to get me to reduce my clinical work. Then he continued with Linda Ganderson, and wasted what seemed like hours following a red herring about my not having seen her at the twenty-eight-week visit – which turned out to be because she was on holiday. I found it hard not to betray my irritation as he slowly worked out all the dates and entries. Mr Harvey spent some time questioning me, and Professor Howie helped me out when I was getting tired.

Then Mr Kennedy began on the AU case, going over and over the notes, for more than five and a half hours. I did not feel confident of having reassured Mr Harvey that I had weighed up the risks. I also hoped that Professor Howie had accepted that, in view of her poor labour pattern, I thought the risk of entrapment of the aftercoming head was negligible after two hours of good contractions. I mentioned that I thought the cause of death was idiopathic thrombocytopenic purpura.

Day 18. Wednesday, 26 February

The *Guardian* headline was ‘Stillborn baby’s mother not seen often enough’, and *The Times* had ‘Savage tells why she let mother attempt labour’ and quoted my reply: *an understanding through her own body that this baby was not going to come out.*

We continued with the AU case. Mr Kennedy tried to discredit my assessment of the depth of her feeling about avoiding a Caesarean section, using the 1980 notes about her first pregnancy, and how she had accepted the senior registrar’s advice then.

Finally we got to Denise Lewis, and Mr Kennedy concentrated on the instructions I gave about inducing her labour as evidence of my inability to communicate. Then he asked me to speculate as to how I would be able to work again at the London Hospital if I was cleared. I did not think that this had anything to do with the panel and appealed to the chairman, but he allowed Mr Kennedy to continue this line of argument. Finally, I lost patience with him. *I said, I am sorry, Mr Kennedy, but I think that you are wasting time... I do not think I am incompetent. I think these five cases are not perfectly managed. I have admitted fault at certain points, but beyond that I will not go.* He persisted: *This has arisen out of disharmony in the division, has it not, really?* I looked at him in surprise: *You have said so, Mr Kennedy*. I said I would be happy to compare my practice with my colleagues, but I did not want to speculate about what might happen when the panel reported. John Hendy intervened to suggest that I could be asked about specific assurances. I suggested that an enquiry into the Division of Obstetrics and Gynaecology was what was needed – and perhaps the enquiry panel would like to take that on. There was laughter in the room; both obstetricians threw up their hands in horror, and I heard someone saying ‘no’. Finally, Mr Kennedy tried to suggest I could not work with the junior staff. I replied, *If the will to work together is there, there is no reason why we should not have a perfectly satisfactorily functioning department.*

My cross-examination was over. John Hendy took up the last point and drew the panel's attention to my letter to Professor Grudzinskas of 5 March 1984 where I had urged that the professor find 'three wise persons' to help the department to function more productively. John clarified one or two points, and then my evidence was over. I hoped I had got across the principles of management of these cases, even though the way they were cared for was less than ideal.

My supporters had noticed the other side passing round the *Daily Mirror*, and at the lunch break they bought a copy and passed it to us. We read: 'A new competition: spot the accused!' They had worked out deliveries per session from the figures introduced on 7 February and compared them with the perinatal mortality rates. These showed that I delivered more babies than my colleagues per session but had fewer deaths. When these figures had been introduced at the enquiry, the professor was recalled to comment on them just before I started my evidence. Mr Harvey said to him, *Would you not agree though, professor, that in actual fact when you are dealing with such small numbers in this day and age that actual perinatal mortality rates, because they are so small, can fluctuate quite widely because of the small numbers involved. If you reduce the argument ad absurdum on F* (the letters refer to the pages of graphs) – *and I'm sure this is a totally wrong interpretation – it could be alleged if you look at C that for example under Mrs Savage that the perinatal mortality rate has fallen still further in a period of time when in fact Mrs Savage has been suspended. You could draw all sorts of stupid conclusions from that which would be totally erroneous.* Gedis replied, *Chairman, I must agree. I would add that to calculate a perinatal mortality rate based on 235 confinements and attribute that to no 7* (the computer code for the professor) *might be a useful pilot exercise, but I cannot draw very much from that. I would also add that if one looked at the maternal mortality rates in the period 1983 or 1984 one would find that my name was linked with all four maternal mortalities in one particular year.*

I knew what he had been trying to say, that with such small numbers the differences between the perinatal mortality rates of individual consultants might be due to chance. However the work load as expressed in the *Daily Mirror* table did show some clear and significant differences. Underneath the table it said: 'Clue – the accused obstetrician is the only one who has ever had a baby!' After the tension of the last week I found it very funny.

Chapter 13

Expert Witnesses for the Defence

> ***I can say without hesitation that if the worst five of my own cases over the period of a year were put under a microscope, it would be possible to create a dossier similar to that of Mrs Savage. I believe the same could be done of every consultant obstetrician that I have ever worked with.***
>
> Peter Dunn, Reader in Child Health, Bristol University

Dr Iain Chalmers, Director of the National Perinatal Epidemiology Unit, Oxford: The first of our expert witnesses to give evidence was Dr Iain Chalmers, who decided to train as an epidemiologist after obtaining his MRCOG in 1973. Brian Raymond took him through his evidence, and Mr Kennedy intervened several times to complain that he was 'leading', or that his evidence was 'irrelevant', saying that there was no dispute about differences in practice. I thought there may well not be any differences in theory, but in practice that was the nature of my colleagues' disagreement with me: their apparent lack of tolerance towards a different viewpoint.

Iain made the distinction between 'standard practice' or 'accepted practice' which was what doctors did, but which might not be based on good evidence and gave as an example the stilboestrol story. This synthetic oestrogen was used widely in the USA between the 1950s and late 1960s to treat threatened abortion. Then in 1969 it was found to have caused vaginal cancer in a small proportion of the women born to mothers given this treatment. Yet it had continued to be used and was *accepted* practice. *Acceptable* practice, on the other hand, was that which was based on sound evidence.

Brian asked him whether there was 'unified' practice in relationship to some of the issues in the five cases: investigation and treatment of anaemia, length of second stage, IUGR and Caesarean section. His answers were thoughtful and based on scientific work that had been done, or he admitted the profession's ignorance because of research that had not been done. He also said that one could not make a realistic assessment of competence on the basis of an unrepresentative sample of a person's work.

When Mr Kennedy rose to cross-examine him there was an air of tension and his questions were acid in tone. And they became more so as Iain refused to be drawn into making statements other than those he felt were right, and in his quiet but firm way refused to be led into unscientific argument.

You ought to recognise your own fallacies as scientists is the point really, said Mr Kennedy after the stilboestrol story had been given as an example. Iain replied, *By all means refer to it as science if that is helpful. What I am saying is that there is a need for humility amongst all doctors, including research workers like me, in the light of the record of unintended mistakes that have been made in the past, made in the best faith and with a firm belief that they were doing good by the people who came to them for help, but which nevertheless in the long run turned out to be harmful. What I am saying is that if one wants to protect the patients that come to doctors from those unintended mistakes in future and now, then we must be careful before accepting opinion without evidence.* Mr Kennedy looked at him and asked, *Do you say that is wrong? And Iain said, Yes, I do. I say that it is wrong to accept opinion without evidence when people's livelihoods are at stake.* Mr Kennedy looked irritated: *If you are not careful you are making noises like a trade unionist!* This was another moment when our side of the room was united against Mr Kennedy. For him it was so clearly a terrible thing for anyone to be an articulate trade unionist!

There were moments of humour when, for example, Mr Kennedy read out some of the instructions about the induction of Denise Lewis, and Iain said, *You have got a lot more written between your lines than I have got on mine, actually.* There was laughter from behind me, and even the panel members smiled.

Turning to IUGR, Mr Kennedy did his best to trip Iain up. However, Iain said that, firstly, the whole question of how IUGR was defined was confused and, secondly, the evidence that you could use to determine who was at high risk of IUGR was heavy smoking and a previous baby who was growth-retarded, not weight at booking. This contrasted with Professor Dennis's evidence the next day. (We had not anticipated that the prosecution case would take more than a week, and as Iain was due to go abroad on 10 February the prosecution allowed him to appear between two of their witnesses.) As regards scanning, routine ultrasound had been shown to identify more babies who were growth-retarded, but not to have any effect on the outcome of the pregnancy. However, some people wanted to be sure that the intervention once IUGR had been diagnosed did more good than harm.

Mr Kennedy looked more and more displeased as the morning wore on, and finally he said, *But there cannot be any question that the prudent practitioner keeps the matter under lively review.* Iain replied pleasantly, *Oh, I am sure that is right.*

Sarcastically Mr Kennedy ended his cross-examination: *It is nice that we can agree. So, really, at the end of the day what you are telling the committee is this: what can we be certain of in this wicked world?* Iain answered steadily, *I have given you some examples. I would be very happy to go on giving you examples of things where I am certain. What I am saying is that there is an awful lot of uncertainty around, and we need to deal with that in a way that is credible.* In his re-examination Brian Raymond remarked, *That I understand, but to use your own words, the committee and nearly all of us are hamstrung.* His glasses flashing, Kennedy interrupted him again: *That is not a question, that is a speech.*

Afterwards Brian and John said to me that Iain had given me a textbook example of how to respond to cross-examination. He had not lost his temper despite the tone of some of Mr Kennedy's questions. He had stuck to his point and not allowed Mr Kennedy to extrapolate from his replies things which he had not meant, and he had thought carefully about the way he answered. I hoped I would be able to do as well.

Dr Marion Hall, Consultant and Honorary Senior Lecturer, Aberdeen: Marion Hall from Aberdeen was the second of our expert witnesses and took her place at the table on Wednesday 26 February, Day 18, a fortnight later. Mr Kennedy had spent so long pursuing irrelevant points and minuscule details in the notes in an attempt to find something to strengthen his case, that there was considerable pressure of time, as Marion had to be back in Aberdeen on Thursday afternoon. John Hendy therefore took her fairly rapidly through her evidence-in-chief. Brian had prepared statements from all our experts dealing with the original fifty-nine charges, and their overall comments as to whether there was evidence for a finding of incompetence. These were given to the panel members either the night before or when the witness came to give evidence.

Several important points were made. Crude weight was not a risk indicator for IUGR – weight for height was more useful, and Linda Ganderson was not in this risk category. Women's own feelings were important in relation to Caesarean section. Consultants were not expected to be governed by the same arbitrary rules as medical students or doctors at the beginning of their careers. In the case of Susan Payne there was no risk to mother and child. Ms X had been managed perfectly correctly. IUGR was difficult to diagnose, and the criticisms that I should have informed my covering consultant were nonsensical – she had worked out that about ninety women might at anyone time be under suspicion of IUGR, although Peter Howie questioned this vigorously. Finally, John read from her statement, *'If asked to advise as to whether Mrs Savage should be reinstated, I can only say that there is no basis at all in the information before me upon which she should even have been suspended, and I have no hesitation in recommending her immediate reinstatement.'* She answered firmly, and some indignation crept into her voice, *Yes, I think it remarkable she was suspended on this basis. If the professor... felt that he had problems with his relationship with Mrs Savage in respect of her academic work, then it is entirely proper for him, as he is head of the department, to give her instructions about how to conduct her academic work, but he is less clinically experienced than she is, and it is not part of his duty to look after her clinical competence, and I find it very surprising that the Health Authority should have accepted the cases being dredged up in this way and brought up as evidence of incompetence. I think it has been a quite improper way of conducting proceedings.*

Mr Kennedy rose to his feet – a gleam in his eye, his opening question was hostile in tone – because she had used the word 'dredge' he implied she was not an objective witness. Mr Conlin asked that we went into camera, as he put it to her that the cases had been raised at meetings by the junior staff – which John Hendy rose to dispute.

When we resumed the public session, Marion commented reasonably on the habit Mr Kennedy had of looking directly at the panel when he thought he had made a good point or asked a question, the reply to which he wanted the panel to pay particular attention to. Mr Kennedy replied *I am terribly sorry. I do not mean to be rude.* In her soft Scottish voice, Marion said, *It came across rudely.* Mr Kennedy looked surprised – I suppose he was not used to being challenged about his manner in court. *In that case I apologise now and I apologise for the times when I shall offend again.* (But not, I thought, for the previous times.)

The next morning Mr Kennedy concentrated almost entirely on the AU case. I found it almost unbearable as he put different questions to Marion, points which I had answered, or, where I had admitted I was at fault, different theoretical possibilities. I could hardly keep quiet. It was worse than being cross-examined myself.

When discussing the point as to whether or not Mrs U was going to return to Bangladesh, which later he stated was a 'footling point', Marion said, *I do not know that it is really very appropriate to ask for a firm commitment of: 'Are you going back to wherever you came from?' at 4 o'clock in the morning. I mean, it would sound like a rather hostile question.* Everybody in the room laughed. *You obviously go in for early discharges in Aberdeen. Surely it is absolutely essential if you are going to take into account the woman may go to Bangladesh?* Marion replied, *No... her knowledge of the local population would be that there is a fair degree of movement to and fro... if that is quite common, then I think that would have to be taken into account.* Mr Kennedy's own viewpoint came out clearly: *Some of us might have thought there was rather more 'to' than 'fro'. Nowadays an increasing number of people from the Third World are settling and making their homes here, so that the general tendency is that the non-indigenous population of this country is increasing?* The second half of this question was almost lost as the people behind me responded to his 'to than fro' by a low hiss. Mr Kennedy responded to the audience's reaction defensively, *You have only got to shut your eyes and think how many brown faces you saw in England fifteen years ago. The answer was many less than today.* One gained the impression he did not think the change was for the better.

He continued pressing Marion about all sorts of tiny details of the management of the AU case, and his manner was condescending and sceptical by turn. He insisted on using the argument that it took an hour to get a Caesarean done at Mile End, despite my evidence that in an emergency that was not so. He and those of my colleagues who insisted on using the poor anaesthetic service at Mile End to attack me were responsible for the headlines the next day: 'Hospital accused of birth delays' in the *Guardian* and, in *The Times*, 'Hospital "should not deliver babies"'.

Marion Hall had responded to his questions by saying that, *Any labour ward which is not able to respond quickly and do a Caesarean section in fifteen minutes should not be delivering babies*, and to a later statement about the anaesthetic arrangements, *But if it is the case that they are administering epidurals without a live-in anaesthetist, then they should be closing the hospital, or else they should have a live-in anaesthetist.* It really upset me to have Mile End downgraded in the way that Mr Kennedy kept on doing, and I thought that the money being used on this enquiry would have paid the salaries for several years of the four anaesthetic registrars said to be needed to provide a proper service.

Last question: is there anything that you have heard, or that has been put to you that has altered your view about Mrs Savage's competence? Marion replied, Since coming here, do you mean? Yes. John waited. There was a pause – then she said strongly, and with some emotion, *No, no. I mean, I have been distressed to hear her being accused of lying, because my impression is that she is honest to a fault.* Mr Kennedy brought us back to the law: *That is nothing in point.* Mr Beaumont agreed: *That is not to do with competence.* Mr Kennedy: *That comes from having a public enquiry.*

I didn't think he had understood the point. It was not the publicity, it was the behaviour of doctors, even if it was being done through their legal mouthpiece, that upset Marion Hall. Was it because she was a woman that she had expressed some emotion? Is this why women are so often seen as a 'problem' in professions like medicine and law?

I thought of Marion ringing her children the evening before to make sure that they had got the supper sorted out, how she was chair of their division, involved in local politics, had got her MD, and as an NHS consultant was more involved in research than many academics I knew. And I echoed the views expressed by one of my supporters. Why can't we have more people like that in obstetrics – direct, caring and yet up-to-date and professional? Why wasn't she a professor?

Mr John McGarry, Consultant Obstetrician from Barnstaple: John is above average height, with glasses and slightly curly hair. He never rushes into things, but speaks quietly and slowly. He has a great sense of humour, and told the enquiry panel that, having been a senior lecturer and gone up the academic ladder, having done his professor's work for five years and observed what professors do, he had decided to become an NHS consultant because he liked practical obstetrics and he liked dealing with patients.

Mr Kennedy spent almost a day trying to get him to condemn my management of the AU case, and suggested that he was not impartial because of his comments about some of the 'behind the scenes' behaviour. As the hours went by I saw John, steady as a rock, stone-walling the questions. John's obvious sympathy for women came across strongly, and when Mr Kennedy accused me of misleading the parents by saying the woman would not deliver soon instead of never, he replied, *What she is in the business of doing there is what we all do every day – she is giving the lady some hope.*

His own experience of personally delivering over 150 breech babies vaginally had led him to believe that the risk of entrapment of the aftercoming head was overemphasised in the books, and that if the progress of labour was smooth and descent was steady, the risk was negligible. He shared care in all his cases with GPs and midwives, and said that the relationship between GP and obstetrician was the most important factor in deciding on the pattern of care. Also as he had got older he had become less worried about anaemia and he did not treat it unless it fell below 8 Gms. Neither did he use prophylactic iron and folic acid.

He was an unshakable witness. At the end of the day one of the women said to me, 'We have all decided to go to Barnstaple to have our next babies', and one of my friends, a grandmother, said, 'That includes me – what a lovely man!'

We had not met on Friday 28 February; but the lawyers had agreed both to an extra week and extended hours as everyone wanted to get the enquiry over with.

That weekend I had been really depressed. I did not read the transcripts which came about a week after the evidence and were read through by Brian and John, who took note of points which they had not marked in their own daily notes of the case. When I had asked the BMA legal adviser how long it usually took for the panel to report after a 112 enquiry, he had said two weeks. Even though Brian was sceptical because nobody seemed to know much about this procedure, I had held on to this timing. John Hendy had floated the idea with the chairman when the lawyers and panel met that they could announce the verdict at the end of the enquiry and give the written report later. Mr Beaumont had said that this would be ready for the July or September Health Authority meeting. I could not believe that I would have to wait so long – I turned on the answerphone, I ignored the post which needed answering, the untidy house, and read two novels to cheer myself up and put the whole business out of my mind.

The support group who had maintained a rota of women to attend the enquiry, and had brought the mobile creche once so mothers with young children could come, had arranged to lobby on what we had thought would be the last day, Friday 7 March, with a disco at Oxford House in Bethnal Green in the evening to celebrate the end. Now we were going to work on the Saturday as well, and thinking about Mr Kennedy's slowness in cross-examination I sometimes wondered if we would get all our witnesses in.

Dr James McGarry, Consultant Obstetrician and Gynaecologist, Southern Hospital, Glasgow: The fifth and last week began. Monday was bitty; Professor Taylor came to give evidence while John McGarry was still being cross-examined. Then Dr James McGarry was called to give evidence. He is a quietly spoken man in his late fifties, with a strong sense of justice. He had written a statement after he had read the affidavits about the way the affair had come into being. The statement was a model of clarity, common sense and fairness, and his responses to the detailed charges reminded me of the respect that my Glaswegian teachers in Nairobi had expressed for him both personally and as someone who had taught them. Because we were so short of time, John was not going through these statements line by line. Dr McGarry spoke with his usual quiet authority. He did not think that this method of analysing five cases out of context was a valid way of assessing competence, and originally had made no comments on the five cases at all in his statement:

> It is suggested that an enquiry will allow debate about the five cases. The prospect is an absurdity. Two entirely different questions will be inextricably confused. The first question, the management of the five cases, will quickly become the management of three cases or even one case and will finally dissolve into conflicting opinions. The second question, that of Mrs Wendy Savage's right to retain her post and to be compensated for the damage done to her reputation by her suspension, will be settled in Mrs Savage's favour in less than five minutes...

He had written that on 28 October 1985 and now we were in the fifth week of this interminable enquiry. John Hendy asked him, *Do you see anything in any of these cases which would justify her removal from practice as an obstetrician either temporarily or permanently?* Dr McGarry looked up towards the panel and said in a firm voice, *Absolutely not*. Because we were running so short of time, John Hendy concentrated on the most contentious points, one of which was the allegation that my management of Mrs U was dangerous. Dr McGarry spoke of the deep impression that the fear of entrapment of the head had on obstetricians, but added that, *In general I would say that the difference between the size of the fetal trunk and the fetal head is not such that it would be at all common for the baby to be born and the head arrested at the pelvis brim*. On the other hand, he took the view that if a Caesarean is going to be done, the earlier it is done the better, although the problem of women wanting to do things their own way was not one he was familiar with in the Southern General Hospital.

When Mr Kennedy stood up, his voice had taken on a totally different tone. Gently, almost obsequiously he said, *I think it revolts you to be discussing these things in public* – Dr McGarry shook his head – *or offends you. Revolts is too strong a word?* Dr McGarry said in an almost inaudible voice, *No, that is not the nature of my objection*. He answered Mr Kennedy's next few questions briefly with 'yes' or 'no' before we went into private session again.

Then after a short break, Mr Kennedy continued his cross-examination. On and on it went. James McGarry gave his thoughtful answers, like a doctor in an academic forum, and Mr Kennedy, naturally, dissected them to score his legal points. In relation to Susan Payne Dr McGarry said that after two hours he would have done a Caesarean section. I remembered John reminding the panel that it did not matter if the individual obstetrician would not have done something in that particular way – it was a question of whether the practice was within acceptable limits – but then he went on to say: *And the other reason which I hinted at – and it is not necessarily very good science – I think that those of us who tend to be conservative about our use of Caesarean section have got to be careful: we must be aware of getting conservatism a bad name. That is, if you push too far in every instance for what might be achieved safely but on occasion it might turn out badly, then the criticism which would be used against one would be quite strong...* My eyes filled with tears – I pushed past Brian and John, meaning to go to our room and have a good cry. As I reached the door I could hear that most people were still in the room drinking tea. I didn't want to cry there – I stood outside, swallowing my tears, out of sight of the panel and the press and the other side.

I kept thinking over the details of the Us' case and of the ordeal that my witnesses were being put through. After about five minutes – it felt like hours – I went back to my seat. Although I wished that I had done things differently in the U case, I was not going to lose sight of the principle behind the management, that if a woman wants to attempt a vaginal delivery or experience labour I will go along with that, as long as she and the baby are healthy. I will not put the options in such a way that really the woman has no choice.

The Paediatric Evidence

The three paediatricians were very impressive and very different in their approaches. Professor Campbell from Aberdeen was very soberly dressed, solid and understated. He gave evidence first and said that the most likely cause of baby U's death was idiopathic thrombocytopenic purpura (a rare cause of bleeding in the newborn baby due to lack of platelets, cells which help the blood to clot), which I will call ITP for short. Although in response to Professor Howie's question he conceded that a multifactorial cause – that is a tentorial tear and platelet deficiency – was possible, on balance he thought it unlikely. He said that there was no evidence that the baby's death had any relation to what happened during the pregnancy. John Hendy asked on Monday afternoon, 3 March, if the Health Authority would withdraw the charge that my management had caused the death of the baby – which, as he pointed out, had been widely reported. Mr Kennedy said he would have to take instructions about this, but the charge was never withdrawn.

Dr Hey from Newcastle was a complete contrast to Professor Campbell: he wore a roll-necked sweater, a sports jacket and open-toed sandals. He gave his evidence rapidly, almost bubbling over with words, ideas and enthusiasm about his subject. Mr Kennedy, having been very polite to Professor Campbell who does a lot of medico-legal work for the Medical Protection Society, looked at Dr Hey with an air of distaste and leapt upon his use of the word 'wolfed' (in his description of the baby's milk intake) in an effort to throw doubt on his evidence. However, Dr Hey has a thorough grasp of neonatal paediatrics and Mr Kennedy was unable to shake him scientifically. Dr Hey was very careful to say that one could not prove the cause of death, but the balance of probabilities led to it being a lack of platelets as the primary cause, with the most likely reason for this being ITP.

He confirmed what Professor Campbell had not had time to elaborate on, that Baby X had no skull fracture visible on the films.

In the case of Linda Ganderson, Dr Hey told the panel that each obstetrician is likely to have two deaths every three years, which mirrored her case. The only differences were that the notes were of a much higher standard than those he had seen in the Northern Regional Perinatal Survey where most of the cases were completely missed, whereas in Linda's case the IUGR had been picked up, and she had been admitted to hospital.

Peter Dunn, the Reader in neonatal paediatrics at Bristol was heard on Wednesday 5 March, Day 22 of the enquiry. Tall and loose-limbed, he looked too big for the chair at the witnesses' table. He was an excellent witness and, like all our expert witnesses, his vast clinical experience and theoretical knowledge was impressive. He had also discussed the U baby's blood results with the director of his regional blood transfusion service, whereas Gordon Bourne, John Dennis and Gedis Grudzinskas hadn't even discussed them with their local haematologist before accusing me of causing the baby's death. All three of them said ITP was uncommon, occurring in one baby in 5,000. Edmund Hey had reviewed the literature and found that 12 per cent of these babies die, that is about one in 40,000 births. Peter Dunn also said he had seen two cases similar to this in thirty years.

As far as the theory about a tentorial tear was concerned, Peter Dunn saw perhaps, one case a year in Bristol. In Baby U's case, the mild birth asphyxia (found in 25 per cent of babies born by Caesarean section) and the good condition of the baby for twenty-four hours after birth made the diagnosis of this type of tear exceedingly unlikely.

I wondered whether, if we had had a perinatal meeting, a diagnosis of ITP would have been reached. And why was it that we never had enough time for the junior staff or ourselves to go to the library and do a literature search? We must also involve other people – because the haematologist might well have been able to reach this diagnosis, and then the parents would not have had so much suffering.

When John Hendy turned to Baby X, Mr Kennedy rose to his feet and said he had spoken to Dr Harris, the London Hospital paediatrician who had looked after Baby X and Baby U. He had never thought Baby X had had a fracture. I thought of the *New Society* article, headed 'Incompetent health authority': it was all of seventeen months after the birth and into the fifth week of the enquiry before they conceded this. During his evidence we had been given the Baby X notes, and suddenly I saw Ms X's labour CTG. I had a quick look: the transient tachycardia (abnormally rapid heart rate) that had been reported by the midwives at 8 p.m. was there, but the rest of the trace was normal. I handed it to Brian, who gave it to Mr Dibley in the coffee break.

Gordon Stirrat, Professor of Obstetrics and Gynaecology, University of Bristol: Gordon Stirrat is serious and thoughtful; another Scot, he seemed to me to be the same sort of person as Peter Howie. In his evidence-in-chief he did not withdraw from his own position about AU, but had this to say: *I am very aware of the aversion to Caesarean section amongst particularly the Bengali community. We have such a community within Bristol... the aversion to Caesarean section goes beyond, in one sense, what we might call reason... I can certainly see that that was an important force in the decision to try to achieve vaginal delivery... I have a recent example of a Bengali woman under my care... She came into my hospital in labour, and was obviously, as time went on, in obstructed labour... Progress was not being made, so Caesarean section was counselled, over a lot of resistance, although... counselling had taken place beforehand, and the baby actually was fit and well... The community midwife... reported to me on Friday of last week that she was very concerned about that woman because the husband was now rejecting his wife – she thought the husband was rejecting his wife because she had been a failure... the midwife then reminded me of another case... again from the same community, and the woman had a Caesarean section for reasons which were absolutely cast-iron... That was two years ago. This woman is now in one of our local long-stay mental hospitals, and the psychiatric opinion is that the triggering factor in a woman who was predisposed to this anyway was the Caesarean section and her husband's response to the fact that she had Caesarean section, so two cases have recently been borne in on me in which a proper decision to carry out a Caesarean section has very severe effects in one case and possibly horrifying effects in another, so I am very aware of the problems.*

Gordon Stirrat said he thought the criticisms of the management of Denise Lewis's anaemia were *absurd*, and she did not have severe pre-eclampsia in June. In answer to John's question about my competence in relation to her he replied, *In no way, shape or form can she be described as incompetent in this regard. If it were, I suggest that the majority of obstetricians are similarly incompetent.* In Ms X's case there was no incompetence, and with Linda Ganderson it was regrettable that I had missed her at thirty-six weeks. But on admission, Gordon Stirrat said, *Intervention at that point could have resulted in a live birth.* He looked at the AU traces and confirmed that there was no evidence of fetal distress. Finally... *I, really, honestly, reading these notes, found it quite incomprehensible that a claim of incompetence was being made in the context of these five cases... one cannot possibly make a diagnosis of incompetence based on one case. If that is the way... then questions must be asked about every obstetrician who is practising in this country today'. I certainly would not like... five cases picked out to be viewed by a tribunal such as this. I would be quite embarrassed.* I looked at Mr Kennedy. He was staring at him with that detached expression.

John went on: *If the management of these cases does demonstrate incompetence, what implications do you see for obstetricians?* Gordon Stirrat replied, *Very, very serious implications for the whole of obstetrics in this country. It would be a decision which would move us very significantly towards the defensive medicine position which we are only too well aware of from across the Atlantic... There is no single body of practice which is agreed within obstetrics in this country, and one has to ask why that is... There are basic scientific facts about so many of our practices that are lacking. We are practising on the basis of our training, our experience, such scientific knowledge as is available. If I had to encapsulate my job, it is as a risk assessor.* Mr Kennedy asked a lot of questions, but his heart was not in it.

The Tower Hamlets General Practitioners

Tony Jewell, who is Denise Lewis's GP; Felicity Challoner, who has been a house officer on my firm as part of the East London Vocational Training scheme; and Katy Simmons, who had worked as an SHO with Peter Huntingford, as a locum registrar for me and was now doing her trainee year for general practice at South Poplar Health Centre, gave evidence on Day 23 of the enquiry.

Felicity, obviously a caring doctor, was very quiet, and I found her evidence moving. She said she had never had any difficulty in understanding my instructions and had found no great differences at her level between my practice and that of my colleagues. In cross-examination, Mr Kennedy had modified his tone towards her. In a fatherly manner, he asked her if she remembered any controversial cases from her six months. Two, she replied. He only wanted to know about mine. I was impressed by the candid way in which she explained how she and the senior registrar had not diagnosed a breech in labour. In fact, the baby died soon after birth because it had Potter's syndrome (a congenital abnormality incompatible with life).

Katy Simmons, with her Newcastle accent, slightly off-beat but respectable clothes, was refreshingly frank, caring and alive. She confirmed that there were no difficulties in communication, and said she had learnt more in four months working for me than in all her other obstetrics and gynaecology posts together.

Tony Jewell was another excellent, thoughtful witness. His handling of Denise Lewis's antenatal care, and his reference to her healthy twins seen in his baby clinic showed that he was a better-than-average doctor. He spoke for the GPs and mentioned that his own wife and several other GPs and their partners had chosen me as their obstetrician – hardly a mark of incompetence.

Professor Ron Taylor, United Medical School of St Thomas's Hospital and Guy's Hospital: By the time that Ron Taylor took the stand for the second time on Thursday afternoon, everybody was exhausted. Mr Kennedy, however, was back on fighting form and started off with an attack on Ron's affidavit, in which he had sworn that Professor Grudzinskas had said his first task was to change his senior lecturer. Ron Taylor repeated the advice given to him by Professor Ian Donald when he himself had been appointed – that it would take ten years to get his department the way he wanted. How sad, I thought, that Gedis did not take this advice. Ron's quiet voice, with his slight Liverpool accent, his relaxed position at the table and his humour, lightened the atmosphere. He and one senior registrar looked after 1,000 women a year out of the 3,500 delivered at St Thomas's Hospital – so much for Professor Dennis and my impossible workload! His tolerance was so obvious in everything he said, and his clinical experience in particular with reference to vaginal breech delivery came across clearly. He said he would be very happy to have me working in his department, and he ended, *Certainly, I couldn't remotely apply the term 'incompetent' to the handling of these cases.* John asked him: *If the question was 'Is Mrs Savage safe to return to practice tomorrow?' what would your answer be?* Ron's answer: *Yes, certainly.*

Mr Kennedy worked hard, and the phrase 'vaginal delivery at all cost' was used at one point. Ron answered reasonably, despite the tone of some of Mr Kennedy's questions, but we were all glad when the day was over.

Day 24. Friday, 7 March

I went to buy five dozen roses for the Support Group who I knew would be lobbying. I had never had so many flowers in my life, and I thought it was time I gave some back. The shop wrapped them individually and I was nearly late. Everybody was standing outside, including BBC News cameras as I tried to park my son's beat-up Jaguar. I distributed the roses. And then we were inside the chamber for the closing speech for the prosecution. In Kennedy's closing speech I did not recognise myself as this terrible ogre of whom the junior staff were terrified, who could not communicate, and was *convinced of the advantages of vaginal delivery to a point where she subordinates the patient to that wish;* in addition, I was a *crusader with perhaps a sharp temper,* which was one of Kennedy's most memorable criticisms, and a person *with that grave defect of character which is an inability to recognise fault in one's self.* He accused me of lying, of being unable to communicate with the junior staff, and then right at the end he brought up the fact that I had not called Peter Huntingford. The reason that I had not done this was because I thought that he would not be seen as an objective expert witness, having been my professor – and now even this was thrown back at me!

John and Brian were quite pleased, indicating that if the opposition resort to character assassination it means they know they have no case, and I was quite surprised at how detached I felt from this speech. I suppose that if you do not respect a person it does not matter what he or she says and you do not believe that reasonable people are going to be influenced.

As we finished early, I suggested that the panel members visit Mile End. Gedis had another engagement, so I took them round with one of the administration people and the new Mile End midwifery sister. Ironically, in the labour ward we met the midwife who found that Baby U was ill when she came on duty, and on the post-natal ward the sister involved in Susan Payne's first labour. I felt quite sad going round my hospital, but the nurses were glad to see me, and I wanted to be back at work.

Day 25. Saturday, 8 March

It was a beautiful sunny day; it felt like spring, and I hoped this was a good omen. The chamber was packed, as lots of people who worked during the week were now able to come. Mr Badenoch rose, apologised for Mr Kennedy's absence, and brought in another point about competence depending on the consultant's ability to lead a team, i.e. to be a captain.

John Hendy disposed of this later intervention as *legal mumbo-jumbo* and opened his speech with a story about a film in which the hero had bought an Old Bailey kit and found himself, when he had put it together, in the dock in No. 1 court. He invited the panel to tear down the edifice that had been erected over the last five weeks and get back to the atmosphere of a coffee room in a busy hospital. His speech was on a different level from Mr Kennedy's – he defined incompetence, he referred to the various legal definitions, he destroyed all of the new case by reference to evidence in the enquiry using the day, and page and paragraph numbers. I was very impressed by the way he marshalled the evidence together and presented such a good case.

We ate lunch, and afterwards John invited the panel to give us the verdict then and there – and write their reasons at leisure. He presented a letter from the GPs asking for this. I knew that the DHA had also supported a rapid verdict but, although we had the impression that the obstetricians were willing to agree, Mr Beaumont was not. John tried again. The chairman said that they would retire, but if they did not reappear within a minute, we could assume that they had refused our request... and then the lawyers were called in to see them.

I felt sorry for Gedis Grudzinskas, alone on the opposite side of the room. His counsel had deserted him, and there was not one of his colleagues with him – as had been the case for most of the five-week enquiry. Apart from the Us' solicitor, only twice had there been a woman on those benches: the wife and an ex-pupil of Mr Badenoch's. I wondered how he felt after five weeks away from his work. He left on his own.

I had got some champagne to celebrate the end of the enquiry, and I went and got the bottle and the glasses. Brian and John came back – they had been offered lukewarm gin and tonic. We all drank to what we felt was a moral victory, and I drank to Brian and John, who had worked so hard for me – and for justice.

That night we went out for a celebratory dinner: the legal team, Luke Zander, and Sam Smith, and their wives, and Sue Hadley and Heather Reid from the support group; Katy Simmons came later; (Felicity Challoner was working for her Diploma in Child Health, and Tony Jewell had another dinner party; Ron Taylor was up in Scotland). We had a great party. It was Brian's idea, and the right thing to do, as the anticlimax of having to wait four months for the result was terrible.

Chapter 14

The Long Wait

'But this second acquittal isn't final either,' said K., turning away his head in repudiation. 'Of course not,' said the painter. 'The second acquittal is followed by the third arrest, the third acquittal by the fourth arrest, and so on. That is implied in the very idea of ostensible acquittal.' K. said nothing. 'Ostensible acquittal doesn't seem to appeal to you.'

Kafka, *The Trial*

The day after the enquiry ended I flew to Liverpool to open a Women's Health Bus. It was sad to see the devastation of this once-thriving city, but the women were terrific. I felt at home in the informal atmosphere, wearing my dungarees after five weeks in a tailored tweed suit. Returning to London, it felt strange on the Monday not to be going to Addison House. Doing something for long enough can make it begin to feel normal. The atmosphere had been so intense – reading the transcripts in the evenings – it became my whole life. I almost missed it! It was the same with my suspension. Sometimes I felt that not practising as a doctor was the way it was going to be for ever.

I looked at the pile of unanswered mail that had come during the enquiry. I had started off well, filing it in my 'support' folders and sending out a standard letter of thanks, but after the first ten days when the transcripts began coming, I had got behind. It cheered me re-reading all the letters and I was amazed to find that there was over £2000 in personal donations to the Appeal Fund. I felt humbled by the people who, despite living on supplementary benefit, had written enclosing small sums. I could not let them all down, but I felt emotionally volatile. Some days I was buoyed up by the feeling that we had fought the battle well: other days I felt depressed. The wait seemed interminable.

During the enquiry, Dr Noel Olsen, a community physician in Hampstead, had been rapidly collecting the 250 signatures needed to hold an extraordinary general meeting of the Medical Defence Union to discuss why they had decided not to support me. Before this was done the MDU Council met and decided to pay my legal costs. I felt very cheered by this but hoped the public would not think I had been raising money under false pretences. Tony Jewell, the Chairman of the Appeal Fund, put out a press statement which announced Sam Smith's sudden death and stated that the £60,000 raised to pay my legal fees would be banked until I was satisfactorily reinstated. If there was any money left the donors would be contacted.

In March, and after many publishers had expressed an interest, I made the decision to write this book. I had not anticipated how, when I sat down at the Amstrad, I would relive the whole experience. Often I was overtaken by the emotions I had not had time to feel before, and I cried or felt too depressed to write anything for days. I had not thought it would have been so difficult as I had all the documents to hand, but the memories that came flooding back kept on disconcerting me.

Waiting for the Report

On 3 June, Brian wrote to Mr Beaumont pointing out that in order for the report to be considered by the DHA at their meeting on 10 July as promised, it needed to be in our hands by mid-June. The circular gives the accused doctor two weeks to check the first part of the report, the facts, for accuracy, and once this is returned the panel then issue the second part – the findings or, in my case after the 'trial', the 'verdict'. Obviously the DHA members would need time to read and digest this before their meeting to decide about my reinstatement. Mr Beaumont replied on 5 June but gave no date. By mid June, when there was no sign of the report, we asked the Support Group if there was any chance of postponing the march which had been planned to coincide with the DHA meeting. Plans were too far advanced, however, as the posters had been printed and advance publicity was unstoppable.

As the time dragged on we became more and more convinced that we were not going to have the report in time for the meeting. However, a journalist who had spoken to Mr Beaumont told us that the latter had said that having read Part 1 it would be clear what Part 2 was going to be. My answerphone worked overtime, referring the press to Brian, and the pressure mounted as we got to the end of June.

Through the legal grapevine we were given an ongoing progress report on the timing of the report. The first part was finally ready at lunchtime on Wednesday 9th. Brian took the train to Rugby at 1 p.m. to pick it up and I went to the first Dorothy Russell Memorial Lecture at the London Hospital that afternoon. She had been a distinguished neuropathologist, a London Hospital graduate and Professor of Pathology. I forced myself to try and concentrate. At 5 p.m. I rang Brian. 'We've won,' he said and he had already set in motion the contingency plan for a press conference if the report was as clearcut as it had been rumoured to be. I went and joined the neuropathologists, neurologists and neurosurgeons for salmon and strawberries and white wine, but I was too excited to eat and left at 5.45. I rushed to Brian's office to read the report. Brian opened some champagne, and photocopied the first and last parts which we had decided to give out at the press conference the following day. John Hendy called in at about 10 p.m. and had the last glass of champagne. I wondered if all those who talk about the only winners being the lawyers knew how many hours both Brian and John had put in during the enquiry.

Thursday, 10 July 1986

The following morning I drove to the press conference at Queen Mary College Student Union. Although the media had been following the case throughout the whole saga, over the last fortnight interest had reached fever pitch. The Support Group Committee were already there preparing for the evening cabaret planned for after the march and, as we started, with the TV cameras whirring behind their blazing lights, Sue Hadley and Heather Reid presented me with a beautiful bunch of flowers. Brian began with a carefully prepared speech. When had he written it? He must have spent hours on it after we had left his office the previous night. 'The nightmare is over. The attempt to accuse Wendy of incompetence has been shot down in flames. The women of Tower Hamlets will soon have back among them the obstetrician they want.' He had counted up the separate charges, fifty-nine were listed, fifty-five were found to be invalid or insubstantial, and in four instances there were criticisms of my management which did not amount to incompetence.

I had not prepared a speech. I began by thanking all those who had helped and supported me, saying how relieved I was that the panel had cleared me of incompetence. 'I feel I have been vindicated, although I have never said that my work was free of errors.' The criticisms that were made were all, bar one, accepted by myself as errors in the comments I gave to the chairman in 1985. After the press conference various television and radio journalists asked me to do interviews. We finished about 1 p.m. and I drove to Whitechapel to put some wine in the refrigerator for after the march, and then back again for the march itself.

It was a lovely sunny day but not too hot. There were balloons and babies, women wearing the new badges 'Women need Wendy', several local GPs and Ian Mikardo and Jo Richardson, two of the MPs who had supported me throughout the long suspension. Photographers were jostling for position as we started the march led by Ian Mikardo and myself. It was extraordinary to be at the front, with all the photographers walking backwards, traffic being slowed down and hundreds of people with babies and pushchairs and a band. It both cheered and saddened me, as I saw so many of my patients amongst them whom I'd not been able to care for all these months.

The march continued to Vallance Road gardens, where the police unceremoniously asked the meths drinkers, who were sitting peacefully in the sun, 'to move on' – the only thing that marred the day – and everyone sat down and produced picnic teas, bottles of milk and the kids played on the swings. When the party broke up I had a small celebration with my sister and other close supporters before going on to the cabaret at Queen Mary College. It was a very good party – the feminist groups who entertained us were amusing and professional and the food from the Punjab cooked by one of my patients and from Somalia cooked by women from the Maternity Services Liaison Scheme was delicious. Everyone was there: Brian and John and their wives, all the members of the support group, students, and people from the trades council and local council, journalists and general practitioners, midwives and nurses, women who had had babies and those who had been gynaecological patients of mine – it was a friendly and happy occasion and I felt welcomed back into the community.

The newspapers all carried the story the next day, many placing it on the front page. It was interesting to see how seriously the media had taken the whole struggle which could so easily have been reduced, as one headline put it, to a 'Savage Squabble'.

The Second Part of the Report

Over the weekend Brian and I went through the report, checking it carefully. We met on Tuesday to compare notes and on Wednesday 16 July the few typing errors and interpretations about which we differed were delivered to Mr Beaumont.

On 20 July, the *Observer* carried an article, 'Savage faces ban on comeback'. It suggested that the second part of the report would 'make circumspect comments about the case which would embarrass the Health Authority and, unexpectedly, Mrs Savage herself'. Brian had replied to this firmly: 'Members of the panel would be stepping outside their powers if they made any comments. If the Health Authority fail to reinstate Mrs Savage they will be punishing the innocent victim and rewarding those who made false accusations against her.' Once again the rumour and gossip circuit seemed to have been working overtime and when I was interviewed for the Today programme on the Tuesday I could deduce from the questions I was asked what a panel member had been saying to the press 'off-record'.

On Monday 21 July Brian heard from Mr Beaumont that the second part of the report, including our copy, had been sent to the DHA on Saturday 19 July. I went over to the district offices to collect it. I knocked on the door of Mr Alway, the new general manager. Sitting in the room were Mr Cumberlege, Mr Alway at his desk, and another official. I explained why I had come; Mr Cumberlege said he had been called from a 'luncheon engagement' to see the report, which he was just reading. Mr Alway said I could have a copy, and I sat down to read it. No incompetence, so no disciplinary action. Relief flooded through me. However, because of the implications for patient care the panel had made some observations:

> 10.2 These matters of concern are referred to in part one of the report. In broad terms they can be categorised as
>
> a) poor working relationships between Mrs Savage and some other consultants.
>
> b) poor communication between medical staff.
>
> c) unsatisfactory cross-cover arrangements between obstetric consultants.
>
> 10.3 We do not seek to apportion responsibility for those matters in any way. We recognise and respect the genuine differences of opinion and deeply held views of the individual consultants. A practical solution would be to separate the obstetric units at Whitechapel and Mile End. This could be achieved by Mrs Savage and another consultant (perhaps a new appointment) being responsible for Mile End, whilst the other present obstetric consultants would be responsible for Whitechapel.
>
> 10.4 We also recommend that when unfamiliar methods of management are being employed, the consultant concerned should be closely and personally involved at all stages.

Mr Alway told me that the DHA would release this to the press the following day at 2 p.m. Mr Cumberlege confirmed that a special DHA meeting would take place on Thursday 24July. I left – it seemed unreal – a certificate of competence at last. I went to see a senior member of the hospital consultant staff. 'We are back to where we were in April 1985,' he said. I answered 'except £250,000 poorer, and my patients deprived of my services for all that time'. I felt depressed. Although we had won, the battle would continue. I had admitted mistakes, but it seemed it was too much to expect that anyone else would publicly. I could see the reluctance to face the issues that had caused this debacle. A satisfactory result, justice had been done, banish the 'odd-one-out' to Mile End. I could see that this was a pragmatic solution, but was it right that this small group of men could get away with the damage that they had caused? The last hurdle lay ahead: would the DHA recommend my reinstatement? It seemed a foregone conclusion, but after the last fifteen months I would not believe it until I heard it.

The Health Authority brought out the result on Wednesday, the day of the Royal Wedding. It was duly reported that Mr Cumberlege was going to propose that I be reinstated, and ask the Authority to ratify a proposal, which had been discussed at a previous meeting, that an advisory panel of eminent persons be set up to consider the observations of the panel.

That afternoon Brian and I went to see Mr Alway and the new solicitor representing the North East Thames Region. We read the press release. I was pleased about the recommendation for reinstatement, but slightly alarmed at yet another panel of enquiry. After the meeting we wrote a letter to the DHA making it crystal clear that I was not prepared to remain suspended indefinitely whilst another panel decided how to get the obstetricians in Tower Hamlets to work together.

The Authority met the following day at 4.30 p.m. We had arranged with Mr Alway that we would wait in my office in Walden Street where we would be telephoned once the result was known. The call came at 6.15. Brian and I walked round the back of the London Hospital and in the side door to avoid any lurking cameras. Mr Alway came and told us the good news. The Health Authority had voted unanimously to reinstate me. The enquiry panel had been agreed: Dame Alison Munro who had chaired the Maternity Care in Action DHSS working party, a representative from the RCOG, and Mr Alway himself. They would prepare a report for the DHA meeting on 11 September 1986 which would enable me to be back at work by mid-September. Brian made some arrangements about the press conference which was scheduled for 7.30 that night. I thanked Mr Alway and we left, almost unable to take it in that it was finally over. At the same time there was a feeling of unreality – was it really over? – and an awareness that there was still another panel to convince.

Back in my office I did a phone-in programme and then we set off for the press conference. It had already started and Mr Cumberlege was answering questions, with Mr Alway on his left and Jean Richards on his right. Mr Cumberlege saw me standing at the back, ‘Do come and sit down, Mrs Savage, I do hate to see a woman standing.’ I could feel the women behind me almost ready to burst into shouts of rage. I sat down about a yard from Jean Richards and observed the session. Someone asked Mr Cumberlege if he thought it had been right to suspend me; he mentioned the rigidity of the procedure, how in two two-hour meetings he had made the decision and weighed things in the balance. Had he expected the public support? Yes, he had taken that into consideration. I looked at him in disbelief.

The press were pretty kind to Mr Cumberlege, I thought. Amongst other things he said that Mr Bourne had no connection with Tower Hamlets – technically true, but what about our joint Academic Department which meant I met regularly with him, what about his training of the professor and the lecturer? Could he not have said that with hindsight it might have been better to consult someone less closely connected? Someone asked about the proposal that I work at Mile End and how this departed from the district’s plan; ‘India was partitioned in 1947,’ he replied. A gasp of amazement rose from the supporters in the back of the room. Linda Lewis, a BBC reporter, asked why he had refused to appear in front of the TV cameras and he explained that he didn’t like the way he looked on the television screen. He continued: ‘I prefer steam radio.’

Mr Cumberlege drew the press conference to a close and we moved to another room where Mr Alway had agreed to do a TV interview. Brian and I then answered questions. I said how delighted I was with the result, that even if the response from the public had not surprised Mr Cumberlege it had astounded and impressed me, and that I thought it a sad comment that after being a chairman of various boards for thirty years in the NHS it had taken an enquiry costing an estimated £250,000 to convince him that doctors held different opinions. Brian spoke strongly: 'The decision that Mrs Savage is not incompetent clearly has implications for those who said she was. They have their consciences to examine.' Radio 4 and LBC then wanted interviews and finally about 9.30 it was over. We went to a pub opposite the London Hospital where we celebrated somewhat more modestly than at the end of the enquiry.

The next day Brian and I made an appointment to discuss our submission to the Munro enquiry panel. The battle had been won, but the terms of the peace had yet to be agreed. The Governors of the London Hospital Medical College had an emergency meeting, and the Dean Elect wrote to me on 28 July suggesting I work at Mile End, thus avoiding the issue. The situation reminded me of the article by Anthony Clare, Professor of Psychological Medicine at Bart's in the *Daily Telegraph* on 12 July: 'Throughout all this the London Hospital Medical College stood aloof, although one of its professors was publicly accusing one of its senior lecturers of incompetence. A better example of the current spinelessness of much of academic medicine would be hard to find.' He ends his article: 'the hushed silence of the medical profession in the face of such a lamentable farce (with one or two admirable exceptions) was one of the most depressing aspects of a most depressing tale. But if there is a moral and I suspect there are a few, it is that if doctors yield their right to regulate themselves up to administrators, managers and lawyers, then such claim as they have to be a profession disappears. And they should not be surprised if the dignity, the standing and the respect that a profession commands disappears with it.'

Chapter 15

Birth and Power

> ***The public has the right to expect a great deal of the medical profession in relation to our standards of professional conduct and practice. We have always set very high standards for ourselves and must surely continue to do so, knowing as we do how easily this vital public trust, which we value so highly, can be damaged.***
>
> Sir John Walton, General Medical Council report, 1984

The fifteen months of my suspension from my post at the London Hospital and the subsequent enquiry has been a terrible waste of NHS funds. It has damaged relationships between the GPs and obstetricians in Tower Hamlets and it has reduced, both at the service level and personally, choice for women in the district, especially those women who want a woman obstetrician and gynaecologist. It has prevented over a hundred medical students from being taught by a woman with a different approach to the subject, and it has damaged the reputation of the London Hospital, its Medical College and those doctors involved. Yet I do not accept 'the only winners have been the lawyers'.

The debate about obstetric care has been widened and women have had the opportunity to see that obstetricians can hold radically different views about how childbirth is managed. The women in Tower Hamlets have found a voice and a way of putting their views forward. The three major childbirth consumer organisations, the NCT, AIMS and Maternity Alliance have come together publicly for the first time and an ongoing 'think tank' on maternity care is going forward. Midwives have been strengthened in their battle to regain professional autonomy. Chairmen of Regional Health Authorities have started moves to change the disciplinary procedures for doctors, and some individual doctors have begun to fight against their demoralising, long drawn-out and expensive suspensions.

There are at least six important issues arising from my suspension:

- Birth and Power – who controls childbirth?
- What kind of services do women want – and who is going to decide on the kind of care that is offered to them?
- Accountability – of the District Health Authority and of doctors.
- Incompetence – how is it defined? How does one measure it?
- Disciplinary procedures for doctors in the NHS – can they be improved?
- Academic freedom and the role of professors and senior lecturers.

The issue of birth and power is one which arouses strong emotions, because birth is a profoundly moving experience for all those who participate in the drama, whether as the person who should be the central point of the whole event, the woman, or the person who should be in a supporting role, the midwife or doctor.

Birth arouses primitive and elemental feelings within us, reawakens unconscious or conscious memories in connection with our own beginnings and those of our siblings. It reminds us of death as well as life, and the awareness of the tragedies which do still occur is not far from the surface.

Throughout history women have controlled birth in most cultures, and still do in many parts of the Third World. In the developed world men-midwives began to take over the control of birth in the eighteenth century. In the twentieth century the power of the obstetrician has risen to unprecedented heights. In the last forty years we have seen in this country a complete take-over of the whole process of birth by obstetricians, 88 per cent of whom are men at consultant level, where hospital policies are dictated. Only 1 per cent of women still have their babies at home, whereas before the Health Service almost half of all women delivered in their own homes. Midwives were responsible for the care of the majority of women and worked independently.

This major change in childbirth patterns in society has been followed by increased medicalisation of birth and rising rates of intervention, without good scientific evidence that these high rates are necessary. It is true that childbirth is safer than ever before, and that a woman is more likely to have a live baby than ever before, but the relationship between these improvements and many of the changes that have taken place in the 'management' of childbirth have not been properly evaluated and in particular, the fall in perinatal mortality is probably as much related to improved living standards, and easier access to contraception and abortion, as to neonatal intensive care and high technology in obstetrics – although for an individual woman these may make all the difference between a successful outcome and losing her baby.

In particular, antenatal care has not been subjected to rigorous analysis, and yet it has been accepted as essential to a good outcome. Fetal monitoring became widespread before its effectiveness was tested by a valid trial; induction of labour reached 40 per cent a decade ago, with no evidence that this high rate was necessary or even useful. And now the seemingly inexorable rise in the rate of delivery by Caesarean section is justified by some obstetricians for the sake of the baby, but although in some instances this is valid, in others the benefit is not proven.

Although obstetricians justify their takeover of birth by reference to the improved outlook for mother and baby, and although there have been many advances for which women are grateful, there are still a large number of situations about which doctors lack adequate information to say which is the best course of action. My philosophy, in which I am not alone, of involving the woman in the decisions about her care, means that the obstetrician must relinquish some power. Accepting that the woman should have control over her own fertility by means of access to contraception and abortion on her terms, not those of the medical profession, and understanding that the woman should have choice about the way her pregnancy and labour is conducted, seems to be deeply threatening to some obstetricians – of both sexes. Such demands also challenge that power which has been based on a way of looking at evidence which proves the virtues of hospital or interventionist obstetric care over the traditional home-based, non-interventionist practice of midwives.

Although women may not have analysed their dissatisfaction with the care that they have received during childbirth, many hundreds have responded to my suspension by writing letters which show clearly that they do see this issue as a struggle for the control of birth. Women – and the feminist movement – must involve themselves in this battle before we reach the situation in the USA where midwifery is illegal in most states, and where over 24 per cent of women were delivered by Caesarean section in 1985.

What kind of services do women want and who is going to decide on the kind of care that is offered to them? This is part of the wider issue about the way services are provided in the NHS: whether doctors and nurses are the best people to make decisions about what patients need and want, or whether administrators, either as non-practising doctors or as general managers with no medical background, should decide on grounds of efficiency alone. Sometimes when one looks at the cuts one feels that the ultimate hospital, as far as some planners are concerned, would be one which had no patients and thus required no revenue to run it!

My own feeling is that there needs to be a partnership between the consumers and the providers, both medical and administrative. It is too easy for the professionals to become distant from the reality of patients' feelings. For example, doctors and midwives feel at home in hospitals, the surroundings are familiar, we know all the people, we have the pleasure and satisfaction of having accomplished worthwhile work in the building, and it is hard for us to see the place as an outsider does, frighteningly impersonal, overlarge, filled with remote people in a rush – and often associated with unhappy memories of illness or death. The routine, the forms, the technology may make some people feel secure but others feel lost and depersonalised – the very size overwhelms them. In this frame of mind understanding explanations becomes difficult, and the patient is acutely sensitive to attitudes and the way things are said and done.

There are two reasons why this debate is particularly contentious in obstetrics and gynaecology. Firstly, the majority of consultants are men, whereas the consumers are all women. Secondly, many of these women are not ill, they are seeking help and advice about how to avoid pregnancy, or how to get pregnant, how to obtain an abortion or what is best for themselves and the baby if they decide to embark on a pregnancy. Pregnancy is not an illness; it is a very important part of a couple's life together or a woman's life if she decides to go it alone. Women need help to achieve the kind of birth they want – about which many of them, even young women or those with little formal education, often have strong views. The role of the doctor is that of a counsellor rather than that of an authoritarian, trained professional, and this is very hard for some doctors to accept – especially the majority of male obstetricians.

This issue – of who decides on the type of care that a woman gets, the place that she delivers, the importance of her own views – has recurred over and over again in the letters that I have had from women. I think that obstetricians have to take a hard look at the way they are delivering services to women, and join with them in planning for the future so that women have more say, and sterile confrontation is avoided.

The third issue is that of accountability. How is it possible that the Chairman of the Health Authority and a handful of doctors could set in motion an enquiry costing an estimated £250,000 at a time when the impoverished district of Tower Hamlets is cutting beds and services? To whom is the Chairman of the District Health Authority accountable? To the people of Tower Hamlets? To the DHSS? To the North East Thames Regional Health Authority? To anyone? The Early Day Motion calling for his resignation was signed by over a hundred MPs in the fortnight between the publication of the first part of the report on 10 July and when Parliament rose on the 25th, but at the press conference on 24 July Francis Cumberlege seemed satisfied with his performance in this matter. He expressed no regret over the cost of the enquiry, nor the damage done to services.

To whom are the rest of the members of the DHA accountable? To the people of Tower Hamlets? To the bodies of whom they are nominees, but not representatives, i.e. the University of London, the Regional Health Authority, the London Borough of Tower Hamlets? The Local Medical Committee of GPs, the Medical Council of the London Hospital, or to none of these bodies? The whole system seems to lack any mechanism for assessing the performance of a Health Authority except in one way – can they keep within their budget?

To whom are hospital consultants accountable for the quality and organisation of their services? To the new General Managers? To the DHA? To the DHSS? To the GMC? To their patients or to no one except themselves? As medicine is a self-regulating profession, in which, quite rightly, clinical autonomy is jealously guarded so that doctors have the right to decide what kind of treatment is best for an individual patient, to whom are doctors accountable – their professional colleagues as represented by the various Royal Colleges?

How does one define incompetence in a specialty like obstetrics where there is a wide spectrum of opinion about the best way to look after pregnant women? The legal definition which John Hendy adopted, based on the 1974 NHS reorganisation, was that if the management lay 'within the broad limits of acceptable medical practice' the action could not be said to be evidence of incompetence. Secondly, even if an action was outside these broad limits there had to be more than one deviation. Incompetence must be a continuing state not an isolated event. But what is acceptable practice as far as the professional is concerned? Does this differ from what women think is acceptable practice? Is there good scientific evidence for many of the things that we do in obstetrics – indeed in all branches of medicine? How much of accepted practice (based on opinion and current working methods) is acceptable practice, which should, as Iain Chalmers said in his evidence at the enquiry, be based on good scientific evidence?

Then there is the question of disciplinary procedures for doctors working as consultants in the NHS. Naturally there has to be a mechanism for dealing with doctors who cannot fulfil their duties because of mental or physical illness, dependence on drugs or alcohol, or who abuse their position in relation to patients either emotionally or sexually. Some of these matters can be dealt with through the GMC, and the doctor usually continues to practise until his or her case has been heard.

Occasionally a doctor may be appointed who has not been properly trained, or he or she may become incompetent for one of the reasons listed above. Clearly, for the protection of patients, this person cannot be allowed to practise if he or she is unfit to do so, and suspension is sometimes used as an emergency measure to allow time for the responsible administrative doctor to assess the situation. There is only implied power to suspend, not a well-defined procedure in any of the regulations relating to the employment of consultants.

The procedure used to investigate doctors in whom professional misconduct is suspected, HM(61)112 is virtually unchanged from the 1951 circular drawn up three years after the Health Service began. It is expensive and time-consuming, and although suspension is not part of the HM(61)112 procedure, and the Beaumont Panel stated that 'it was not within their terms of reference', it appears that in practice suspension is frequently used concurrently, which is damaging to the doctor, deprives the NHS of his or her services and adds to the expense if a locum is employed.

HM(61)112 does not conform to modern employment law in which, if an employee is at fault, he or she must be warned verbally and then in writing. In this case the accused doctor is not told that there is any doubt about him or her until a *prima facie* case has been established to the satisfaction of the Chairman of the Health Authority, who is usually a lay person. It gives no guidance on how to gather evidence or how to obtain expert independent medical advice in the case of incompetence, or how widely the chairman should consult before taking any action. Usually the enquiry is held in private and the 'confidentiality' which is maintained in public allows gossip to thrive and thus damage the doctor's reputation even if he or she is later exonerated by any enquiry.

Lastly, there is the issue of academic freedom and the position of senior lecturers within the medical schools. In private many academics will recount the difficulties that they have had with their professors and this, in addition to the uncertainty about academic salaries and poor fringe benefits, makes many doctors who would be good academics choose NHS contracts and greater independence. In time this is bound to lead to poorer training of our medical students and a lowering of standards of doctors. This is an issue that should concern the universities, who cannot pass all the responsibility for standards to the medical schools while retaining all the pomp and status for themselves.

Academic freedom, the right to express opinions, is necessary if we are going to train doctors who can think; and the silence of so many makes the outspoken support of Professor Taylor, Luke Zander and Iain Chalmers, as well as the expert evidence given by those who undertook the unpleasant task of appearing at the enquiry, especially noteworthy.

Many of the letters I have received, as well as the medical and lay press articles and radio and TV programmes, have mentioned one or more of these issues and I think the public debate which followed my suspension has already had positive effects.

The Future

If the dissatisfaction with the way maternity services are provided is to be overcome it is important that obstetricians, midwives and women meet together to discuss how best to use resources and what women want. Their conclusions must then be backed up by research.

The establishment of a study group by the RCOG might enable women to voice their requests in a forum which could lead to change throughout the country, but it needs to be supported by obstetricians as well.

Midwives need to organise and regain their professional autonomy, and take over more of the normal pregnancies and labours. This would please women, especially those with a religious objection to male doctors, and would improve the job satisfaction for midwives. This would also give the obstetrician more time to evaluate what she or he is doing and more time would be spent teaching the junior staff, in particular on the labour ward.

Women need to be more involved in planning local services and they also need to put their requests in a form that administrators can understand. It is a positive gain in Tower Hamlets that the Support Group have started looking forward and are producing a Women's Health Charter which will be presented to the DHA when it is finished.

Changes need to be made in the statutes relating to the appointment of consultants and the way that Health Authorities are formed to increase the representation of consumers. The present system is not democratic and as far as consultant posts are concerned, the influence of a few people, often nearly at the age of retirement, means that the present system is perpetuated.

Incompetence is not a major problem amongst doctors practising in Britain as the training process is rigorous but also fairly personal. But how are doctors taught about assessment in medico-legal cases? Is this an area in which a regular practical session could be provided by the RCOG on the steps necessary to write a report, on what evidence is needed and in what circumstances doctors should agree to do this task, and on the need to understand the breadth of medical opinion? Here some basic legal knowledge could be learned before rather than in the course of a case.

Disciplinary procedures for hospital consultants need to be re-examined by the medical profession in conjunction with experts in employment law. The defence organisations should re-examine the way in which they advise doctors in dispute and see if a better system could be devised.

The medical profession also needs to look at its institutions, and see whether by sharing the power and responsibility, a broader band of doctors would take on the burdens of committee work, examinations, medico-legal work, postgraduate education and other administrative tasks. This would allow those at the top to think and respond to situations such as my suspension, and the incredible waste of public money which followed it. Doctors in senior positions, by ignoring the outcry from their GP colleagues and my patients, despite their appreciation of the injustice of this act and their suspicion that I was not guilty, have threatened the concept of the profession as a self-regulating one. We need to find a way to be more honest and less bureaucratic.

I hope that this book, by adding to knowledge of this whole affair, will help us to go forward and make changes which will be of benefit to both women and the medical profession. Ultimately these issues affect everybody, because the way a society deals with birth affects the whole fabric of that society and sets the scene for the next generation.

Appendix I

1. Susan Payne

1. If the normal treatment for slow or no progress during the second stage of labour in a breech presentation in a prima gravida, namely Caesarean section, was not to be pursued, then a consultant assessment within two hours of the commencement of the second stage of labour should have been undertaken with subsequent consultant assessment and direction being provided personally.
2. Syntocinon should not have been used to augment the second stage of labour.
3. (i) Mrs Savage should not have made a judgement on the telephone that the diagnosis of full dilatation was wrong in the absence of clinical observations of her own to support this disagreement with the reported findings of those on the ward;

   (ii) If Mrs Savage did not trust the combined judgement of her juniors, and/or if (as she says in her comments, page 23 (c)), the registrar was to her an unknown quantity, she should not have left matters in that registrar's hands, in particular when disputing the diagnosis, without herself attending.
4. The second stage of labour was allowed to continue for an inordinately long time, namely over 8 hours, in particular having regard to the footling breech in a prima gravida.
5. Mrs Savage's course of management in this case was idiosyncratic, quite outside the limits of normal management, and potentially hazardous to the unborn child.
6. By her assertion that the successful outcome proves her assessment of risk to have been correct, Mrs Savage:

   (i) demonstrates a lack of insight into the potential for danger which was inherent in her management, and

   (ii) propounds an approach to obstetrics which allows risk taking judged ex post facto by fortunate result.

2. Linda Ganderson

1. This patient was unsuitable for continuation of shared care once growth retardation was suspected. Mrs Savage continued the shared care notwithstanding this suspicion.
2. At 30 weeks gestation intra-uterine growth retardation should have been recognised as the probable diagnosis, but was not.
3. IGR [IUGR] having been so recognised, the patient should have been admitted to hospital for full investigation and inpatient treatment at 30 weeks, namely on 27 February, or at the latest on 12 March 1984, on both of which dates Mrs Savage saw her.
4. The patient was referred back to the sharing GP on 12 March 1984 with Mrs Savage's reference to 'possible' IGR [IUGR] and/or 'wrong dates'. In the premises, the GP was inadequately informed and Mrs Savage delegated to the GP assessment and decision-making which was properly Mrs Savage's responsibility and for which

the GP had not the necessary level of training or expertise, as Mrs Savage well knew.

5. Having thus referred the patient back to the GP, Mrs Savage failed to ensure that the patient's progress was monitored expertly and adequately, so compounding the errors above referred to, with the result that the patient was not thereafter seen by Mrs Savage and/or hospital specialist staff for 4 weeks and was not admitted until 18 April 1984.
6. At the time when the patient was admitted on 18 April the junior staff and covering consultant had not been adequately informed by Mrs Savage and/or by the GP with whom Mrs Savage shared the patient's care as to the fact of severe growth retardation and weight loss.
7. The severity of growth retardation was not recognised by Mrs Savage and/or the GP with whom she shared the care of this patient, and their determination to continue this inappropriate management unnecessarily prejudiced the outcome.

3. AU

1. (i) A purported 'trial of labour' was ordained by Mrs Savage and attempted when there were known contraindications which taken singly, but more importantly together, should have altogether precluded any such attempt;

   (ii) In the light of all the known contraindications to 'trial of labour', and the attendant risks, it was an improper exercise of Mrs Savage's specialist obstetric role to opt to use 'two hours of good labour... to show her that she was not going to be able to deliver vaginally'. (Mrs Savage's comments, page 20 at (e)).
2. (i) The known history of the patient should have compelled an early decision, made in advance of the onset of labour, that there must be an elective Caesarean section as the only safe course;

   (ii) In the absence of the decision for elective section, a section should have been performed very much earlier in the course of labour and by 4.00 a.m. at the latest;

   (iii) Mrs Savage compounded the dangers inherent in the failure to decide on elective section, and non-performance of timely section during labour, by administering syntocinon (a potentially dangerous drug used for the purpose of strengthening uterine contractions) when she did not herself believe that the baby could safely be delivered vaginally;

   (iv) Giving instructions to continue syntocinon but 'to watch the fetal heart carefully and perform immediately Caesarean section if deceleration continued to occur' Mrs Savage failed to ensure such immediate Caesarean section, despite decelerations continuing to occur, until 1.20 p.m. and did not do the section herself, but should have done.
3. (i) The necessary discussion and explanation of the need for elective section should have, but did not, take place well in advance of the onset of labour and should have included, but did not, clear advice about the necessity for that course in the interests of mother and child outweighing the natural preference of the parents for normal labour and vaginal delivery;

(ii) Having failed to discuss and recommend elective section at the early stages of the pregnancy and to make all reasonable efforts to secure informed agreement thereto, elective Caesarean section should have been recommended at the stage in late pregnancy when the fetal lie was found to be unstable with the baby presenting by breech in a patient with a Caesarean scar whose earlier Caesarean had been carried out for disproportion and whose baby Mrs Savage now estimated to be larger than that of the first pregnancy (all of which matters should have been explained);

(iii) The discussion process between the consultant team and the parents whereby the parents ought to have been enabled to participate in, understand and jointly agree the likely necessity for intervention was delayed and inadequate, with the result that the parents were not in a position during labour to make an informed decision;

(iv) The parents' expressed wish, following Mrs Savage's examination of the patient at 12.15 p.m., to have 'another couple of hours effort towards vaginal delivery' should not have been encouraged but should have been the subject of clear warnings as to the known dangers.

4. (i) Syntocinon augmentation was contraindicated but commenced on Mrs Savage's instructions at 9.30 a.m.;

   (ii) Whatever the alleged reasons for commencing syntocinon it should not have been continued after Mrs Savage's examination of the patient at 12.15 p.m.;

   (iii) Knowing, as she did, that the patient had received epidural anaesthesia and that syntocinon had been commenced, she ordered the drug administration to continue as aforesaid, despite her own allegedly clear instructions about the management of labour given to the juniors and her own express view that – 'epidural is contraindicated in a woman with a uterine scar in which syntocinon is given' – Mrs Savage's comments, page 18 (b).

5. Mrs Savage disregarded at the time, and continues to disregard in her comments on the case, the conclusive evidence of pelvic disproportion.

6. Mrs Savage delayed the decision to undertake emergency Caesarean section notwithstanding her knowledge that, by reason of the geography and organisation of the hospital facilities, there was a predictable delay between any decision to do a section and its performance of up to 45 minutes.

7. Mrs Savage, having embarked on a course of management which was wholly outside normally accepted practice and carrying with it well known attendant risks, should have been, but was not, personally involved in the important later and more dangerous stages.

8. By her irrational management and continuing failure to appreciate and act appropriately upon a manifestly deteriorating situation throughout the progress of labour, Mrs Savage instigated management which resulted in prolonged and strong uterine contractions in the presence of disproportion and thus, on the balance of probabilities, caused the baby's death or alternatively contributed to the fatal outcome.

4. Denise Lewis

1. Shared care with the GP was inappropriate for this abnormal pregnancy with a known potential for the development of complications.
2. (i) Having regard to the patient's previous history of anaemia and the fact of multiple pregnancy, the development of anaemia was not investigated satisfactorily or early enough;

   (ii) Having decided against prophylaxis against predictable anaemia, Mrs Savage failed to inform her covering colleague, Mr Oram, of the potential problem.
3. When iron injections were administered in late May 1984 it was too late to be effective by the time of delivery.
4. (i) Despite severe pre-eclampsia, Mrs Savage decided upon induction in the presence of twin breeches which was a wrong decision;

   (ii) Caesarean section should have been carried out electively.
5. (i) Mrs Savage gave instructions at 6.30 a.m. that induction of labour should commence 'that day' on the basis of incomplete and/or inadequate assessment of the patient's true condition;

   (ii) Mrs Savage acted as aforesaid notwithstanding her contention made in her comments at page 13(h) that, had she assessed the woman vaginally herself, she would not have induced her with an unfavourable cervix and with a breech 4 cm above the spine.
6. Induction having been decided upon, it was continued for 11 hours which was much too long, in particular having regard to her own awareness that the breech was high.
7. (i) In the light of all the known features of this lady's pregnancy and labour and her previous history, this was a high risk pregnancy. In the circumstances, Mrs Savage:

   (a) did not adequately brief her junior staff;

   (b) did not ensure her own regular and complete information on progress by telephone or otherwise;

   (c) was absent when her own idiosyncratic plan for management dictated that she should be present herself to carry that plan into effect.

   (ii) Mrs Savage absented herself as above without ensuring appropriate consultant cover and without informing her consultant colleague that he was indeed required to cover this serious problem case in circumstances where she had provided for her juniors an inappropriate, confusing, and potentially dangerous plan of management.
8. In the light of the known history of this pregnancy and labour, Mrs Savage should acknowledge, but persists in her refusal to acknowledge, that a potentially dangerous condition of pre-eclampsia was present and required immediate steps to effect delivery which were not taken.
9. In the premises Mrs Savage is at fault in seeking by her comments to lay blame at the door of her colleagues and juniors.

5. X

1. A trial of labour was the appropriate management for this teenage prima gravida of short stature (4 ft 10 ins) who had sought late termination, but the procedure followed was not a trial of labour.
2. Notwithstanding that, after 11 hours in the labour ward, the cervix was 5–6 cms dilated, and after 12 ½ hours the blood pressure was 150/100, and the fetal heart rate was over 160, labour was permitted to continue for a further 6 ¾ hours before Caesarean section was advised by Mrs Savage.
3. Mrs Savage gave instructions at 2.45 a.m. for emergency section in an obstructed labour with technical difficulties of delivery inevitable, without herself attending to perform the operation or ensuring that staff of seniority and experience were present and available to undertake it.

6. Generally

1. Taken together, the five cases show a consistent aberration of clinical judgement, thereby exposing the patients to unnecessary and unjustifiable risks.
2. The historical sequence of the five cases indicated a failure to recognise and/or analyse adequately or at all the areas of legitimate concern and/or failure in the light of such analysis to modify her approach accordingly.
3. By her responses to the criticisms made of her conduct of the five cases, Mrs Savage:

   (i) indicates an unwillingness and/or inability to recognise genuine causes for concern affecting patient safety;

   (ii) demonstrates a readiness to avoid and shift personal consultant responsibility for such shortcomings as she is prepared to acknowledge existed.
4. Mrs Savage's conduct and approach as aforesaid was and is not such as meets the standards reasonably required of a senior lecturer at a major teaching hospital, and carries with it the serious risk of:

   (i) confusing junior staff and/or midwives and/or undermining their confidence in, and/or their adherence to reasonable criteria for safe practice;

   (ii) undermining the consistency in standards for safe obstetric practice which such a hospital ought to teach, establish and maintain;

   (iii) jeopardising the continuity of care which reasonable conformity in such standards between consultants is designed to ensure.

Appendix II

General Conclusions of the Panel's Report

We do not agree that the five cases, even if they should properly be taken together, reveal a consistent aberration of clinical judgment. In only one of the cases, AU, did Mrs Savage make a clinical judgment (the suitability of syntocinon in the presence of a breech, a scar and a small pelvis) which went close to the bounds of acceptable practice. We are satisfied that as soon as there were signs that the potential risks in that management could become real rather than theoretical Mrs Savage's advice finally convinced the parents that they should agree to a Caesarean section. We do not agree that, taking the 5 cases together, Mrs Savage's patients were exposed to unnecessary and unjustifiable risks, subject to the qualifications expressed above in respect of the individual cases.

We do not agree that there is any historical sequence of the five cases. Their only connection is that they all took place within a period of about 13 months. In that 13 month period Mrs Savage dealt with many hundreds of other cases, and we have heard no suggestion that complaints could have been made in any of them. In the one other case, that of Y, that we have heard something of, we did not form the view that Mrs Savage acted wrongly in any way. In our view, in all these cases where Mrs Savage has been, to some degree, at fault she has recognised it and tried to analyse it to prevent it happening again. She applied that principle to one case, that of LG, in which the fault was not her own and immediately took steps to see that the error, which had occurred, could not recur.

We do not agree that by defending herself against criticisms which she felt to be unjustified Mrs Savage showed any unwillingness and/or inability to recognise genuine causes for concern affecting patient safety. We recognise that those responsible for the criticisms themselves genuinely felt concern. However, a genuinely felt concern is not necessarily a justified concern. We have indicated in the preceding chapters which concerns we consider to have been justified, and to what extent. We also find that Mrs Savage had an equally genuine concern for patient safety at all times.

We do not agree that Mrs Savage seeks to avoid and shift personal consultant responsibility. She seems to us to recognise that she is broadly responsible for all patients in her care. It does not follow from that, however, that she must necessarily accept personal responsibility and blame for everything which might go wrong in connection with a patient, nor for every mistake which may be made by another person helping to care for the patient. In our view that principle should be applied even more strongly when the issues are not simply about consultant responsibility, but about a consultant's competence, which is a far different and more fundamental thing. A consultant could be personally responsible for mistakes without his competence necessarily being called into question. That principle must also apply where the consultant was not personally responsible for a particular mistake.

We do not agree that Mrs Savage's conduct was, or is, not such as meets the standards reasonably required of a senior lecturer at a major teaching (or any) hospital.

We do not agree that Mrs Savage's conduct and approach carry with them any risk of confusing junior staff and/or midwives. Such persons must understand that in obstetrics, as in all medicine, there is often more than one valid way to deal with a particular situation. We have heard no evidence of sufficient weight that Mrs Savage's criteria for safe practice are unreasonable, nor that Mrs Savage has sought to affect, or even unconsciously affected, any person's adherence to reasonable criteria for safe practice.

We have heard no evidence of sufficient weight to indicate that Mrs Savage's general standards for safe obstetric practice are lower than those of anyone else at the London Hospital. We have heard no evidence to justify the charge that Mrs Savage's conduct (or approach) undermined the consistency of standards in the London Hospital.

We have had no evidence to indicate that any failing of continuity of care as between Mrs Savage and any other consultant can be blamed on Mrs Savage more than any other person.

Index

Ackroyd, Briony 114
Advisory, Conciliation and Arbitration Service (ACAS) 142
Allison, Julia 180
All-Party Parliamentary Group on Maternity Services 176
Alway, John 5, 10,
American College of Obstetricians and Gynecologists (ACOG) 43
Antenatal care 29, 51, 190
Armstrong, Paul 12, 20
Association for Improvements in Maternity Services (AIMS) 2, 28, 31, 176, 180, 182
Association of Radical Midwives (ARM) 172, 176
Athena Project 159
Atlay, Bob 5
Audit Commission 2, 28
Ayling, Clifford 78, 191

Balaskas, Janet 176
Beaumont, Sir Christopher (Beaumont Enquiry) 8, 10, 11
Beech, Beverley 30, 32, 176, 179
Beedham, Trevor 14, 18
Berry, Colin 7, 18
Bevan, Aneurin 68, 80
Bousquet, Pauline 112
Brahams, Diana 112
Brew, Richard 12
Bristol Royal Infirmary Enquiry 2, 23, 60, 78, 191, 201
British Medical Association (BMA) 7, 111, 135
British Medical Journal (BMJ) 43, 83, 84, 125
Brown, Alfred 133

Caesarean Section Rate (CSR) 27, 30, 31, 59, 94, 172, 189
Calman, Kenneth 93
Calvert Committee 165
Canada 95, 134, 136–8, 143, 157
Chalmers, Iain 22
Changing Childbirth 28, 174, 176, 187
Chard, Tim 12, 19, 20
Chaudhury, Roy 112
Chief Medical Officer (CMO) 2, 61, 83, 93, 96, 111, 113, 200, 201
Clark, Helen 45
Clarke, Kenneth 62, 110
Clarkson, Brian 165
Cochrane Report 133
Cohen, Michael 166
Commission for Audit and Health Improvement (CHAI) 2
Committee on Professional Performance 94
Confidential Enquiry into Maternal Deaths (CEMD) 88
Council for Healthcare Regulatory Excellence (CHRE) 61
Cranbrook Committee 27
Cronk, Mary 176
Crossman, Richard 69, 80
Cumberlege Report 1, 29, 31, 62, 173, 188

Daly, Helena 112
Darnell, Sir Royce 112
Davies, Sir Michael 165
Day, Patricia 65, 67, 70, 76
Diggory, Peter 7, 9
District Health Authority (DHA), accountability of 62–3
Djahanbakhch, Ovrang 20, 21
Dobson, Frank 62
Donald, Ian 5
Donaldson, Sir Liam 83, 109, 111, 113, 114, 139
Donley, Joan 31, 32, 45
Donnison, Jean 179, 180
Drife, James 63, 83, 134
Dutch system 199
Dyer, Claire 1

Education Reform Act 162
Edwards, Nadine 183
Ellis, Sir John 5
Empey, Duncan 17, 18
Everington, Sam 7
Eversley, John 31, 63, 65

Fairey, Mike 15
Flint, Caroline 176
Floyer, Mike 5
Fowler, Norman 2, 110
Francome, Colin 19

Gaskin, Ina May 172
General Agreement on Trade in Services (GATS) 158
General Medical Council (GMC) 2, 9, 21, 22, 60, 61, 63, 84, 86, 88, 93–5, 106, 112–115, 139, 149
Gillie, Oliver 172
Goodyear, Michael 116, 133
Gorsky, Martin 80
Griffiths, John (Report) 73, 162,163
Grudzinskas, Gedis 10, 13, 16, 18, 20, 21
Guilliland, Karen 55

Haines, Michael 16
Hardman, Victoria 6
Hare, John 7
Hartgill, John 10, 11
Hatch, David 83
Health Overview and Scrutiny Committees (HOSC) 62
Healy, David 157
Hendy, John 7, 116, 117, 119, 125, 158
Hibbs, Pam 18
Hillier, Sheila 21, 202
Hoffenberg, Sir Raymond 133
Home births 28, 29, 30, 31, 36, 43, 60, 174, 180, 182, 185
Hudson, Chris 12
Huntingford, Peter 19

Hutton, John 128

Independent Midwives Association (IMA) 176
Irvine, Sir Donald 22, 60, 93, 95

Jacobs, Harry 23, 111
Jarratt Report 162
Jewell, Tony 9

Kendall, Bob 22
Kennedy, Sir Ian 21
Kitzinger, Sheila 176
Klein, Rudolf 65, 67, 70, 76
Knight, Dame Jill 114

Lancet, The 7–9, 11
Ledward, Rodney 95
Leigh, Irene 202
Leighton, Jane 5
Leys, Colin 31
Litigation 31, 60
London Hospital Medical Council (LHMC) 8

McGarry, John 18
McKelvie, Peter 7
Maclean, Anne 156, 161
MacNaughton, Sir Malcolm 8, 10, 11
MacVicar, John 7
Mallinson, Ann 10
Manero, Elizabeth 176
Marek, John 112
Medical Defence Union (MDU) 14, 18, 112
Medical Research Council (MRC) 29
Medical Women's Federation (MWF) 159
Middlesex University 19, 201
Midwives 1, 14, 27, 29, 31, 36–9, 43, 45–55, 171–6, 181–5, 188, 189, 191–4
Moore, Michael 7
Morrison, Herbert 68
Munro, Dame Alison (Munro panel) 5, 7, 8, 9, 10, 11, 21, 158

Nairne, Patrick 67
National Audit Office (NAO) 114
National Care Standards Commission (NCSC) 2
National Childbirth Trust (NCT) 3, 28, 31, 36, 176, 182
National Clinical Assessment Authority (NCAA) 2, 113, 114
National Clinical Assessment Service (NCAS) 2, 89, 93, 95, 114, 123, 124, 140, 141
National Health Service (NHS) 31, 59, 62, 65–80, 85–90, 101, 102, 109–16, 119, 124, 127, 132, 138, 172
National Institute for Clinical Excellence (NICE), 30, 36, 102, 183, 190
National Patient Safety Agency (NPSA) 2, 191
National Service Framework for Children, Young People and Maternity Services (NSF) 187
Neale, Richard (Enquiry) 63, 78, 95, 96
New Zealand 32, 45–55
New Zealand College of Midwives (NZCOM) 47–54
New Zealand Medical Association (NZMA) 46–52
New Zealand Nurses Association (NZNA) 45
Newland, Adrian 21
NHS and Community Care Act 110

O'Connell, Bridget 112, 113
O'Donnell, Michael 21, 22
Olivieri, Nancy 157
O'Neill, Baroness Onora 61, 200, 201
Oram, David 5

Patel, Naren 17
Pathasundaram, Vythilingam 13, 15, 16, 19, 21
Patient Advisory and Liaison Service (PALS) 63, 79
Patient and Public Investment Forums (PPI) 79–80
Patients' Association 21
Peel, Sir John (and Peel Report) 27, 180
Perinatal Mortality Rate (PMR) 27, 28, 41, 55, 172
Poloniecki, Jan 134
Private Finance Initiative (PFI) 62, 67
Public Accounts Committee 113

Quebec model of revalidation 95

Raymond, Brian 13, 14, 15
Regional Medical Officer (RMO) 109–111
Richie, David 202
Robinson, Jean 21, 182, 184
Rosenthal, Marilynn 137
Royal College of Midwives (RCM) 28, 31, 174
Royal College of Obstetricians and Gynaecologists (RCOG) 5, 6, 8, 10, 11, 12, 14–17, 18, 19, 30, 36, 63, 83, 88, 89

Salkind, Mal 8, 10, 11, 202
Sandall, Jane 32, 187
Savage, Wendy 5–24, 27, 37–8, 59, 65–6, 69–70, 77–8, 93, 109, 152, 157, 171, 199, 203–5
Schafer, Arthur 157
Scotland, Alastair 14
Sedgemore, Brian MP 112
Shaw, George Bernard 134
Shipman, Harold 60, 106, 115, 134
Short Committee (and Report) 27, 28
Skidmore, David 120–1
Smith, Dame Janet 61, 83
Smith, Sam 19
Society of Clinical Psychiatrists 112
Society to Support Home Confinement 182
Stephens, Mark 16
Steyn, Lord 120,128
Stirrat, Gordon 17
Stone, Ian 2
Storrs, Robert 179

Strong, Roy 99
Sweden 137
Swinnerton-Dyer, Peter 167

Taylor, Ron 21, 96, 99
Tew, Marjorie 182
Thatcher, Margaret 161,162
Timmins, Nick 1
Tomlin, Peter 23, 111
Tower Hamlets District
Health Authority (DHA) 1,
63, 69–73

Ultrasound 29
USA 27, 30, 31, 37, 194

Veitch, Andrew 1
Virago Press 5

Wagner, Marsden 32, 35
Walton, Lord 22
Warner, Lord 71
Weston, Ruth Sharples 183
Whyte, Margaret 182
Williams, Norman 7
Williamson, Colwyn 166
Williamson, Lorne (LW) 10–
12
Wingate, David 202
Winston, Lord Robert 20
Winterton Committee (and
Report) 1, 28, 187
Women's Health Care
Research Unit 20
World Health Organisation
(WHO) 30

Zander, Luke 7, 60, 199

Other Titles in the **Middlesex University Press Health Series**

Caesarean Birth in Britain: Revised and Updated

A book for health professionals and parents

Wendy Savage, Helen Churchill, Colin Francome

ISBN 978 1 904750 17 8 / 1 904750 17 6

Price £18

Caesarean Birth in Britain presents expectant parents, educators and health professionals with the facts and figures, and documents a number of important changes which have occurred in obstetrics since the original book was published in 1993. Using data from a nationwide survey of obstetricians, the authors offer a comprehensive analysis of what has changed and ask at what cost.

Vaginal Birth After Caesarean

The VBAC handbook

Helen Churchill and Wendy Savage

ISBN 978 1 904750 21 5

Price £6.99

Vaginal Birth After Caesarean presents pregnant women and health professionals with all the necessary information regarding options for birth following caesarean delivery. The handbook provides suggestions for constructive ways to achieve vaginal birth after caesarean (VBAC) when this is the right option. The book includes several successful VBAC stories.

How to Avoid an Unnecessary Caesarean

A handbook for women who want a natural birth

Helen Churchill and Wendy Savage

ISBN 978 1 904750 16 1

Price £6.99

How to Avoid an Unnecessary Caesarean is aimed mainly at pregnant women and health professionals. The book provides case studies and suggestions for constructive ways to avoid unnecessary caesareans.

Health Policy Reform: Driving the Wrong Way?

A Critical Guide to the Global 'Health Reform' Industry

John Lister

ISBN 978 1 904750 45 1 / 1 904750 45 1

Price £25

Health Policy Reform: Driving the Wrong Way? focuses on the main structural, managerial and policy changes that have been taking place within the world's health care systems since the early 1990s. It questions whether these 'reforms' are driven primarily by the health needs of the wider population or, in fact, by non-health considerations – the financial, ideological and political concerns of governments and global institutions. This text contains up-to-date facts and case studies making this a valuable reference work on health care reform and health policy.

Female Genital Mutilation

Treating the Tears

Haseena Lockhat

ISBN 978 1 898253 90 7 / 1 898253 90 0

Price £15.99

Female Genital Mutilation: Treating the Tears deals with the topical and controversial issue of female circumcision. A thoroughly researched and academic work, it aims to raise awareness not only of the physical but also the psychological effects of this procedure. Female Genital Mutilation (FGM) has re-surfaced in the UK since the 1980s following the migration of people from FGM-practising countries. Various professionals nationwide are likely to encounter girls and women who have been either circumcised or are 'at risk' of being circumcised, as such this is a useful reference for those working in the health and social care industry.

Ordering Information

To order any of the above titles, please visit **www.mupress.co.uk**